Emergency Laparoscopy

Ferdinando Agresta •
Fabio Cesare Campanile •
Gabriele Anania •
Carlo Bergamini
Editors

Emergency Laparoscopy

Springer

Editors

Ferdinando Agresta
Department of General Surgery
Azienda ULSS19 del Veneto
Adria (RO)
Italy

Gabriele Anania
Department of Morfology, Surgery and Experimental Medicine
School of Medicine
University of Ferrara
Ferrara, Italy

Fabio Cesare Campanile
Ospedale San Giovanni Decollato Andosilla
AUSL Viterbo
Civita Castellana (VT)
Italy

Carlo Bergamini
Careggi University Hospital
Florence, Italy

ISBN 978-3-319-29618-0   ISBN 978-3-319-29620-3 (eBook)
DOI 10.1007/978-3-319-29620-3

Library of Congress Control Number: 2016938912

Printed on acid-free paper

This Springer imprint is published by Springer Nature
The registered company is Springer International Publishing AG Switzerland

" . . . I swear by Apollo the physician, and Aesculapius, and Health, and All-heal, and all the gods and goddesses, that, according to my ability and judgment, I will keep this Oath and this stipulation—to reckon him who taught me this Art equally dear to me as my parents, to share my substance with him, and relieve his necessities if required; to look upon his offspring in the same footing as my own brothers, and to teach them this Art, if they shall wish to learn it, without fee or stipulation; and that by precept, lecture, and every other mode of instruction, I will impart a knowledge of the Art to my own sons, and those of my teachers, and to disciples bound by a stipulation and oath according to the law of medicine . . . " (Hippocratic Oath)

To all our masters who have taught us that the real proof of the evidence is the everyday life!

To all the surgeons who daily test the value of the evidence!

Ferdinando Agresta
Fabio Cesare Campanile
Gabriele Anania
Carlo Bergamini

Foreword

Emergency represents one of the most debated fields of surgery, but concurrently it is one of the most interesting. Experience, technology, and availability of paramedical support are often not adequately widespread in hospitals; thus, still to date laparoscopy is not common in emergency settings. Yet, the dogma "laparoscopy as the last diagnostic step and the first therapeutic act" should be clearly impressed in emergency surgeons' minds. For this reason, when I was President of the Italian Society of Surgical Endoscopy (S.I.C.E.), I embraced enthusiastically the proposal of an update of the guidelines about emergency laparoscopy, which we had already published a few years before. Hence, we could be again first in line in Europe about this topic. The update was mandatory, due to the fast advances and improvements in the emergency field. Thanks are due to my friends Ferdinando Agresta, Fabio Cesare Campanile, Carlo Bergamini, and Gabriele Anania for their brilliant contribution. In my opinion, this volume represents a considerable update for the surgeon already trained in laparoscopic approach to emergencies, as it offers a valid appraisal of the efficacy of laparoscopy in the different abdominal emergencies, along with a cost-effectiveness evaluation. Moreover, this volume should represent a helpful tool and an incentive to improve for the unexperienced surgeon, in order to identify the proper treatment of several emergencies. Sustainability and efficacy currently represent hot topics in every field, and in this light we all have to work together to implement the correct use of laparoscopy even to satisfy economic needs. Finally, thanks are also due to Springer, for its usual careful editing and for the wide distribution that it will provide to this project not only in the surgical field.

Francesco Corcione
President of the Italian Society of Surgery
(SIC), Naples, Italy

Foreword

Laparoscopic surgery has been the main innovation in surgery over the last 25 years. After the first laparoscopic cholecystectomy performed by Mouret in France in 1987, and after the initial distrust, laparoscopic surgery has rapidly spread throughout the world. From treating benign and relatively simple techniques such as gallstones, it has gone to treat malignancies and also increasingly complex techniques. Technological development of all laparoscopic surgical instruments has allowed surgeons to perform surgery in emergency also in critically ill patients, offering them the opportunity to get all the well-known advantages given by laparoscopy: the intraoperative ones, where the main advantage is to be able to explore, wash, and drain with a minimal incision all abdominal areas in order to reach a complete diagnosis, and the postoperative ones including fewer postoperative hospital stay, less postoperative pain, early intestinal functioning, and less use of analgesics. Even in emergency laparoscopic surgery, rapidly it has been moved from treating patients with simple illnesses, such as cholecystectomy and appendectomy, to situations technically more complex, such as bowel obstruction, perforation, and trauma. In an area as complex as laparoscopic surgery, especially the emergency one, it seems quite impossible for a single surgeon to gain the necessary experience in order to standardize both indication and technique. This book must be considered the result of the not only Italian experience in the field of laparoscopic emergency. It seems to me a useful and unique setup on the subject: a possibility offered to all laparoscopic surgeons to try to achieve a standardization in such a delicate matter as surgical emergencies.

Diego Piazza
President of the Italian Society of Community
Hospital Surgeons (ACOI), Catania, Italy

Foreword

Emergency surgery and laparoscopic surgery have been traditionally considered as sharing opposite features. Indeed, while minimally invasive procedures were supposed to be more complex and to need a longer operative time in order to achieve a better outcome in terms of quality of life, on the other side the urgent surgery might not afford to be too much time-consuming for obvious reason of immediate need of intervention. Thus, several conditions, such as occlusion, trauma, abdominal sepsis, intestinal infarction, have been traditionally considered as contraindications to laparoscopy since the time of the beginning the mini-invasive surgery era.

But these two faces are nowadays converging together. Indeed, the Research of the last years has gradually been overlapping them in a single mode and a single approach where both the attitudes find their own space, according to absolutely rigorous and well-defined criteria of indication.

The very ambitious aim of this book has been to treat, in a very critical and analytical way, this subject of the feasibility and safeness of this process of fusion between emergency surgery and laparoscopy, in most of the critical surgical conditions. This has been carried out from time to time with a careful examination of the pros and cons in the application of the available minimally invasive techniques in emergency conditions, as it has derived from a careful and deep review of the literature, according to the inviolable principles of the Best Practices and the Evidence Based Medicine.

The result is a vision at the same time very modern, up to date, but also judicious in this delicate "alliance" between emergency surgery and laparoscopy, thus balancing the recklessness sometimes too technically daring of the mini-invasivity "at all costs," and the attitude too impetuous and invasive of the emergency surgeons, who may feel justified by the situation of immediate danger to avoid the complex and delicate procedures of the laparoscopy.

This text can be truly considered a Must for those who wish to read up on where you can and where you cannot make this transition from the two oppositional faces of the coin toward a single one, where these two aspects of laparoscopy and emergency approach are fused together as a unique feature of the modern Surgery.

Andrea Valeri
President of the "Italian Society for Endoscopic Surgery and New Technologies" (S.I.C.E), Florence, Italy

Preface

"...The development of new instruments and the refinement of established techniques will lead to the expansion of minimally invasive surgery to new areas of interest for general surgeons. However, one must realize—and accept, that minimally invasive surgery only represents a different technique that offers an alternative to open surgery. The indication for surgery are similar for both minimally invasive surgery and open surgery... It is important for all general surgeons to keep up with this trend and become an integral part of the revolution in medicine that the advent of minimally surgery has wrought..." (H.S. Himal: Minimally invasive (laparoscopic) surgery. The future of general surgery. Surg Endosc 2002;16:1647–52).

Without any doubts, there are three truths in this never old editorial. The first is the expansion of laparoscopy to wider areas of surgical interest, such as the emergency. The second is that this expansion must follow the same rules of the open approach. Third, surely the most important: every surgeon should have the "laparoscopy" in his/her background as an indispensable tool. Let us go back to the first: expansion. Laparoscopy has always been mentioned as a revolution and might be the only true revolution in surgery in the recent past. Revolution because it has changed the way we think and act as surgeons. Again, revolution because the scientific community has not easily accepted it and agreed about its fields of applications. Finally, today any surgeon cannot disregard the right value of laparoscopy, either when it is accepted as the "gold standard" procedure or when its outcome is similar to that of the open approach, and its potential therapeutic value has yet to be proven. However, nowadays, after the revolution *"...as doctor and surgeons our mission is to treat patients to the best of our knowledge and expertise. The exponential knowledge eruption and the nearly daily skill-related technology advances in minimal invasive surgery make it more than ever mandatory that we, surgeons and doctors, humbly examine, analyze and objectively audit our own practice... we have to recognise and discard our acquired biases, and base our diagnostic procedures and surgical therapy on "hard" evidence..." (Fingerhut A. Do we need consensus conferences? Surg Endosc 2002;16:1149–1450).*

Therefore, the mission of each surgeon has two aspects that cannot be separated: as clinicians we have to give our patients the best possible treatment, and as scientists we are committed to examining our data to find out the "hard evidence." However, the "hard evidence" needs to be continuously reassessed and updated because our knowledge is always expanding and the renewal of the technology we use is constant.

We are forced to keep up with the times, continue confronting each another, and study. We are supposed to review and update our knowledge, first through the recognition of our limitations and bias, under the light of the scientific evidence, universal “compass” that guides us in the open surgery as in laparoscopy.

The duty of every surgeon to keep abreast also with the daily evolution of laparoscopy must be paid in every hospital, whether small or large. This is the main idea that has driven us, editors and authors, to write this book.

In 2011, with the same group, we had updated the milestone 2006 EAES consensus conference guidelines about emergency laparoscopy. We did it sharing our experience and knowledge with all the other actors of the emergency surgical theater: anesthesiologists, emergency room physicians, radiologists, nurses, and patients. Time continues to move on, and a tremendous amount of literature data is the result of the constant evolution of our profession. For this reason, we decided to stop again, “quite rightly,” to use Fingerhut’s words, as we did yesterday, and to review what we had done 4 years ago in light of the latest evidence on the topic that every surgeon has to face daily: the emergency.

The principal idea of this update is to offer to all our colleagues and students the possibility to have almost on one hand all the actual evidence about emergency laparoscopy. Like 4 years ago, we wish to state again: “*Every surgeon has generally developed a fine ability to decide the best approach according to a personal evaluation of her/his own experience, taking into account the clinical situation, her/his proficiency (and the experience of the team) with the various techniques and the specific organizational setting in which she/he is working. This book has been developed bearing in mind that every surgeon could use the data reported to support her/his judgment*” (Agresta F, Ansaloni L, Baiocchi GL, Bergamini C, Campanile FC, Carlucci M, Cocorullo G, Corradi A, Franzato B, Lupo M, Mandalà V, Mirabella A, Pernazza G, Piccoli M, Staudacher C, Vettoretto N, Zago M, Lettieri E, Levati A, Pietrini D, Scaglione M, De Masi S, De Placido G, Francucci M, Rasi M, Fingerhut A, Uranüs S, Garattini S. Laparoscopic approach to acute abdomen from the Consensus Development Conference of the Società Italiana di Chirurgia Endoscopica e nuove tecnologie (SICE), Associazione Chirurghi Ospedalieri Italiani (ACOI), Società Italiana di Chirurgia (SIC), Società Italiana di Chirurgia d’Urgenza e del Trauma (SICUT), Società Italiana di Chirurgia nell’Ospedalità Privata (SICOP), and the European Association for Endoscopic Surgery (EAES). Surg Endosc. 2012 Aug;26(8):2134–64).

Adria, Italy — Ferdinando Agresta
Civita Castellana, Italy — Fabio Cesare Campanile
Ferrara, Italy — Gabriele Anania
Florence, Italy — Carlo Bergamini

Note to the Reader

The authors of this book adopted the following methodology for literature search and appraisal: the primary objective of the search was to identify all clinical relevant randomized controlled trials (RCT) and meta-analysis. Afterward, other reports, population-based outcome studies, case series, and case reports have been also included. A systematic review based on comprehensive literature search has been made on PubMed according to the following criteria: *Limits Activated*: *Humans*, *Clinical Trial*, *Meta-Analysis*, *Practice Guideline*, *Randomized Controlled Trial*, *Review*, *English*, *All Adult*: *19+ years*, *published in the last 20 years*. *Search details*: [((“*laparoscopy*” [*MeSH Terms*] *OR* “*laparoscopic*” [*All Fields*]) *AND* (“*condition-specific key word*” [*MeSH Terms*] *OR* “*condition-specific key word*” [*All Fields*])) *AND* (“*humans*” [*MeSH Terms*] *AND* (*Clinical Trial* [*ptyp*] *OR Meta-Analysis* [*ptyp*] *OR Practice Guideline* [*ptyp*] *OR Randomized Controlled Trial* [*ptyp*] *OR Review* [*ptyp*]) *AND English* [*lang*] *AND* “*adult*” [*MeSH Terms*] *AND* “2010/25/*11*” [*PDat*]: “*2015*/10/*31*” [*PDat*])]. Then, limits regarding language, age, and publication date and study type have been removed, to search for additional papers. Cross-link control was performed with Google Scholar and Cochrane library databases. The full text paper was obtained for all relevant articles. The papers have been selected and classified on the basis of the highest level of evidence, design of the study, and most recent publication. The 2011 Oxford hierarchy for grading clinical studies according to levels of evidence (LoE) has been used (http://www.cebm.net/index.aspx?o=5653). Studies containing severe methodological flaws have been downgraded as necessary. For each intervention, the validity and homogeneity of study results, effect sizes, safety, and economic consequences have been considered.

Contents

A Worldwide Overview of Emergency Laparoscopic Procedures

1

Carlo Bergamini, Ferdinando Agresta,
Fabio Cesare Campanile, and Gabriele Anania

1.1 Introduction

Laparoscopy has become a common procedure in elective surgery worldwide. Actually, it can be considered the preferred surgical approach in various diseases, due to its sure advantages. The last decade has been characterized by the increasing numbers of surgeons trained to a high standard in minimally invasive surgery and by the validation of laparoscopic procedures in emergency surgery. However, despite the undisputed advantages of laparoscopy (such as the shorter hospital stay, the faster recovery, and the less morbidity), the advances in technology, and a structured training for young surgeon that have stimulated the spread of the laparoscopic procedure in the world, the perception has hovered for many years that laparoscopic surgery should remain the preferred approach only in case of elective fields.

1.2 Notes on Diagnostic Laparoscopy

In the last decade, fortunately, we assisted to a major diffusion of laparoscopic procedures also in the emergency field that have led to an evidence-based validation

C. Bergamini (✉)
Careggi University Hospital, Florence, Italy
e-mail: drcarlobergamini@gmail.com

F. Agresta
Department of General Surgery, Azienda ULSS19 del Veneto, Adria (RO), Italy

F.C. Campanile
Ospedale San Giovanni Decollato Andosilla, AUSL Viterbo, Civita Castellana, VT, Italy

G. Anania
Department of Morfology, Surgery and Experimental Medicine, School of Medicine,
University of Ferrara, Ferrara, Italy

F. Agresta et al. (eds.), *Emergency Laparoscopy*,
DOI 10.1007/978-3-319-29620-3_1

of emergency laparoscopic surgery: it was in 2006, in fact, when the European Association for Endoscopic Surgery (EAES) published its consensus statement on laparoscopy for abdominal emergencies concluding that "...available evidence clearly demonstrates the superiority of a laparoscopic approach in various emergency situations" [1]. Furthermore, it is interesting to note that these guidelines outline the role of emergency abdominal laparoscopy as a diagnostic tool as well, allowing the resolutions of preoperative diagnostic doubts besides the treatment of the underlying disease.

Different pathologic conditions are responsible for various acute abdominal situations; in particular, the most common cause of acute abdominal pain is the nonspecific abdominal pain (NSAP), followed by acute appendicitis, acute biliary disease, and bowel obstruction or diverticulitis. Despite noninvasive diagnostic procedures (ultrasonography and CT scan) help surgeon to establish a preoperative diagnosis, in most of the cases these are not completely accurate and conclusive about many authors [2–6]. On the contrary, the rate of diagnostic accuracy of laparoscopy is variable from 89 to 100 % in international literature [1, 6–9].

Concerning the trauma setting, prior to ultrasonography and CT scan, laparotomy for abdominal trauma was negative and nontherapeutic in approximately one-third of cases [10]. Nowadays, laparoscopy has a dominant role in well-selected traumatic patients as a diagnostic tool or therapeutic tool in repairing injuries to the diaphragm, liver, or spleen and limited gastrointestinal injuries.

1.3 Notes on Lap Cholecystectomy

Laparoscopic approach actually is generally considered to be a gold standard for cholecystectomies, and the safety of this procedure has also been proved in case of acute cholecystitis. In the last decades, the number of cholecystectomies increased worldwide. However, even if several national guidelines suggest laparoscopic cholecystectomy as a standard of care, it is surprising to find in some national reports that acute cholecystitis is treated in 50 % of cases. In a population-based study conducted in the USA, from January 2000 through December 2005, there were an estimated 2.5 million patients with acute cholecystitis. Among these patients, fewer than half underwent cholecystectomy and, among them, the 85 % was treated with a laparoscopic procedure while the 15 % with an open procedure [11]; however, this study did not consider the patients who underwent delayed cholecystectomy after the conservative resolution of the cholecystitis. On the other hand, in a study conducted in the USA on 4011 patients, early laparoscopic cholecystectomy was performed in 38.0 % of patients and delayed laparoscopic cholecystectomy in 62.0 %. In this study, authors state that laparoscopic cholecystectomy for acute cholecystitis in patients older than 65 years with significant comorbidities is associated with shorter postoperative stay and no increase in postoperative complications or conversion to open cholecystectomy [12].

On the contrary, in Denmark, among 28,379 patients who underwent cholecystectomy between 2006 and 2009, a laparoscopic procedure was performed in

97.7 % [13]. When surgery is performed laparoscopic cholecystectomy represents the treatment of choice for acute setting with more than 80 % of the operations done with a laparoscopic approach.

1.4 Notes on Lap Appendectomy

Acute appendicitis represents the greatest cause of emergency surgery; in fact, 250,000 operations are performed every year in the USA [14]. Open appendectomy has been the standard procedure for acute appendicitis for more than 100 years. It was in 1983 when Semm [15] reported the first video-assisted laparoscopic appendectomy in an adult patient, and since then the acceptance of laparoscopic appendectomy by surgeons was quite slow if compared to cholecistectomy. Laparoscopy for acute appendicitis, fortunately, has spread widely in the last 10 years. In a national audit conducted in Italy, for example, results confirm the trend of the dissemination of LA to peripheral district hospital: in fact, it is practiced in 93 % of Italian hospitals, and the percentage is increasing [16]. In a national survey conducted in Germany, results show that the technical infrastructure for laparoscopic appendectomy was provided in all units, but only in 79 % of units laparoscopic technique was the standard approach for appendectomy [17]. In a national survey conducted in Massachusetts, among 2565 patients with appendicitis, 90.1 % of appendicitis patients underwent some intervention. Of these patients, 15.3 % underwent open appendectomy and 72.9 % underwent laparoscopic appendectomy; meanwhile, 1.9 % underwent radiologically guided drain placement [18].

While the laparoscopic approach for appendectomy is widely diffused in the majority of countries and represents a standard of care, in other countries this technique is still in the process of development and diffusion. In a nationwide population-based study conducted in Taiwan, the proportion of patients undergoing laparoscopic appendectomy was lower (13.3 %) than that of patients receiving open appendectomy for acute appendicitis. Nevertheless, the frequency of laparoscopic appendectomy increased over time, passing from less than 1 % in 2001 to 37.2 % in 2008 [19]. In a survey of Polish pediatric surgeon, the low rate of laparoscopic appendectomy in Poland (33 % of cases) is confirmed: these data suggest that laparoscopic appendectomy still remains far from being a standard in that country [20].

1.5 Other Lap in the Urgency Setting

The role of laparoscopy in the diagnosis and treatment of many other acute gynecological disorders is fundamental, due to the nonspecific clinical presentation of both diseases in the majority of cases. Similarly, there are many causes of acute pancreatitis and a large spectrum of clinical presentation, and even if laparoscopy is unnecessary for diagnosis, it plays a key role in the management of necrotizing pancreatitis.

It was in 1990 when Mouret et al. [21] reported the first laparoscopic repair of a perforated peptic ulcer and actually this technique is universally accepted. A laparoscopic approach is indicated also in case of complicated diverticulitis as well as in case of small-bowel obstruction due to adhesions.

Small-bowel obstruction (SBO) requiring adhesiolysis is a frequent and costly problem in the USA: in 2005, 119 per 100,000 hospitalized patients had adhesiolysis-related disease [22].

Open adhesiolysis is accepted as the standard surgical intervention for adhesive SBO, but since the first successful laparoscopic adhesiolysis performed in the early 1990s, many small-scale studies have found this procedure to be feasible and safe. In a systematic review of 29 studies with a total of 2005 patients undergoing laparoscopic treatment of acute SBO, O'Connor et al. found that 64 % of the operations were completed without conversion to an open procedure with a postoperative morbidity of 14.8 % and mortality of 1.5 % [23]. A recent study in the USA performed on a total of 9619 patients who underwent adhesiolysis between 2005 and 2010 demonstrated that only 14.9 % of operations for SBO were performed laparoscopically with a significant reduction in 30-day mortality, major complications, and incisional complications associated with laparoscopic adhesiolysis compared with open adhesiolysis for the treatment of acute SBO [24]. Laparoscopy, furthermore, plays an important role in the diagnosis and in the management of acute mesenteric ischemia because it is relatively quick, is well tolerated, and if necessary can be performed at the bedside in the intensive care unit or emergency room [25].

1.6 Lap Emergency Surgery in Developing Countries

While the spread of laparoscopy in emergency surgery is a standard practice in most of the countries of the world, open surgery unfortunately remains the standard of care in developing nations. The introduction of laparoscopy in resource-poor areas has been a topic of debate; in fact, within poor countries surgical services are concentrated almost wholly in cities and priority is given to surgical abdomens, severe trauma, and other potentially fatal pathologies that do not have laparoscopic indications [26]. There are few studies in the literature about this topic, but they demonstrate the use of laparoscopy in emergency surgery in most countries of the world. A study conducted in Pakistan [27], for example, demonstrates that also in a developing country early diagnostic laparoscopy is a safe procedure with high efficacy. In this study, authors excluded the use of diagnostic laparoscopy in trauma patients because of the nonavailability of technical expertise at all times. In another study conducted in Nigeria [28], in which authors explain their experience in laparoscopic appendectomy, emerges the fact that the development of laparoscopic surgery in this country is slow if compared to other developing nations like India, but, at this moment, in some institutions surgeons with a basic training in minimal access surgery who perform most of the operations with a good outcome are present. Another Nigerian study [29] conducted on pediatric patients demonstrated that laparoscopy has been used to perform cholecystectomies, appendectomies, and also adhesiolysis for intestinal obstruction due to adhesions. Authors conclude stating that laparoscopic surgery technique is feasible in developing countries despite scarce resources.

While the use of laparoscopy in emergency surgery is still under development in few countries and widely used for appendectomies or diagnostic laparoscopy, in a recent systematic review and meta-analysis conducted by Li et al. [30], a comparison between laparoscopy and laparotomy in the management of abdominal trauma was performed. Authors analyzed 64 studies (countries included China, Finland, Turkey, Brazil, Russia, the USA) including 9058 patients with abdominal trauma. The type of abdominal trauma reported mainly involved gastrointestinal injury, spleen injury, hepatic injury, pancreatic injury, mesenteric injury, and omentum majus injury (most of the studies enrolled patients with multiple injuries). Moreover, laparoscopy was used as a screening, diagnostic, or therapeutic tool. Authors conclude by stating that laparoscopy is effective and superior in the treatment of abdominal trauma than conventional open laparotomy if patients have appropriate indications.

In conclusion, laparoscopic surgery represents a valuable standard of surgical care for most of the country, for both diagnostic and therapeutic intent, in most abdominal emergencies and it surely has improved our management of surgical emergencies being an essential part of our clinical and therapeutic approach.

References

1. Sauerland S, Agresta F, Bergamaschi R, Borzellino G, Budzynski A, Champault G et al (2006) Laparoscopy for abdominal emergencies: evidence-based guidelines of the European Association for Endoscopic Surgery. Surg Endosc 20(1):14–29
2. Salem TA, Molloy RG, O'Dwyer PJ (2005) Prospective study on the role of the CT scan in patients with an acute abdomen. Colorectal Dis 7(5):460–466
3. Andersson RE (2011) Routine ultrasound and limited computed tomography for the diagnosis of acute appendicitis: a surgeon's perspective. World J Surg 35(2):295–296
4. Golash V, Willson PD (2005) Early laparoscopy as a routine procedure in the management of acute abdominal pain: a review of 1,320 patients. Surg Endosc 19(7):882–885
5. Kirshtein B, Roy-Shapira A, Lantsberg L, Mandel S, Avinoach E, Mizrahi S (2003) The use of laparoscopy in abdominal emergencies. Surg Endosc 17(7):1118–1124
6. Domínguez LC, Sanabria A, Vega V, Osorio C (2011) Early laparoscopy for the evaluation of nonspecific abdominal pain: a critical appraisal of the evidence. Surg Endosc 25(1):10–18
7. Agresta F, Mazzarolo G, Ciardo LF, Bedin N (2008) The laparoscopic approach in abdominal emergencies: has the attitude changed? A single-center review of a 15-year experience. Surg Endosc 22(5):1255–1262
8. Champault G, Descottes B, Dulucq JL, Fabre JM, Fourtanier G, Gayet B et al (2006) Laparoscopic surgery. The recommendations of specialty societies in 2006 (SFCL-SFCE). J Chir (Paris) 143(3):160–4
9. Hori Y (2008) Diagnostic laparoscopy guidelines: this guideline was prepared by the SAGES Guidelines Committee and reviewed and approved by the Board of Governors of the Society of American Gastrointestinal and Endoscopic Surgeons (SAGES), November 2007. Surg Endosc 22(5):1353–1383
10. Renz BM, Feliciano DV (1995) Unnecessary laparotomies for trauma: a prospective study of morbidity. J Trauma 38(3):350–356

11. Csikesz N, Ricciardi R, Tseng JF, Shah SA (2008) Current status of surgical management of acute cholecystitis in the United States. World J Surg 32(10):2230–2236
12. Haltmeier T, Benjamin E, Inaba K, Lam L, Demetriades D (2015) Early versus delayed same-admission laparoscopic cholecystectomy for acute cholecystitis in elderly patients with comorbidities. J Trauma Acute Care Surg 78(4):801–807
13. Harboe KM, Bardram L (2011) The quality of cholecystectomy in Denmark: outcome and risk factors for 20,307 patients from the national database. Surg Endosc 25(5):1630–1641
14. Addiss DG, Shaffer N, Fowler BS, Tauxe RV (1990) The epidemiology of appendicitis and appendectomy in the United States. Am J Epidemiol 132(5):910–925
15. Semm K (1983) Endoscopic appendectomy. Endoscopy 15(2):59–64
16. Vettoretto N, Gobbi S, Belli F, Corradi A, Mannino L, Ricciardelli L et al (2012) Diffusion of laparoscopic appendectomies in Italy: a national audit. Minim Invasive Ther Allied Technol 21(2):101–107
17. Dingemann J, Metzelder ML, Szavay PO (2013) Current status of laparoscopic appendectomy in children: a nation wide survey in Germany. Eur J Pediatr Surg 23(3):226–233
18. Madore JC, Collins CE, Ayturk MD, Santry HP (2015) The impact of acute care surgery on appendicitis outcomes: results from a national sample of university-affiliated hospitals. J Trauma Acute Care Surg 79(2):282–288
19. Yeh C-C, Wu S-C, Liao C-C, Su L-T, Hsieh C-H, Li T-C (2011) Laparoscopic appendectomy for acute appendicitis is more favorable for patients with comorbidities, the elderly, and those with complicated appendicitis: a nationwide population-based study. Surg Endosc 25(9):2932–2942
20. Golebiewski A, Czauderna P (2015) The role of laparoscopy in the management of pediatric appendicitis: a survey of Polish pediatric surgeons. Wideochirurgia i inne Tech małoinwazyjne = Videosurgery other miniinvasive Tech/Kwart Pod patronatem Sekc Wideochirurgii TChP oraz Sekc Chir Bariatrycznej TChP 10(1):101–106
21. Mouret P, François Y, Vignal J, Barth X, Lombard-Platet R (1990) Laparoscopic treatment of perforated peptic ulcer. Br J Surg 77(9):1006
22. Scott FI, Osterman MT, Mahmoud NN, Lewis JD (2012) Secular trends in small-bowel obstruction and adhesiolysis in the United States: 1988–2007. Am J Surg 204(3):315–320
23. O'Connor DB, Winter DC (2012) The role of laparoscopy in the management of acute small-bowel obstruction: a review of over 2,000 cases. Surg Endosc 26(1):12–17
24. Kelly KN, Iannuzzi JC, Rickles AS, Garimella V, Monson JRT, Fleming FJ (2014) Laparotomy for small-bowel obstruction: first choice or last resort for adhesiolysis? A laparoscopic approach for small-bowel obstruction reduces 30-day complications. Surg Endosc 28(1):65–73
25. Iberti TJ, Salky BA, Onofrey D (1989) Use of bedside laparoscopy to identify intestinal ischemia in postoperative cases of aortic reconstruction. Surgery 105(5):686–689
26. Farmer PE, Kim JY (2008) Surgery and global health: a view from beyond the OR. World J Surg 32(4):533–536
27. Rubbia A, Faryal GA, Javeria I, Roohul M (2015) Role of diagnostic laparoscopy in patients with acute or chronic nonspecific abdominal pain. World J Laparosc Surg 8(April):7–12
28. Mshelia NM, Obiano SK, Guduf MI, Gital YS (2014) Our experience in laparoscopic appendectomy in Federal Teaching Hospital, Gombe. World J Laparosc Surg 7(December):111–115
29. Misauno MA, Ojo EO, Uba AF (2012) Laparoscopic paediatric surgery: a potential for paradigm shift in developing countries. Afr J Paediatr Surg 9(2):140–2
30. Li Y, Xiang Y, Wu N, Wu L, Yu Z, Zhang M et al (2015) A comparison of laparoscopy and laparotomy for the management of abdominal trauma: a systematic review and meta-analysis. World J Surg 39(12):2862–2871

Acute Calculous Cholecystitis

2

Fabio Cesare Campanile, Domenico Giannotti, Ferdinando Agresta, Nereo Vettoretto, and Rao Ivatury

2.1 Introduction

Acute calculous cholecystitis is one of the most common conditions faced by a general surgeon. Cholecystectomy is the most common digestive operation and about 30 % of them are performed after an acute cholecystitis [1]. Still, many aspects about its treatment are controversial and common practice often differs from the indications provided by the literature.

The disease itself is very heterogeneous: the degree of inflammation may vary from a self-limiting to a life-threatening form; furthermore, associated conditions often impose a deviation from the most common course of action, and the general status of the patient has a relevant impact on both the severity of the illness and the treatment outcomes.

Such heterogeneity should correspond to a tailored approach, able to grant the more appropriate treatment to every single patient; however, the literature is devoid of clear indications about how to adapt the clinical pathway to the diverse scenarios, the parameters to stratify the risk of surgery in this population are not clear, the most commonly adopted risk scores are not validated for the acute cholecystitis, and no instrument is available to select the best course of action in different situations [2,3].

F.C. Campanile (✉) • D. Giannotti
AUSL Viterbo, Ospedale San Giovanni Decollato Andosilla, via Ferretti 169, 01033 Civita Castellana, VT, Italy
e-mail: campanile@surgical.net

F. Agresta
Department of General Surgery, Azienda ULSS19 del Veneto, Adria (RO), Italy

N. Vettoretto
Montichiari Surgery Department, ASST Spedali Civili di Brescia, via G. Ciotti 154, 25018 Montichiari, BS, Italy

R.R. Ivatury
Virginia Commonwealth University, Richmond, VA, USA

F. Agresta et al. (eds.), *Emergency Laparoscopy*,
DOI 10.1007/978-3-319-29620-3_2

The available guidelines provide a very valuable support for the daily surgical practice; however, their recommendations are affected by the lack of literature evidence about several crucial aspects.

We will try to examine the controversial clinical issues about acute calculous cholecystitis, analyzing the evidence supporting the guidelines and the most recent scientific literature data.

2.2 Diagnostic Issues in the Acute Calculous Cholecystitis

The diagnosis of acute calculous cholecystitis relies on a combination of local, systemic, and imaging signs. A systematic review by Trowbridge [4] suggested that no single clinical finding or laboratory test carries sufficient weight to establish or exclude acute cholecystitis. In 2006, based on these results, the European Association for Endoscopic Surgery (EAES) suggested that the presence of acute right upper quadrant pain for more than 6 h along with ultrasound evidence of acute cholecystitis (the presence of gallstones with a thickened and edematous gallbladder wall, positive ultrasound Murphy's sign, and pericholecystic fluid collections) could achieve a high diagnostic specificity. The demonstration of gallstones without clear imaging cholecystitis should be supported by one or more of the following: temperature above 38°, leukocytosis greater than 10,000/dL, and C-reactive protein higher than 10 mg/L [5]. The 2012 update of those guidelines maintained the validity of those criteria [6].

In 2007, the Tokyo Guidelines (TG07) proposed a similar set of criteria that quickly became widely adopted worldwide [7, 8]. The Tokyo Guidelines Revision Committee reported that 92.1 % sensitivity and 93.3 % specificity was achieved when those criteria were adopted in clinical practice. Their last revision (TG13) is reported in Table 2.1; the imaging findings necessary for the definite diagnosis are detailed in Table 2.2.

Table 2.1 TG13 diagnostic criteria for acute cholecystitis[a]

A. Local signs of inflammation, etc.
(1) Murphy's sign and (2) RUQ mass/pain/tenderness
B. Systemic signs of inflammation, etc.
(1) Fever, (2) elevated CRP, and (3) elevated WBC count
C. Imaging findings
Imaging findings characteristic of acute cholecystitis
Suspected diagnosis: One item in A + one item in B
Definite diagnosis: One item in A + one item in B + C

[a]RUQ, right upper abdominal quadrant, CRP, C-reactive protein, and WBC, white blood cell

With kind permission from Springer Science+Business Media: Yokoe M et al. (2013) TG13 diagnostic criteria and severity grading of acute cholecystitis (with videos). J Hepatobiliary Pancreat Sci 20:35–46. ©Japanese Society of Hepato-Biliary-Pancreatic Surgery and Springer 2012, Table 1 [8] (modified)

Table 2.2 TG07 Imaging findings of acute cholecystitis[a]

Ultrasonography findings
Sonographic Murphy sign (tenderness elicited by pressing the gallbladder with the ultrasound probe)
Thickened gallbladder wall (>4 mm; if the patient does not have chronic liver disease and/or ascites or right heart failure)
Enlarged gallbladder (long axis diameter >8 cm, short axis diameter >4 cm)
Incarcerated gallstone, debris echo, and pericholecystic fluid collection
Sonolucent layer in the gallbladder wall, striated intramural lucencies, and Doppler signals
Magnetic resonance imaging (MRI) findings
Pericholecystic high signal
Enlarged gallbladder
Thickened gallbladder wall
Computed tomography (CT) findings
Thickened gallbladder wall
Pericholecystic fluid collection
Enlarged gallbladder linear high-density areas in the pericholecystic fat tissue
Tc-HIDA scans
Non-visualized gallbladder with normal uptake and excretion of radioactivity
Rim sign (augmentation of radioactivity around the gallbladder fossa)

[a]With kind permission from Springer Science+Business Media: Hirota M et al. (2007) Diagnostic criteria and severity assessment of acute cholecystitis: Tokyo Guidelines. J Hepatobiliary Pancreat Sci 14:78–82. ©Springer-Verlag Tokyo 2007 [7] (modified)

2.3 Laparoscopic or Laparotomic Surgery for Acute Cholecystitis?

Early after the introduction of laparoscopic surgery, acute cholecystitis was considered a contraindication for mini-invasive surgery: laparoscopic cholecystectomy in the acute inflammatory phase of cholecystitis required uncommon dexterity and experience for those early times, and a higher complication rate was reported [9, 10].

In later years, the increased experience and progressive acquisition of the required skills allowed us to safely complete a laparoscopic cholecystectomy even in the most severe acute conditions. All the recent guidelines consider laparoscopic cholecystectomy as the gold standard for the treatment of acute calculous cholecystitis [6, 11–13]. Nevertheless, practice pattern varies. Most patients, at least in the western world, receive laparoscopic cholecystectomy [14, 15]; however, many do not undergo surgery [16, 17] and almost 50 % of all complicated acute cholecystitis worldwide are still operated by laparotomy, as shown by the CIAO and CIAOW studies [18, 19].

Therefore, it is quite important to examine the clinical advantages reported in the literature in favor of the laparoscopic approach.

2.3.1 Laparoscopic Cholecystectomy for Acute Cholecystitis: The Evidence

The superiority of laparoscopic cholecystectomy in the treatment of acute calculous cholecystitis has been mainly demonstrated in four randomized controlled trials (RCTs) [20–23]. They show that laparoscopic cholecystectomy is associated with faster recovery and shorter hospital stay. They also indicated that the morbidity of the laparoscopic approach was not higher, as initially supposed, but actually lower. However, a full demonstration of a statistically significant reduction in the complication rate could only be obtained by the meta-analysis just recently published by Coccolini et al. [24]. This study took into consideration both randomized and non-randomized researches; however, some of the outcomes could be separately analyzed on the basis of RCTs data only. In this way, it was possible to demonstrate, with the highest level of evidence, that laparoscopic cholecystectomy in acute cholecystitis carries a lower risk of complications. Mortality also appeared lower in the laparoscopic group but the data were available only for non-randomized comparative studies. Among the complications, wound infection, pneumonia, and bile leakage deserved a separate inquiry: the wound infection and pneumonia rate favored laparoscopic surgery, while the bile leakage did not differ significantly between the two groups. These data represent a strong support for the role of laparoscopic cholecystectomy as the gold standard in the treatment of the acute calculous cholecystitis.

The interpretation of the results about faster recovery and postoperative length of stay deserves a word of caution. As a matter of fact, the evaluation of these parameters is partially subjective, and it cannot be excluded that the improved outcome of laparoscopic surgery be related to an expectation bias of the medical staff rather than to real clinical and physiopathologic changes. The trial by Johannson [21] was designed to avoid this bias and included a blind assessment of the outcomes: both patients and postoperative care staff were unaware of the surgical access received by the patient because the wounds were kept concealed at all times. Still a reduced hospital stay could be shown.

One of the RCTs [22] demonstrated a reduction in the surgical trauma and immunosuppression by measuring serum C-reactive protein and tumor necrosis factor-α (TNF-α) secretion of peripheral blood mononuclear cells.

If the data of the RCTs with their meta-analysis constitute the strongest evidence in support of the laparoscopic approach also in the acute setting, the findings reported by the large observational studies provide an insight into the reality of the everyday practice. In 2008, Csikesz conducted a population-based analysis on the USA National Hospital Discharge Surveys about more than one million cholecystectomies performed for acute cholecystitis from 2000 through 2005. The study confirmed that laparoscopic cholecystectomy is associated with lower morbidity, mortality, and shorter length stay. Open surgery was associated with a 1.3-fold increase in perioperative morbidity (95 % CI 1.1–1.4) after adjusting for patient and hospital factors [14].

2.4 When to Operate an Acute Cholecystitis? A Question of Timing

The optimal timing for surgical interventions in an acute cholecystitis is difficult to determine and controversial; most of the recent literature is devoted to this aspect.

In the pre-laparoscopic era, several randomized controlled trials had shown the superiority of early versus delayed open cholecystectomy: early surgery was associated with lower morbidity and shorter hospital stay [25–28].

As we underlined in section "Laparoscopic or Laparotomic Surgery for Acute Cholecystitis?," right after the introduction of laparoscopic surgery the skills to manage an acute cholecystitis by laparoscopy were uncommon, and the condition was considered to be a contraindication for mini-invasive cholecystectomy. The safety of laparoscopic surgery in the acute phase of the disease was questioned [9], and, again, practice evolved in favor of delayed laparoscopic cholecystectomy as an alternative to immediate open surgery: initial antibiotic treatment and resuscitation followed by elective laparoscopic surgery about 6 weeks after the acute attack.

Later, after having developed the necessary experience, the performance of mini-invasive cholecystectomies even in the acute phase of the disease became more and more common, and trials comparing early versus delayed laparoscopic cholecystectomy were possible.

2.4.1 The Evidence Supporting Early Laparoscopic Cholecystectomy

A systematic review of the literature found 15 randomized controlled trials comparing early versus delayed laparoscopic cholecystectomy [29–43], analyzed in several meta-analyses [1,44–49].

The definitions of "early" and "delayed" differ among the trials; however, most of them take into consideration patients operated on less than 72 h or less than 7 days from the onset of symptoms as "early"; their treatment is planned at least 6 weeks after the initial diagnosis in the "delayed" groups. Here, we do not mean to analyze in detail this large amount of literature; however, all the studies agree that early laparoscopic cholecystectomy is superior because it reduces the total hospital stay (due to the two episodes of admission) without a significant difference in the complication or conversion rate. One of the meta-analyses shows that the rate of bile duct injury, the most feared complication, seems to be even higher in the delayed treated patients but the difference was not statistically significant [1]. The same review also revealed that 18.3 % of the patients included in the delayed groups, in five RCTs, had to undergo emergency surgery in the interval period for either non-resolution or recurrence of symptoms before their planned operation [1]. The conversion rate was 45 % in this subgroup.

A very large population-based study confirmed those findings on 10,304 acute cholecystitis patients who did not undergo cholecystectomy on the first admission. The probability of a gallstone-related event was 14 % at 6 weeks and 29 % at

12 weeks. At 1 year after discharge the likelihood of an acute gallstone-related episode raised to 29 %. Of these events, 30 % were for biliary tract obstruction or pancreatitis [50]. A Swedish study found that 6.1 % of patients discharged without cholecystectomy had emergency surgery in the 2-year study period [16].

Other recent and large population-based studies sustain early surgery and show that morbidity (included common bile duct injuries) is lower in the early treated patients [51–53].

These data further support the practice of early laparoscopic cholecystectomy.

Despite the growing evidence in favor of it, the optimal time to perform early laparoscopic cholecystectomy is still not clear. Is there any difference if the operation is performed at 24, 48, and 72 h after the onset of symptoms or even later? Can we establish a threshold of delay after which cholecystectomy can no longer considered "early" and surgery had better be deferred to a later date (delayed)?

The already mentioned Cochrane review [1] performed a subgroup analysis comparing the data obtained from the trials that included only patients treated less than 4 days from the onset of symptoms to those including also patients with a longer delay, and did not find any statistically significant difference between them.

Once again, population-based study helps to clarify the issue. In 2011, Banz et al. examined the outcome of 4113 patients divided into six different groups according to their preoperative length of stay (adopted as a surrogate measure of the onset of symptoms): operated on the day of admission, on the following day, 2, 3, 4 or 5, 6 days later, or afterwards. There was no significant difference between preoperative length of stay and postoperative morbidity or mortality. However, the longer was the preoperative stay and the higher were the operative times and the conversion rate [51]. Their work did not include any risk adjustment, but similar results were reported by Brooks et al. on the American College of Surgeons National Surgical Quality Improvement Program database [54]. Their risk-adjusted analysis showed an increasing morbidity for cholecystectomies performed from the day of the admission to 4 days later (from 6 to 19 %) even if they could not demonstrate a statistical significance. In their 2015 paper, Zafar et al. used propensity score matching techniques to account for severity differences in a very large (95,523 patients) population-based series from the Nationwide Inpatient Sample (NIS). They demonstrated that surgery performed within the first 48 h of presentation was associated with the lowest complication, length of stay, mortality, and hospital cost. In fact, patients who had surgery during days 2 through 5 and days 6 through 10 had increasingly worse outcomes than those undergoing surgery on days 0 through 1. They could show statistically significant differences for mortality (OR = 1.26; 95 % CI 1.00–1.58 and 1.93; 95 % CI 1.38–2.68) and postoperative infections (OR = 0.88; 95 % CI 0.69–1.12 and 1.53; 95 % CI, 1.05–2.23) for days 2 through 5 and days 6 through 10, respectively. Also significant were the differences for pneumonia, UTI, and postoperative length of stay. Their extensive analysis took also into consideration the adjusted mean hospital cost, and showed it to increase from $8974 (days 0–1) to $17,745 (days 6–10). The analysis by each incremental day demonstrated the optimal time of surgery to be within the first 48 h of presentation. As already mentioned, the relevant size of the series allowed to properly assess the differences in the rare event of perioperative death: the lowest risk-adjusted mortality was found for surgery performed within 1 day or 2 days of presentation (0.36 % and 0.37 %, respectively), and sudden increase in mortality appeared from day 3 and later (0.45 %, $P = 0.01$). It is interesting to point out that mortality for surgery performed on day 0 was higher (0.42 %) than later. The authors explain the finding with the higher probability of under-resuscitated patients among those operated on the day of the admission [55].

Then, laparoscopic cholecystectomy should be performed as early as possible after the onset of symptoms, and preceded by an adequate resuscitation.

A recent large randomized controlled trial compared laparoscopic cholecystectomy performed within 24 h of admission versus surgery between 7 and 45 days after initial diagnosis [40]. This trial demonstrated that the morbidity rates were lower in the delayed than early laparoscopic cholecystectomy group and the length of hospital stay was 5 days shorter.

In conclusion, several RCTs and their meta-analyses show that laparoscopic cholecystectomy in the first 7 days after the diagnosis is preferable for its reduced length of stay, while morbidity is similar if the operation is performed after 6 weeks; on the other side, one trial reports that cholecystectomy between 7 and 45 days carries a higher morbidity rate. Therefore, we can affirm that laparoscopic cholecystectomy is safe within 7 days from the diagnosis but, outside that window, is probably better to wait until the 6th week. Large and sophisticated retrospective studies demonstrate that, within the 7 days of diagnosis, the earlier the operation the better the outcome and, ideally, laparoscopic cholecystectomy should be performed within the first 48 h of presentation.

Of course, it is just the case to underline that some of the above examined data use the time of diagnosis or day of admission as surrogate indicators of the onset of symptoms because the knowledge of the real beginning of the latter was not easy to determine; it can be assumed that the symptoms occur just before the hospital admission but this is not always the case. The everyday clinical practice has to keep into consideration this variability.

2.5 Laparoscopic Cholecystectomy in Particular Conditions

If the gold standard role of laparoscopic cholecystectomy for acute cholecystitis in the general population is well clarified by the above reported evidence, still a few particular conditions deserve a separate review. Are the above described principles applicable in every case irrespective of the severity of the inflammation and the local conditions? Are there groups in which a different conduct may be more appropriate?

2.5.1 Severe Cholecystitis

Is laparoscopic surgery indicated for empyema, perforated or gangrenous cholecystitis (severe cholecystitis)? Local inflammatory changes can be a real challenge for

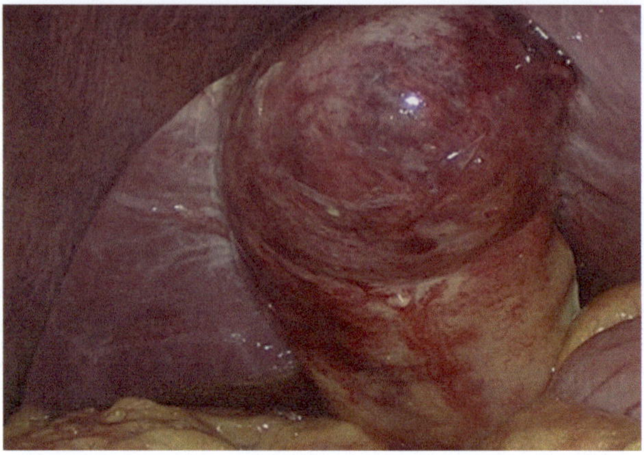

Fig. 2.1 A case of severe cholecystitis: gallbladder empyema

any surgeon, and the question of safety of laparoscopy in these extreme conditions needs to be addressed.

The EAES guidelines published in 2012 stated that empyema, perforated or gangrenous cholecystitis do not preclude the indication for laparoscopic cholecystectomy [6]. However, the Tokyo guidelines incorporate severe cholecystitis in Grade II of their classification (moderate cholecystitis), likely to be associated with increased operative difficulty (Fig. 2.1). Therefore, they advocate more cautious indications with a major propensity for gallbladder drainage and delayed surgery [8].

As a matter of fact, some of the RCTs mentioned in section "Laparoscopic Cholecystectomy for Acute Cholecystitis: The Evidence" specifically included patients with severe cholecystitis [20, 23], and a systematic review of observational series of severe cholecystitis did not show an increase in local postoperative complications despite a threefold conversion rate [56]. In their case-series, Nikfarjam et al. did not find any difference in the complication rate between the gangrenous and non-gangrenous cholecystitis [57].

In addition, some observational reports examined the treatment of severe cholecystitis with the aim to compare open versus laparoscopic surgery. A recent very large retrospective population-based series about gangrenous cholecystitis studied a total of 141,970 cholecystectomies from the 2005–2011 National Surgical Quality Improvement Project Participant User File. The authors extracted 7017 gangrenous cholecystitis. Although they were associated with increased morbidity and mortality compared with the general series of acute cholecystitis, the multivariate logistic regression model demonstrated a significant decrease in overall complication rate (odds ratio = 0.46; $P < 0.001$) for laparoscopic versus laparotomic cholecystectomy, with a lower, although not significant, perioperative mortality (OR = 0.59; $P = 0.12$) [58].

The retrospective investigation by Lo et al. [59] included 74 patients with cholecystitis and gallbladder perforation divided into 3 groups: early open cholecystectomy, early laparoscopic cholecystectomy, and percutaneous gallbladder drainage followed by delayed elective surgery. There were no differences in operative time, blood loss, conversion rate, and morbidity between the groups, but the length of hospital stay was significantly shorter for laparoscopic cholecystectomy. The authors concluded that early LC should be considered the optimal treatment for gallbladder perforation.

If in Lo's study early laparoscopic cholecystectomy compared favorably with both early open and delayed laparoscopic surgery for perforated cholecystitis, other observational reports examined the treatment of different forms of severe cholecystitis, with the aim to compare early laparoscopic surgery versus some kind of delayed treatment. Recently Choi et al., in a retrospective study about gangrenous cholecystitis, compared patients who had early versus delayed laparoscopic surgery, the latter often preceded by percutaneous cholecystostomy. They failed to find a significant difference in the morbidity rate, and the total hospital stay was longer in the delayed group [60]. Similar results were reported by Kwon et al. about gallbladder empyema [61].

Therefore, laparoscopic surgery is not precluded by severe cholecystitis and actually seems to be beneficial in terms of morbidity and hospital stay. Early surgery appears to be advantageous and there is little support for the assumption that deferring the definitive treatment of these conditions may improve the outcome and reduce complications.

Nonetheless, the operation may be extremely demanding in those cases in which the intense inflammation around the Calot's triangle increases the risk of serious complications. When a positive identification of the vascular and biliary structures cannot be achieved with the "critical view of safety" (Fig. 2.2) [62] a laparotomy is advocated. However, conversion not always grants an improved

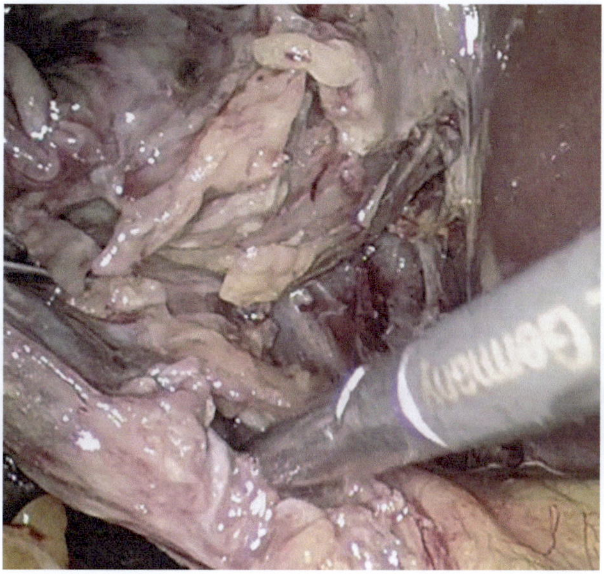

Fig. 2.2 Identification of the "critical view of safety" window in a gangrenous cholecystitis

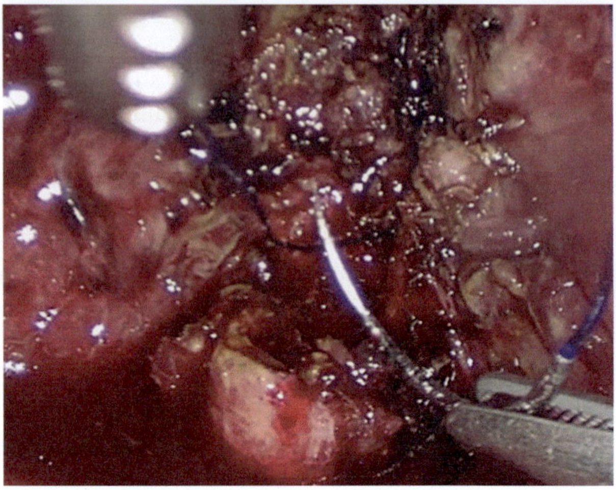

Fig. 2.3 Subtotal laparoscopic cholecystectomy in a patient with "frozen" Calot's triangle: suture of the infundibulum

understanding of the biliary anatomy, and experienced laparoscopic surgeons may proceed laparoscopically with a subtotal (or "partial") cholecystectomy that appears to be a reasonable alternative (Fig. 2.3).

The two most recent systematic reviews about partial cholecystectomy report relatively low morbidity rates, comparable to those of total cholecystectomy in simple cases. Nowadays, most of them are carried out laparoscopically with reduced risk of subhepatic collection (odds ratio OR = 0.4; 95 % CI = 0.2–0.9), retained stones (OR = 0.5; 95 % CI = 0.3–0.9), wound infection (OR = 0.07; 95 % CI = 0.04–0.2), reoperation (OR = 0.5; 95 % CI = 0.3–0.9), and mortality (OR = 0.2; 95 % CI = 0.05–0.9) but more bile leaks (OR = 5.3; 95 % CI = 3.9–7.2) compared with the open approach [63, 64].

2.5.2 Acute Cholecystitis in the Elderly

In a later chapter, we will treat the issue of laparoscopic emergency surgery in the elderly. Here, we will examine some specific aspects concerning acute cholecystitis.

The prevalence of gallstones increases with age and the life expectancy rises worldwide. Therefore, the analysis of the more appropriate treatment modalities in this age group is becoming more and more relevant. In addition, the co-morbidities in the elderly are obviously more frequent and the acute biliary disease itself appears to be more severe in this age group. It does not surprise, then, that age is often considered a risk factor for laparoscopic biliary surgery, particularly in the acute setting, both for morbidity [65, 66] and conversion, [67, 68], but it is very difficult to reach solid conclusions comparing younger versus older patients, because the two age groups are generally not comparable in terms of co-morbidities and functional status.

In the case-series published in 2001 by Decker, cholecystectomy lethality in acute calculous cholecystitis was much higher in the laparoscopic group in patients older than 80 [69]. Lupinacci et al., in their retrospective study, pointed out that the increase in mortality was relevant for cholecystectomy performed in emergency but not for the elective cases [70]. They suggested that, in the aged, laparoscopic cholecystectomy should be performed early after they are found to have symptomatic gallstones, preventing the occurrence of the inflammation, its increased morbidity and mortality risk. Of course, their series had more high risk patients (ASA III and IV) and less laparoscopic cholecystectomies in the urgent (acute cholecystitis) than in the elective groups; these factors can be responsible for part of the worse outcome of the emergency treatment.

Nielsen et al., on the other hand, could demonstrate a significantly worse mortality in the patients older than 80 even if they had a low anesthetic risk (ASA I and II). Their retrospective study showed that the odds for mortality are much higher in the aged (>80) than in the younger groups (65–79 vs. 50–64), with Odds Ratio of 30.86 vs. 5.51 vs. 1 [71].

However, the few observational studies able to compare directly open versus laparoscopic cholecystectomy for acute cholecystitis in the elderly, demonstrated a reduction in hospital stay [72, 73], and morbidity either unchanged [72] or even improved [73] in the patients who had laparoscopic surgery.

Having clarified that mini-invasive cholecystectomy is beneficial even in the aged, one question arises from the above reported data: if it is true that mortality is higher for laparoscopic surgery performed in the acute but not in the elective setting in the elderly group, could delayed cholecystectomy be beneficial at this age?

There is no definitive evidence on this particular aspect. Only a few retrospective cohort studies compare the outcome of early versus delayed cholecystectomy in elderly acute calculous cholecystitis patients. Mortality and morbidity do not appear to be significantly different [74–76]. Furthermore, a recent cohort study showed that recurrent episodes of pancreatitis, cholecystitis, and cholangitis were four times more likely after delayed cholecystectomy, and the conversion rate did not change [77]. These findings are confirmed by a recent population-based study on a sample of the US Medicare Claims Data System. In this analysis, a lack of a definitive surgical treatment at the index admission in the elderly is associated with 38 % gallstone-related readmission rate in 2 years versus 4.4 % in similar patients who had early cholecystectomy and a worse 2-year survival (hazard ratio 1.56, 95 % CI 1.47–1.65) even taking into account patient demographics and co-morbidities [78]. The very large series reported in the study (29,818 Medicare beneficiaries urgently or emergently admitted for acute cholecystitis from 1996 to 2005) showed that most US surgeons are confident in operating elderly cholecystitis patients in emergency: 75 % of the patients aged 66 years and older had an early cholecystectomy (laparoscopic in 71 % of them). The authors conclude in favor of early cholecystectomy for elderly patients to prevent recurrent episodes of cholecystitis, multiple readmissions, and increased costs.

2.6 The High Risk Patient

Acute calculous cholecystitis is a very heterogeneous condition. The severity and complexity of the clinical picture is determined not only by the degree of inflammation and the local conditions but also by the general status of the patient. In the previous chapters we examined the data about laparoscopic cholecystectomy as the definitive therapy of the disease. As a matter of fact, surgery is the gold standard treatment. Nevertheless, quite often, local or general circumstances suggest or even impose a different course of action. The optimal surgical treatment should be examined according to the severity of the disease. In fact, it could be argued that alternative treatment could better fit the needs of patients with reduced functional reserve [2, 3]. Should surgery be avoided in some very high risk patients? Could a delayed treatment be beneficial in some of them? Are there any alternatives to surgery?

The identification of the parameters and instruments to stratify the risk of surgery in this population would be of paramount importance to evaluate the role for alternative therapeutic pathways.

2.6.1 How to Stratify the Risk?

Let's examine the literature to verify if there is any available instrument to select the best course of action in particular high risk groups.

Recently, the Tokyo guidelines attempted to address the acute cholecystitis heterogeneity with a therapeutic algorithm that includes some elements of risk evaluation. Their staging system is based upon severity assessment criteria such as degree of local inflammation and associated co-morbidities, without including any of the most commonly adopted risk stratification scores [11]. However, a retrospective series failed to find any significant benefit following the introduction of their guidelines [79].

Advanced age is often identified as a risk factor for the surgical treatment of acute cholecystitis. We have examined in section "Acute Cholecystitis in the Elderly" the literature about laparoscopic cholecystectomy in the elderly and in particular about the timing for surgery; however, the possibility to compare directly surgical treatment versus an alternative strategy is not available.

In 2006 Yi stratifies the risk in relation to the ASA score, showing a significant difference in morbidity (20 % vs 9.1 %) in patients in ASA III vs ASA I, with no significant differences on the conversion rate, recovery time, and hospital postoperative stay [80].

The only other available comparison of risk assessment scores (ASA, APACHE II, and POSSUM) is limited to the perforated acute cholecystitis. It highlights a significant association of the three scores with morbidity and mortality. Both POSSUM and APACHE II were superior to ASA in risk prediction [81]. However APACHE II is built as an evaluation score in patient admitted to intensive care units, and its use as preoperative risk prediction instrument may be suboptimal. As a matter of fact, a validated score to choose the best treatment in relation to the patient's surgical risk is currently not available.

2.6.2 The Percutaneous Cholecystostomy

A large amount of literature addresses the role of gallbladder drainage (tube cholecystostomy), generally percutaneous, as an alternative to early surgery in septic high risk patients. More than 100 papers have been published in the last few years about this topic. They are generally small case-series of poor quality. Their inclusion criteria, results, and conclusions are largely not homogeneous. The only randomized controlled trial of cholecystostomy versus surgery is under way and not even preliminary results are available [82]. The purpose of gallbladder drainage is decompression of the infected bile, removal of the purulent collection, and solution of the sepsis with an improvement of the clinical conditions. Surgery may be planned at a later date. In particular, the panel of the Tokyo guidelines states that it is known to be a safe option in critically ill patients, and their guidelines consider the percutaneous (or surgical) drainage as mandatory in the severe grade of acute cholecystitis. Its use is also suggested in the moderate grade. However, cholecystostomy has never been proven to be an effective alternative to early surgery, and the evidence on its role is still poor. With all the methodological limits mentioned above, a survey of the literature shows that in-hospital mortality for cholecystostomy varies between 4 and 50 % and its morbidity between 8.2 and 62 %. A recent systematic review performed a particularly detailed examination of 53 papers about gallbladder drainage as an option in acute cholecystitis. It found no evidence to support the recommendation of tube cholecystostomy rather than straight early emergency cholecystectomy even in critically ill patients. Actually, it suggested that cholecystectomy seems to be a better option for treating acute cholecystitis in the elderly and/or critically ill population. The authors include 53 studies with 1918 patients; once again, they warn that the results obtained from the studies reviewed are very heterogeneous. They outline a high success rate of the procedure (85.6 %) with a low mortality directly related to the procedure (0.36 %) but a 30-day mortality of 15.4 %, significantly higher ($P < 0.001$) than after early cholecystectomy (4.5 %), as reported in published series of similar patients [83]. A recent prospective study in high risk patients examined the outcomes of 29 patients treated by percutaneous cholecystostomy and 32 by emergency cholecystectomy. The groups were homogeneous by age and surgical risk, estimated by physiological POSSUM, Charlson, APACHE II, and ASA scores. Eight patients (29.6 %) in the cholecystostomy group required emergency cholecystectomy anyway. The mortality rate was significantly higher in the cholecystostomy group (17.2 % vs nil). The authors concluded that percutaneous drainage appears of little benefit and should be reserved for the patients with surgical contraindication [84]. A large retrospective cohort study, based on administrative databases capturing all emergency department (ED) visits and hospital admissions in a populous area, examined 27,718 acute cholecystitis patients. Of them, 890 (3.3 %) underwent tube cholecystostomy. In-hospital mortality was 5 %, but an additional 18 % had died without surgery. Only 40 % had cholecystectomy within 1 year (due to intercurrent mortality or ongoing contraindications) and 49 % was evaluated in the emergency department or admitted to the hospital for a gallstone-related complication [50].

Therefore, at the moment, tube cholecystostomy, as a bridge to surgery or definitive management of acute cholecystitis, cannot be considered as an established and safe option. More studies are needed.

2.6.3 Endoscopic Gallbladder Drainage

In the attempt to find less invasive solutions in the old-frail patients and those with increased surgical risk, endoscopic gallbladder drainage methods have been proposed. Two techniques have been described: the endoscopic transpapillary (ETGD) and endoscopic ultrasound-guided transmural gallbladder drainage (EUS-GBD).

In the former, endoscopic naso-gallbladder drainage and gallbladder stenting via a transpapillary endoscopic approach are included.

In retrospective studies, endoscopic naso-gallbladder drainage and gallbladder stenting have a technical success rate of 81 % and 96 %, but a clinical success rate of 75 % and 88 %, respectively [85]. However, this technique is not feasible if obstruction or tortuosity of the cystic duct does not allow a guidewire to be advanced into the gallbladder.

As an alternative, a drain or a stent can be placed in the gallbladder by the transgastric or transduodenal route under the guide of endoscopic ultrasound (EUS-GBD). A recent systematic review of the English language literature about this technique collected 155 reported patients with acute cholecystitis treated with EUS-GBD in eight studies and 12 case reports. Their technical and clinical success rates were very high and adverse events were reported only in 8 % of the cases [86]. Of course non-comparative observational studies and case reports carry a very high risk of selection bias and further studies are needed to ascertain the potential role of the endoscopic techniques. Besides, the scarce availability of the technical expertise to complete these procedures is an additional limitation factor.

2.7 Conclusions

Laparoscopic cholecystectomy is the gold standard for the definitive management of acute calculous cholecystitis. It should be performed as soon as possible after the symptoms occurrence. The disease, however, is very heterogeneous as far as degree of inflammation and local conditions are concerned; besides, the general characteristics of the patient (age, associated co-morbidities, and functional status) have a very relevant impact on the disease itself, and surgical intervention may result in increased morbidity and mortality in the elderly, patients with multiple comorbidities, or those with advanced cholecystitis. The management of the disease should be established according to its severity; but reliable and validated instruments to assess the surgical risk and choose the more appropriate therapeutic pathway for each situation are not available. The search for safer and less invasive interventions takes into consideration surgical, percutaneous, and endoscopic methods (single or combined) to achieve the best possible success. However, the evidences about the outcomes of each therapeutic procedure are difficult to evaluate in this heterogeneous context. The quest for the optimal treatment of acute cholecystitis is still ongoing.

References

1. Gurusamy KS, Davidson C, Gluud C, Davidson BR (2013) Early versus delayed laparoscopic cholecystectomy for people with acute cholecystitis. Cochrane Database Syst Rev 6:CD005440. doi:10.1002/14651858.CD005440.pub3
2. Campanile FC, Catena F, Coccolini F et al (2011) The need for new "patient-related" guidelines for the treatment of acute cholecystitis. World J Emerg Surg 6:44. doi:10.1186/1749-7922-6-44
3. Campanile FC, Pisano M, Coccolini F et al (2014) Acute cholecystitis: WSES position statement. World J Emerg Surg 9:58. doi:10.1186/1749-7922-9-58
4. Trowbridge RL, Rutkowski NK, Shojania KG (2003) Does this patient have acute cholecystitis? J Am Med Assoc 289:80–86
5. Sauerland S, Agresta F, Bergamaschi R et al (2006) Laparoscopy for abdominal emergencies: evidence-based guidelines of the European association for endoscopic surgery. Surg Endosc 20:14–29. doi:10.1007/s00464-005-0564-0
6. Agresta F, Ansaloni L, Baiocchi GL et al (2012) Laparoscopic approach to acute abdomen from the consensus development conference of the Società Italiana di Chirurgia Endoscopica e nuove tecnologie (SICE), Associazione Chirurghi Ospedalieri Italiani (ACOI), Società Italiana di Chirurgia (SIC), Società Italiana di Chirurgia d'Urgenza e del Trauma (SICUT), Società Italiana di Chirurgia nell'Ospedalità Privata (SICOP), and the European Association for Endoscopic Surgery (EAES). Surg Endosc 26:2134–2164. doi:10.1007/s00464-012-2331-3
7. Hirota M, Takada T, Kawarada Y et al (2007) Diagnostic criteria and severity assessment of acute cholecystitis: Tokyo guidelines. J Hepatobiliary Pancreat Surg 14:78–82. doi:10.1007/s00534-006-1159-4
8. Yokoe M, Takada T, Strasberg SM et al (2013) TG13 diagnostic criteria and severity grading of acute cholecystitis (with videos). J Hepatobiliary Pancreat Sci 20:35–46. doi:10.1007/s00534-012-0568-9
9. Kum CK, Eypasch E, Lefering R et al (1996) Laparoscopic cholecystectomy for acute cholecystitis: is it really safe? World J Surg 20:43–48; discussion 48–49
10. Russell JC, Walsh SJ, Mattie AS, Lynch JT (1996) Bile duct injuries, 1989–1993. A statewide experience. Connecticut Laparoscopic Cholecystectomy Registry. Arch Surg 131:382–388
11. Yamashita Y, Takada T, Strasberg SM et al (2013) TG13 surgical management of acute cholecystitis. J Hepatobiliary Pancreat Sci 20:89–96. doi:10.1007/s00534-012-0567-x
12. Overby DW, Apelgren KN, Richardson W et al (2010) SAGES guidelines for the clinical application of laparoscopic biliary tract surgery. Surg Endosc 24:2368–2386. doi:10.1007/s00464-010-1268-7
13. Sartelli M, Viale P, Catena F et al (2013) 2013 WSES guidelines for management of intra-abdominal infections. World J Emerg Surg 8:3. doi:10.1186/1749-7922-8-3

14. Csikesz N, Ricciardi R, Tseng JF, Shah SA (2008) Current status of surgical management of acute cholecystitis in the United States. World J Surg 32:2230–2236. doi:10.1007/s00268-008-9679-5
15. Navez B, Ungureanu F, Michiels M et al (2012) Surgical management of acute cholecystitis: results of a 2-year prospective multicenter survey in Belgium. Surg Endosc 26:2436–2445. doi:10.1007/s00464-012-2206-7
16. Sandzén B, Haapamäki MM, Nilsson E et al (2013) Surgery for acute gallbladder disease in Sweden 1989–2006–a register study. Scand J Gastroenterol 48:480–486. doi: 10.3109/00365521.2012.763177
17. de Mestral C, Rotstein OD, Laupacis A et al (2013) A population-based analysis of the clinical course of 10,304 patients with acute cholecystitis, discharged without cholecystectomy. J Trauma Acute Care Surg 74:26–30; discussion 30–31. doi:10.1097/TA.0b013e3182788e4d
18. Sartelli M, Catena F, Ansaloni L et al (2012) Complicated intra-abdominal infections in Europe: a comprehensive review of the CIAO study. World J Emerg Surg 7:36. doi:10.1186/1749-7922-7-36
19. Sartelli M, Catena F, Ansaloni L et al (2014) Complicated intra-abdominal infections worldwide: the definitive data of the CIAOW Study. World J Emerg Surg 9:37. doi:10.1186/1749-7922-9-37
20. Kiviluoto T, Sirén J, Luukkonen P, Kivilaakso E (1998) Randomised trial of laparoscopic versus open cholecystectomy for acute and gangrenous cholecystitis. Lancet 351:321–325. doi:10.1016/S0140-6736(97)08447-X
21. Johansson M, Thune A, Nelvin L et al (2005) Randomized clinical trial of open versus laparoscopic cholecystectomy in the treatment of acute cholecystitis. Br J Surg 92:44–49. doi:10.1002/bjs.4836
22. Boo Y-J, Kim W-B, Kim J et al (2007) Systemic immune response after open versus laparoscopic cholecystectomy in acute cholecystitis: a prospective randomized study. Scand J Clin Lab Invest 67:207–214. doi:10.1080/00365510601011585
23. Catena F, Ansaloni L, Bianchi E et al (2013) The ACTIVE (Acute Cholecystitis Trial Invasive Versus Endoscopic) study: multicenter randomized, double-blind, controlled trial of laparoscopic versus open surgery for acute cholecystitis. Hepatogastroenterology 60:1552–1556
24. Coccolini F, Catena F, Pisano M et al (2015) Open versus laparoscopic cholecystectomy in acute cholecystitis. Systematic review and meta-analysis. Int J Surg 18:196–204. doi:10.1016/j.ijsu.2015.04.083
25. van der Linden W, Sunzel H (1970) Early versus delayed operation for acute cholecystitis. A controlled clinical trial. Am J Surg 120:7–13
26. Lahtinen J, Alhava EM, Aukee S (1978) Acute cholecystitis treated by early and delayed surgery. A controlled clinical trial. Scand J Gastroenterol 13:673–678
27. Järvinen HJ, Hästbacka J (1980) Early cholecystectomy for acute cholecystitis: a prospective randomized study. Ann Surg 191:501–505
28. Norrby S, Herlin P, Holmin T et al (1983) Early or delayed cholecystectomy in acute cholecystitis? A clinical trial. Br J Surg 70:163–165
29. Lai PB, Kwong KH, Leung KL et al (1998) Randomized trial of early versus delayed laparoscopic cholecystectomy for acute cholecystitis. Br J Surg 85:764–767. doi:10.1046/j.1365--2168.1998.00708.x
30. Lo CM, Liu CL, Fan ST et al (1998) Prospective randomized study of early versus delayed laparoscopic cholecystectomy for acute cholecystitis. Ann Surg 227:461–467
31. Davila D, Manzanares C, Picho M et al (1999) Experience in the treatment (early vs. delayed) of acute cholecystitis via laparoscopy. Cir Esp 66:233
32. Chandler CF, Lane JS, Ferguson P et al (2000) Prospective evaluation of early versus delayed laparoscopic cholecystectomy for treatment of acute cholecystitis. Am Surg 66:896–900
33. Johansson M, Thune A, Blomqvist A et al (2003) Management of acute cholecystitis in the laparoscopic era: results of a prospective, randomized clinical trial. J Gastrointest Surg 7:642–645

34. Serralta AS, Bueno JL, Planells MR, Rodero DR (2003) Prospective evaluation of emergency versus delayed laparoscopic cholecystectomy for early cholecystitis. Surg Laparosc Endosc Percutan Tech 13:71–75
35. Kolla SB, Aggarwal S, Kumar A et al (2004) Early versus delayed laparoscopic cholecystectomy for acute cholecystitis: a prospective randomized trial. Surg Endosc 18:1323–1327. doi:10.1007/s00464-003-9230-6
36. Yadav RP, Adhikary S, Agrawal CS et al (2009) A comparative study of early vs. delayed laparoscopic cholecystectomy in acute cholecystitis. Kathmandu Univ Med J 7:16–20
37. Faizi K, Ahmed I, Ahmad H (2012) Comparison of early versus delayed laparoscopic cholecystectomy: choosing the best. Pak J Med Health Sci 7:212–215
38. Mare L, Saadi A, Roulin D et al (2012) Delayed versus early laparoscopic cholecystectomy for acute cholecystitis: a prospective randomized study. HPB 14:130. doi:10.1111/j.1477-2574.2012.00511.x
39. Gul R, Dar RA, Sheikh RA et al (2013) Comparison of early and delayed laparoscopic cholecystectomy for acute cholecystitis: experience from a single center. N Am J Med Sci 5:414–418. doi:10.4103/1947-2714.115783
40. Gutt CN, Encke J, Köninger J et al (2013) Acute cholecystitis: early versus delayed cholecystectomy, a multicenter randomized trial (ACDC study, NCT00447304). Ann Surg 258:385–393. doi:10.1097/SLA.0b013e3182a1599b
41. Verma S, Agarwal PN, Bali RS et al (2013) Early versus delayed laparoscopic cholecystectomy for acute cholecystitis: a prospective randomized trial. ISRN Minim Invasive Surg 2013:1–3. doi:10.1155/2013/486107
42. Ozkardeş AB, Tokaç M, Dumlu EG et al (2014) Early versus delayed laparoscopic cholecystectomy for acute cholecystitis: a prospective, randomized study. Int Surg 99:56–61. doi:10.9738/INTSURG-D-13-00068.1
43. Croo A, De Wolf E, Boterbergh K et al (2014) Laparoscopic cholecystectomy in acute cholecystitis: support for an early interval surgery. Acta Gastroenterol Belg 77:306–311
44. Papi C, Catarci M, D'Ambrosio L et al (2004) Timing of cholecystectomy for acute calculous cholecystitis: a meta-analysis. Am J Gastroenterol 99:147–155
45. Shikata S, Noguchi Y, Fukui T (2005) Early versus delayed cholecystectomy for acute cholecystitis: a meta-analysis of randomized controlled trials. Surg Today 35:553–560. doi:10.1007/s00595-005-2998-3
46. Lau H, Lo CY, Patil NG, Yuen WK (2006) Early versus delayed-interval laparoscopic cholecystectomy for acute cholecystitis: a metaanalysis. Surg Endosc 20:82–87. doi:10.1007/s00464-005-0100-2
47. Siddiqui T, MacDonald A, Chong PS, Jenkins JT (2008) Early versus delayed laparoscopic cholecystectomy for acute cholecystitis: a meta-analysis of randomized clinical trials. Am J Surg 195:40–47. doi:10.1016/j.amjsurg.2007.03.004
48. Zhou M-W, Gu X-D, Xiang J-B, Chen Z-Y (2014) Comparison of clinical safety and outcomes of early versus delayed laparoscopic cholecystectomy for acute cholecystitis: a meta-analysis. Scientific World Journal 2014:274516. doi:10.1155/2014/274516
49. Wu X-D, Tian X, Liu M-M et al (2015) Meta-analysis comparing early versus delayed laparoscopic cholecystectomy for acute cholecystitis. Br J Surg 102:1302–1313
50. de Mestral C, Gomez D, Haas B et al (2013) Cholecystostomy: a bridge to hospital discharge but not delayed cholecystectomy. J Trauma Acute Care Surg 74:175–179; discussion 179–180. doi:10.1097/TA.0b013e31827890e1
51. Banz V, Gsponer T, Candinas D, Güller U (2011) Population-based analysis of 4113 patients with acute cholecystitis: defining the optimal time-point for laparoscopic cholecystectomy. Ann Surg 254:964–970. doi:10.1097/SLA.0b013e318228d31c
52. Pieniowski E, Popowicz A, Lundell L et al (2014) Early versus delayed surgery for acute cholecystitis as an applied treatment strategy when assessed in a population-based cohort. Dig Surg 31:169–176. doi:10.1159/000363659

53. de Mestral C, Rotstein OD, Laupacis A et al (2014) Comparative operative outcomes of early and delayed cholecystectomy for acute cholecystitis: a population-based propensity score analysis. Ann Surg 259:10–15. doi:10.1097/SLA.0b013e3182a5cf36
54. Brooks KR, Scarborough JE, Vaslef SN, Shapiro ML (2013) No need to wait: an analysis of the timing of cholecystectomy during admission for acute cholecystitis using the American college of surgeons national surgical quality improvement program database. J Trauma Acute Care Surg 74:167–173; 173–174. doi:10.1097/TA.0b013e3182788b71
55. Zafar SN, Obirieze A, Adesibikan B et al (2015) Optimal time for early laparoscopic cholecystectomy for acute cholecystitis. J Am Med Assoc Surg 150:129–136. doi:10.1001/jamasurg.2014.2339
56. Borzellino G, Sauerland S, Minicozzi AM et al (2008) Laparoscopic cholecystectomy for severe acute cholecystitis. A meta-analysis of results. Surg Endosc 22:8–15. doi:10.1007/s00464-007-9511-6
57. Nikfarjam M, Niumsawatt V, Sethu A et al (2011) Outcomes of contemporary management of gangrenous and non-gangrenous acute cholecystitis. HPB (Oxford) 13:551–558. doi:10.1111/j.1477-2574.2011.00327.x
58. Ganapathi AM, Speicher PJ, Englum BR et al (2015) Gangrenous cholecystitis: a contemporary review. J Surg Res 197:18–24. doi:10.1016/j.jss.2015.02.058
59. Lo H-C, Wang Y-C, Su L-T, Hsieh C-H (2012) Can early laparoscopic cholecystectomy be the optimal management of cholecystitis with gallbladder perforation? A single institute experience of 74 cases. Surg Endosc 26:3301–3306. doi:10.1007/s00464-012-2344-y
60. Choi SB, Han HJ, Kim CY et al (2011) Early laparoscopic cholecystectomy is the appropriate management for acute gangrenous cholecystitis. Am Surg 77:401–406
61. Kwon YJ, Ahn BK, Park HK et al (2013) What is the optimal time for laparoscopic cholecystectomy in gallbladder empyema? Surg Endosc 27:3776–3780. doi:10.1007/s00464-013-2968-6
62. Strasberg SM, Hertl M, Soper NJ (1995) An analysis of the problem of biliary injury during laparoscopic cholecystectomy. J Am Coll Surg 180:101–125
63. Henneman D, Da Costa DW, Vrouenraets BC et al (2013) Laparoscopic partial cholecystectomy for the difficult gallbladder: a systematic review. Surg Endosc 27:351–358
64. Elshaer M, Gravante G, Thomas K et al (2015) Subtotal cholecystectomy for "difficult gallbladders": systematic review and meta-analysis. J Am Med Assoc Surg 150:159–168. doi:10.1001/jamasurg.2014.1219
65. Kirshtein B, Bayme M, Bolotin A et al (2008) Laparoscopic cholecystectomy for acute cholecystitis in the elderly: is it safe? Surg Laparosc Endosc Percutan Tech 18:334–339. doi:10.1097/SLE.0b013e318171525d
66. Nikfarjam M, Yeo D, Perini M et al (2014) Outcomes of cholecystectomy for treatment of acute cholecystitis in octogenarians. ANZ J Surg 84:943–948. doi:10.1111/ans.12313
67. Yang TF, Guo L, Wang Q (2014) Evaluation of preoperative risk factor for converting laparoscopic to open cholecystectomy: a meta-analysis. Hepatogastroenterology 61:958–965
68. Licciardello A, Arena M, Nicosia A et al (2014) Preoperative risk factors for conversion from laparoscopic to open cholecystectomy. Eur Rev Med Pharmacol Sci 18:60–68
69. Decker G, Goergen M, Philippart P, Mendes da Costa P (2001) Laparoscopic cholecystectomy for acute cholecystitis in geriatric patients. Acta Chir Belg 101:294–299
70. Lupinacci RM, Nadal LR, Rego RE et al (2013) Surgical management of gallbladder disease in the very elderly: are we operating them at the right time? Eur J Gastroenterol Hepatol 25:380–384. doi:10.1097/MEG.0b013e32835b7124
71. Nielsen LBJ, Harboe KM, Bardram L (2014) Cholecystectomy for the elderly: no hesitation for otherwise healthy patients. Surg Endosc 28:171–177. doi:10.1007/s00464-013-3144-8
72. Pessaux P, Regenet N, Tuech JJ et al (2001) Laparoscopic versus open cholecystectomy: a prospective comparative study in the elderly with acute cholecystitis. Surg Laparosc Endosc Percutan Tech 11:252–255

73. Chau CH, Tang CN, Siu WT et al (2002) Laparoscopic cholecystectomy versus open cholecystectomy in elderly patients with acute cholecystitis: retrospective study. Hong Kong Med J 8:394–399
74. Cheng Y, Leng J, Tan J et al (2013) Proper surgical technique approved for early laparoscopic cholecystectomy for non-critically ill elderly patients with acute cholecystitis. Hepatogastroenterology 60:688–691. doi:10.5754/hge121107
75. Ferrarese AG, Solej M, Enrico S et al (2013) Elective and emergency laparoscopic cholecystectomy in the elderly: our experience. BMC Surg 13 Suppl 2:S21. doi:10.1186/1471-2482-13-S2-S21
76. Haltmeier T, Benjamin E, Inaba K et al (2015) Early versus delayed same-admission laparoscopic cholecystectomy for acute cholecystitis in elderly patients with comorbidities. J Trauma Acute Care Surg 78:801–807. doi:10.1097/TA.0000000000000577
77. Cull JD, Velasco JM, Czubak A et al (2014) Management of acute cholecystitis: prevalence of percutaneous cholecystostomy and delayed cholecystectomy in the elderly. J Gastrointest Surg 18:328–333. doi:10.1007/s11605-013-2341-z
78. Riall TS, Zhang D, Townsend CM et al (2010) Failure to perform cholecystectomy for acute cholecystitis in elderly patients is associated with increased morbidity, mortality, and cost. J Am Coll Surg 210:668–677. doi:10.1016/j.jamcollsurg.2009.12.031
79. Lee S-W, Yang S-S, Chang C-S, Yeh H-J (2009) Impact of the Tokyo guidelines on the management of patients with acute calculous cholecystitis. J Gastroenterol Hepatol 24:1857–1861. doi:10.1111/j.1440-1746.2009.05923.x
80. Yi N-J, Han H-S, Min S-K (2006) The safety of a laparoscopic cholecystectomy in acute cholecystitis in high-risk patients older than sixty with stratification based on ASA score. Minim Invasive Ther Allied Technol 15:159–164. doi:10.1080/13645700600760044
81. Ausania F, Guzman Suarez S, Alvarez Garcia H et al (2015) Gallbladder perforation: morbidity, mortality and preoperative risk prediction. Surg Endosc 29:955–960. doi:10.1007/s00464-014-3765-6
82. Kortram K, de Vries Reilingh TS, Wiezer MJ et al (2011) Percutaneous drainage for acute calculous cholecystitis. Surg Endosc 25:3642–3646. doi:10.1007/s00464-011-1771-5
83. Winbladh A, Gullstrand P, Svanvik J, Sandström P (2009) Systematic review of cholecystostomy as a treatment option in acute cholecystitis. HPB (Oxford) 11:183–193. doi:10.1111/j.1477-2574.2009.00052.x
84. Rodríguez-Sanjuán JC, Arruabarrena A, Sánchez-Moreno L et al (2012) Acute cholecystitis in high surgical risk patients: percutaneous cholecystostomy or emergency cholecystectomy? Am J Surg 204:54–59. doi:10.1016/j.amjsurg.2011.05.013
85. Itoi T, Coelho-Prabhu N, Baron TH (2010) Endoscopic gallbladder drainage for management of acute cholecystitis. Gastrointest Endosc 71:1038–1045. doi:10.1016/j.gie.2010.01.026
86. Peñas-Herrero I, de la Serna-Higuera C, Perez-Miranda M (2015) Endoscopic ultrasound-guided gallbladder drainage for the management of acute cholecystitis (with video). J Hepatobiliary Pancreat Sci 22:35–43. doi:10.1002/jhbp.182

Acute Pancreatitis

3

Mario Campli, Alessandra Cerioli, Ari Leppäniemi, Alberto Arezzo, and Carlo Bergamini

3.1 Introduction

"Acute pancreatitis is the most terrible of all the calamities that occur in connection to the abdominal viscera. The suddenness of its onset, the illimitable agony which accompanies it, and the mortality attendant upon it, render it the most formidable of catastrophes."—B. Moynihan, 1925

Throughout much of history, acute pancreatitis (AP) was a mysterious and dramatic disease: delayed recognition, when necrosis had been established, the remote location of the gland in the lesser sac, difficulties in differential diagnosis, and incomplete understanding of the metabolic needs of the seriously ill patients made AP an impossible challenge for surgeons [1]. We actually achieve great advancements of our understanding, but the disease remains problematic.

AP is an inflammatory process of the pancreas with a highly variable clinical course. Most patients experience a mild, self-limiting disease that resolves sponta-

M. Campli, MD
Division of Surgery, "Nuova Itor" Private Health Facility, Rome, Italy
e-mail: mario.campli@gmail.com

A. Cerioli, MD, PhD Candidate
Division of Surgery, "Nuova Itor" Private Health Facility, Rome, Italy

Department of General Surgery, Tor Vergata University, Rome, Italy

A. Leppäniemi, MD, PhD
Second Department of Surgery, Meilahti Hospital, Helsinki, Finland

A. Arezzo, MD
Department of Surgical Sciences, University of Torino, Torino, Italy

C. Bergamini, MD
SOD Chirurgia Generale, d'Urgenza e Mini-invasiva, AOU Careggi, Firenze, Italy

F. Agresta et al. (eds.), *Emergency Laparoscopy*,
DOI 10.1007/978-3-319-29620-3_3

neously or successfully treated with supportive therapy. But no medications exist to treat specifically acute pancreatitis; no actual drugs are available to improve the course of the disease, and this is a big deal for patients going through a severe attack.

Acute pancreatitis and its serious complications are still a tough challenge for surgeons. After an "heroic" age of surgery, nowadays a more cautious attitude is adopted than in the past, with extensive use of laparoscopic and minimally invasive approach, according to the principle that "less is more" in pancreatic surgery.

Due to the high morbidity and mortality of surgical procedures in the course of severe AP, the indications for surgery are strictly regulated: early assessment of the severity and risk stratification are important for well-timed intensive therapy and timely intervention and have been shown to improve prognosis and survival. Currently, AP is not an absolute indication for surgery: only the complications of the disease lead the patient to the operating room to resolve a bowel obstruction, bleeding, ischemia, or to perform drainage of septic/necrotic collections. In the gallstone-related disease, the aim of the surgeon is the clearance of the common bile duct and laparoscopic cholecystectomy with no curative intent but to prevent the risk of recurrence.

Indications, limits, and advantages of surgical treatment will be clarified and specified with the current progress in the knowledge of the natural development and pathophysiology of the disease.

3.2 Classification: Diagnostic and Therapeutic Hints and Tips

During the years many classifications were proposed like Scuro (1984), Marseilles-Rome (1988), and the Atlanta classification, established in 1992 and probably the most frequently used by pancreatologists until its revision. The classification with its empirical conclusions, limits, and gaps was rated more suitable for a retrospective evaluation and for scientific purposes, rather than for a perspective classification of patients. The current Atlanta classification, revised in 2012 [2], is designed to describe AP in a practical way, in order to standardize terminology across specialties, to help in treatment planning, and to compare management and results in different departments and institutions or recruitment in clinical trials. It inserts an additional category to the old classification, providing three classes of acute pancreatitis concerning severity: "mild," "moderate," and "severe." Mild AP is the most common form without organ failure (OF) and local or systemic complications; it does not need an imaging definition and usually resolves in the first week with no risk of mortality. Moderate AP is characterized by the presence of transient OF (less than 48 h) and/or the presence of local complications or exacerbation of comorbid disease and it can eventually require a prolonged specialist care. Its mortality is lower than in the severe form. Finally, severe AP consists in persistent OF (more than 48 h) and represents 15–20 % of cases. If the OF is persistent from the first days, the mortality grows up to 36–50 %. Moreover, morphologically a classification exists, dividing AP into acute oedematous or interstitial pancreatitis and necrotizing that can involve both the pancreas and the peripancreatic tissues, only the peripancreatic tissues (less commonly), and only the pancreatic parenchyma (rarely). Temporally, the AP can be divided into two phases: early, in the first week when only clinical parameters are important for treatment planning, and late, after the first week.

Nevertheless, a consensus about the classification has not been reached yet [3]. In fact, even in 2012 another international multidisciplinary classification has been done as a result of a consultative process among specialists in pancreatic diseases from the entire world [4]. The determinant-based classification provides a set of concise up-to-date definitions of all the main entities pertinent to classify the severity of AP in clinical practice and research and adds a further category in severity classification: the critical one. Complications are classified local or systemic and sterile or infected. Local complications are acute peripancreatic fluid collections (APFC), acute necrotic collections (ANC), pseudocyst, walled-off necrosis (WON), systemic inflammatory response syndrome (SIRS), splenic-portal thrombosis, colic necrosis, gastric outlet dysfunction, and organ failure (OF). OF is defined as a score of two or more for one of these three organ systems (cardiovascular, renal, and respiratory) using the modified Marshall scoring system on the basis of the worst measurement over a 24-h period. APFC contain only fluid and are not or partially encapsulated, develop in 4 weeks in interstitial pancreatitis, and frequently regress spontaneously. ANC contain a mixture of fluid and necrotic material, are not or partially encapsulated, and develop in 4 weeks, usually in necrotizing pancreatitis. Pseudocyst is a fluid encapsulated collection, develops after 4 weeks in interstitial pancreatitis, and also contains necrotic material. WON are necrotic collections, are fully encapsulated, and develop after 4 weeks.

No significant differences were found comparing the two grading systems [5], but surgeons may be slightly more interested in the determinant-based classification, since surgical interventions are indicated only on a few occasions: never in the early stages, unless general complications such as bleeding, bowel ischemia, or perforation; and in the late stages only in case of infected necrosis.

It would be very important to define and stratify the predicted severity of the disease on admission in order to identify potential patients with stones or developing severe AP to set up an aggressive treatment, or a possible transfer to a specialist care [6, 7], but till now it is a challenge to determine the right prediction of AP progression. Furthermore, it is almost impossible to know why a patient remains in mild state of AP or if he could develop complications [4, 8, 9]. Moreover, the improvements in diagnostic image, the better understanding of pathophysiology of the disease, and the development of radiologic, endoscopic, and minimally invasive operative techniques for the management of complications led to a continuous revision of the classifications [8, 10, 11].

Score systems are used to predict hospital mortality and they are a good landmark to classify AP. They are all based on clinical, radiologic, and laboratory variabilities to calculate the severity of the disease. The scores need to be periodically recalibrated to reflect changes in practice and patient demographics. In recent years, many grading systems have been used: Ranson score, Glasgow score, BISAP (Bed Side Index of Severity in Acute Pancreatitis), Balthazar for the valuation of CT images, and even the APACHE II (Acute Physiology and Chronic Health Evaluation) score, which is not specific for AP but rather generically for critically ill patients. In recent comparisons of scoring systems to predict the severity of AP [8, 11], APACHE II score appeared to have highest accuracy for prediction of severe AP, although its predictive accuracy was not significantly different when compared to other scoring systems. Grading systems show a similar predictive accuracy; no simple assessment score capable of reaching maximal utility for prediction of severe AP is still available. They are devised to identify groups of high-risk patients rather than individuals. They work best at the opposite ends of the spectrum (i.e., high negative or positive predictive value in patients with very low or high scores) [12]. An ideal prognostic evaluation system should be simple, noninvasive, accurate, and quantitative, and the assessment methods should be easily applicable at the time of diagnosis [11, 13], but it does not exist. Conversely, application of a severity assessment score is time-consuming and typically requires 48 h to become accurate. Frequently, when a score demonstrates severe disease, the patient's condition is obvious regardless of the score [8, 14]. While they are cumbersome, are not mandatory, and do not help with patient management, they are considered useful tools for risk stratification and to compare the care received by patients with similar risk characteristics in different units, but in the Western World scores for severity assessment of pancreatitis are performed only by one-third of hospitals, and the opinion that the judgment of an experienced surgeon provides evaluation of the disease outcome as good as any severity scoring system is widely spread [8, 14].

The main problem is still the definition of severity, proposed contemporarily by many authors; despite the availability of several clinical and radiological scoring systems, accurate prediction of the AP grade remains uncertain, and a unique reliable classification is still an open matter [9, 15]. Coexistence of several classification systems is a questionable peculiarity that is still waiting for a solution [12, 16].

However, it seems appropriate to deepen understanding of some aspects of the pathophysiology of AP and some diagnostic issues that have considerable implications in refining definitions of the various grading systems and in determining timing and treatment choices.

The proposal takes hold to distinguish between limited and expansive necrosis, considering the spreading of necrosis in various degrees throughout the retroperitoneum and into the small and large mesentery, as there are no anatomical barriers [12]. If expansive, the necrosis cannot be said to be located into a "collection." In CT images it can sometimes be difficult, if not impossible, to distinguish fluid from necrosis. MRI can clearly distinguish fluid from solid components, but in daily practice MRI is not as easily performed as CT. The timing of encapsulation, however, differs markedly among patients and can only be judged on contrast-enhanced CT, rather than according to time from symptom onset. The presence and necrosis extension is not valuable in the first days and it is not directly involved with organ failure and severity. Finally, in the first week a local complication does not require a surgical treatment. The predictive accuracy of CT scoring systems for severity of AP is similar, with no statistically significant differences, to clinical scoring systems. Hence, a CT on admission solely for severity assessment in AP is not recommended because early CT does not reveal any other diagnosis nor any local pancreatic complication and underestimates the presence of parenchymal necrosis in a substantial number of patients [8]. Therefore, CT studies should be reserved only for patients with predicted severe AP by clinical assessment, for those who fail to improve clinically with conservative management, for patients whose diagnosis is unclear, or in suspected severe complication (bleeding, bowel ischemia, or perforation, etc.) [4, 8]. Predicted mild AP on early CT (i.e., low CT scores) does not imply that the patient will not develop clinically severe AP, especially when significant baseline comorbidity is present. The presence of systemic inflammatory response syndrome (SIRS) increases the risk of developing organ failure, essential determinant of severity. SIRS is a clinical condition, but also a diagnostic criterion that can be used to monitor the AP progression [12, 17–19] and, with repetitive monitoring during the first days of admission, to guide treatment decisions.

Infection of necrosis, both pancreatic and peripancreatic, is the primary indication for a specific operative treatment in AP. Extensive research has addressed the possibility of prediction of infected necrosis: several multifactorial scoring systems (e.g., Simplified Acute Physiology Score II—SAPS 2, Ranson and Imrie scores, APACHE II, Balthazar CT severity index—CTSI, and multiple organ dysfunction scores—MODS) and a broad spectrum of biochemical markers (pancreatic proteases and anti-proteases, C-reactive protein, procalcitonin, interleukins, tumor necrosis factor-α—TNF-α, adhesion molecules, serum amyloid A) have been evaluated and systematically reviewed not only for early stratification of severity but for prediction of infected necrosis. Although all these scoring systems have been shown to correlate with morbidity and mortality, it remains difficult to accurately identify on admission or early in the course of their hospitalization individual patients who develop infected necrosis.

Apart from clinical symptoms and blood test findings, a clear diagnostic sign of infected necrosis is represented by gas bubbles within (peri)pancreatic necrosis on CT, with an almost 100 % specificity in the diagnosis of pancreatic infection. However, it is worth mentioning that on rare occasions the presence of gas can indicate the presence of a communication with the gastrointestinal tract. A positive culture of (peri)pancreatic necrosis by image-guided fine needle aspiration (FNA) is not recommended as routine today: FNA should be used selectively when there is no clinical response to adequate therapy or when the clinical and/or imaging features of infection are uncertain [17, 20, 21].

If the pathophysiologic mechanism of necrosis plays a key role in severe AP development, infusion therapy can influence the course of the disease. Massive fluid supplementation to correct or preferably prevent intravascular hypovolemia is commonly accepted as the first step in supportive care, but it may worsen accumulation of fluid in the third space. Development of intra-abdominal hypertension is partly related to the effects of the inflammatory process itself causing retroperitoneal edema, fluid collections, ascites, and ileus, and partly iatrogenic resulting from aggressive fluid resuscitation. Moreover, it is also difficult to differentiate the SIRS of the pancreatitis process itself and the effects of intra-abdominal hypertension. It is likely that the processes exacerbate each other in a multifactorial manner. Raised intra-abdominal pressure causes splinting of the diaphragms, leading to compression atelectasis and hypercapnia. These events, in combination with bilateral pleural effusion, which are common in severe pancreatitis, result in severe hypoxia. The high intra-abdominal pressure with the compression of vessels and viscera further reduces organ perfusion and causes worsening of ischemia, causing multiple system organ failure. At this point, an abdominal compartment syndrome is thus established.

Nowadays, nutritional support is considered a therapeutic measure rather than merely a way to provide calories in a patient with severe pancreatitis. Enteral nutrition through a nasoenteric feeding tube has been shown to reduce organ failure, infected necrosis, and mortality compared with parenteral nutrition. These complications are thought to be mediated by bacterial translocation from the gut provoked by disturbed intestinal motility, bacterial overgrowth, and increased mucosal permeability. Enteral nutrition is believed to stimulate intestinal motility—thus reducing bacterial overgrowth—and is believed to increase splanchnic blood flow, which helps to preserve the integrity of the gut mucosa. The improved outcomes found in the trials following the use of enteral nutrition might also be the result of complications specifically related to parenteral nutrition, such as catheter-related infections [22].

Prophylactic administration of intravenous antibiotics has been used with the aim to prevent infected necrosis and other infectious complications. Several randomized trials have shown that routine use of antibiotics does not prevent infected necrosis. Therefore, antibiotics in AP are indicated in case of proven infection or in case of a very strong clinical suspicion of cholangitis or infected necrosis [14, 22].

Outcome of male patients is worse than those of females [23].

3.3 Mild Pancreatitis

3.3.1 Biliary Pancreatitis

Acute gallstone-associated pancreatitis is initiated and sustained by the passage of stones in the bile ducts. Biliary etiology is the leading cause of AP, 15 cases of gallstone AP per 100,000 persons [24], from one to two-thirds of all pancreatitis depending on the series; when an AP is suspected, an ultrasound scan should always be performed, as well as cholestasis indices. In mild AP, if no common bile duct obstruction but gallstones are detected, laparoscopic cholecystectomy should be performed during the index hospitalization, as soon as pancreatitis symptoms cool off. Although this assumption is widely adopted, a recent Cochrane review failed to demonstrate that early laparoscopic cholecystectomy has a better result, that is, a decreased risk of complications, in comparison with interval cholecystectomy [25] (LE3). For various reasons, the quality of this evidence is poor; anyway the outcome of cholecystectomy is not the only intent to perform an early intervention: between 32 and 61 % of patients with AP are subject to repeated acute episodes.

Recurrent biliary events are common in the first 30 days from index episode, and subsequent attacks could be more severe than the first one [26, 27] (LE3). Delayed cholecystectomy increases risk of readmission for recurrent biliary events, especially recurrent biliary pancreatitis [17, 26, 28–30] (LE2). Therefore, the current recommendation for patients with mild gallstone pancreatitis is to undergo a laparoscopic cholecystectomy during initial hospitalization as soon as pancreatitis has been resolved, before discharge [31]. There is strong evidence that a same-admission cholecystectomy can be performed safely, without increased difficulty or surgery-related complications [32] although a very early cholecystectomy (within 48 h after admission) is contraindicated because patients can still develop pancreatic necrosis or organ failure during this phase of the disease, both representing a surgical contraindication [33, 34]. Routine intraoperative cholangiography at the time of cholecystectomy does not improve outcomes [35]: clinical suspicion of common bile duct stones requests preoperative adequate assessment and possible clearance of bile duct stones with endoscopic retrograde cholangiopancreatography. At the present moment same-admission cholecystectomy in mild biliary pancreatitis is no longer a matter of debate in current guidelines [17, 18, 21], but adherence to the above recommendation is low: in real world early cholecystectomy is not performed for a fairly large proportion of patients [36, 37] often because concerns still exist about an increased risk of cholecystectomy-related complications with this approach. Cholecystectomy during initial hospitalization may also not be feasible because of clinical factors, patient preference, or operating room resources that may be fully. We should also consider the eventuality that some physicians do not follow guidelines. This is not an evidence-based medicine approach, but there are studies showing that patients suffering from pancreatitis and admitted in medical services rather than in surgical wards are treated more conservatively and undergo same-stay cholecystectomy less frequently [38–40] (LE3). This attitude is even more prevalent toward the elderly population: more than half of the patients who do not receive cholecystectomy are never evaluated by a surgeon [41] (LE3).

3.3.2 ERCP and Endoscopic Sphincterotomy

About 20 % of biliary pancreatitis have persistent bile duct stones. Many treatments are available for cholecysto-choledocholithiasis, including laparoscopic, endoscopic, percutaneous, and open traditional techniques, either through a combination of these interventions or by conducting them in a stepwise sequence. But a great number of studies failed to strongly demonstrate the superiority of any technique, and it is unlikely that in the future some rigorous clinical trials will be conducted to compare so many different types of therapeutic options. Therefore, the choice of the best management is often driven by the local presence of professional expertise and resources, rather than by a real superiority of one strategy over another [42]. Nowadays, endoscopic procedures are among the preferred strategies for treatment of bile duct stones. Considered as the least invasive effective technique, they have replaced open choledochotomy as the first intervention for biliary clearance [43].

A real "paradigm shift" has developed, and today associated gallbladder and bile duct stones undergo more often an ERCP and a separate operation than a single open or laparoscopic exploration associated with cholecystectomy [44] (LE3). A recent Cochrane review demonstrates superiority of open bile duct surgery in achieving common bile duct stone clearance, but this statement is based on the evidence available from the early endoscopy age [45]. A recent survey demonstrated that the preferred method of US surgeons for managing common bile duct stones discovered preoperatively is the "sequential" one, ERCP and sphincterotomy followed by laparoscopic cholecystectomy (79–88 % of responders versus 5–8 % preferring laparoscopic common bile duct exploration, and 4–16 % preferring intraoperative or postoperative ERCP) [46].

At present ERCP and endoscopic sphincterotomy are effective in common bile duct clearance and should be performed "as soon as possible" in case of acute biliary pancreatitis to reestablish normal biliary and pancreatic outflow by removal of bile duct stones and/or stenting of the common bile duct. Indeed, there was a debate between those who argued the early use of conservative medical treatment and ERCP only if signs and symptoms suggest an infection (cholangitis) or blockage of the bile duct by a stone (even within the first 24 h of symptom onset according to some guidelines) [22], and those who advise early routine use of ERCP. There is no evidence that early routine ERCP significantly affects mortality and local or systemic complications of pancreatitis, regardless of predicted severity [47] (LE1). Not surprisingly, however, this argument is used to support current recommendation that early ERCP should be considered only in patients with coexisting cholangitis or biliary obstruction: ERCP and endoscopic sphincterotomy have small but not negligible morbidity and mortality, and endoscopists do not perform ERCP without a conclusive evidence of persistent biliary obstruction. Probably a waiting period of 48 h may give more opportunities to a small stone wedged in the papilla of Oddi to pass spontaneously into the duodenum, saving an unnecessary ERCP. A similar waiting period could be useful for a more accurate diagnosis of infection, since cholangitis is difficult to diagnose in patients with severe pancreatitis because of the systemic inflammatory response syndrome [22]. Some authors have recently stressed the uncertainty on the role of routine early ERCP and sphincterotomy in patients with predicted severe acute biliary pancreatitis [12, 48]. The "APEC" trial (ISRCTN97372133), specifically designed to give an answer to this question, will end only in 2017. While the indication for ERCP in case of severe AP is arguable, there is no doubt that it should not be performed in case of mild AP without cholangitis.

Endoscopic sphincterotomy alone may still be considered in poor operative candidates (elderly and frail patients unfit for surgery) [39, 40, 49, 50], but the optimal treatment following sphincterotomy remains early laparoscopic cholecystectomy [30, 51] (LE3).

3.3.3 Non-biliary Mild Pancreatitis

In case of alcohol-related or idiopathic pancreatitis the clinic of the patient becomes paramount: previous acute episodes, serum triglycerides level, serum calcium level, use of drugs or alcohol, abdominal trauma, infective agents, and the possible tumoral differential diagnosis must be considered. In case of idiopathic AP there is no consensus about expecting another AP episode or transferring the patient in a second-or third-level center. IAP/APA guidelines recommend, after negative routine work-up for biliary etiology, echoendoscopy to assess for occult microlithiasis (less than 3 mm stones) or a neoplasia [17]. Eventually, an MRI for pancreas divisum, anatomic variant of Santorini duct, dysfunctional Oddi sphincter, or finally a genetic study are advised. Only aggressive fluid resuscitation and supportive therapy are suggested in non-biliary mild pancreatitis.

3.4 Severe Acute Pancreatitis

Necrosis of the pancreatic parenchyma and/or peripancreatic fat occurs in about 20 % of AP. In the first phase, about 1 or 2 weeks after the onset of symptoms, a systemic inflammatory response syndrome occurs, which is often associated with multiple organ failure. Approximately, half the deaths from necrotizing pancreatitis are caused by multiple organ failure in the early phase. At this stage open or laparoscopic surgery is harmful and contraindicated unless complications. The only permitted surgical indications requiring an emergency laparotomy are acute complications such as abdominal compartment syndrome, bowel ischemia, ongoing acute bleeding, or gastric outlet, intestinal, or biliary obstruction [22, 52] (LE2). During these surgical interventions, drainage of pancreatic collections and/or necrosectomy are not indicated. At this stage pancreatic necrosis is still sterile, but any operative action may increase the risk of developing infected necrosis.

Another problem exists: about 15 % of all patients with predicted mild pancreatitis will progress erratically to severe pancreatitis. Despite the numerous assessment scores, a patient with a mild clinical picture at admission could undergo cholecystectomy and then could develop a severe necrotizing pancreatitis, with high risk of mortality. Prophylactic cholecystectomy in case of severe biliary pancreatitis must be postponed until the clinical recovery: early surgery and severe pancreatitis do not get along.

In the second phase, approximately 30 % of necrotizing pancreatitis develop infection that eventually leads to death if no intervention is performed or if surgery is too long postponed. Infected necrosis is the main surgical indication, while the sterile one can be treated conservatively in most of the cases. In these patients, risk of infection rises because of the downregulation of the immune system that occurs at the end of the first week, when systemic inflammation regresses and a compensatory suppressed inflammatory response takes hold: pathogens can migrate unopposed from the hollow viscera lumen and colonize necrotic tissue in and around the damaged pancreas [53, 54]. No specific drug therapy is available to improve the course of disease, particularly in patients with AP who develop a systemic inflammatory response syndrome early after the onset of symptoms and hence are prone to develop organ failure.

Timing of intervention in patients with severe AP (usually open necrosectomy) has been a debated matter for years. Many series and reviews [12, 22, 55, 56] show that best results are achieved when intervention is performed after about 4 weeks after the onset of symptoms. Delaying surgery affords acute necrotic collections to become walled off while the necrotic tissue liquefies partially during the third and the fourth week, resulting in collections that contain both liquid and solid necrotic material. The encapsulation of peripancreatic collections improves conditions for intervention, facilitates necrosectomy, and thereby decreases the risk of complications such as bleeding and perforation.

Faced with the high morbidity and mortality of an early intervention, postponing surgery when walled-off necrosis occurs improves outcome and decreases morbidity and mortality.

Late open necrosectomy is still an option (the last one) in the treatment of infected pancreatic necrosis. Surgical technique involves a midline longitudinal or a bilateral subcostal incision. The retroperitoneum is entered through the lesser sac to expose the pancreas. In cases that the above approach is not feasible, infracolic approach has been described as an alternative. The blunt dissection is preferred to the formal resection to minimize the incidence of bleeding, fistulae, and removal of vital residual pancreatic tissue. Cholecystectomy can be added to the procedure in cases of biliary pancreatitis. The completion of surgical procedure involves various techniques, from open or closed packing, to continuous irrigation of the lesser sac and retroperitoneum, to planned staged relaparotomies [20]. The latest advancement in the managing of open abdomen is the vacuum-assisted closure, with a packing combined with negative pressure that easily allows repeated laparotomies, prevents abdominal compartment syndrome, simplifies the nursing of patient, and should reduce time to definitive abdominal closure [57].

The need to postpone resorting to surgery led to the proposal of therapeutic maneuvers such as radiology-assisted percutaneous drainage and minimally invasive surgical techniques. These therapies were initially proposed as a bridge therapy to delayed open necrosectomy, but they proved valid alternative measures, resulting in improved patient outcomes.

In 2006, the “PANTER” trial [58] validated the “step-up approach” to severe AP, which utilizes a gradual approach adopting minimally invasive techniques and progressively increases the aggressiveness of the surgical approach that is regulated to the actual need.

Medical management is effective in about two-thirds of patients with sterile necrosis. If patients do not improve on conservative treatment or develop infection, then the first intervention is percutaneous catheter drainage, in about half the cases without any need for subsequent treatments. The minimally invasive nature of the technique allows intervention even in the early phase of severe necrosis, when an open approach could be harmful. Usually, via a retroperitoneal approach through the left flank, 12–30 Fr. catheters are placed with the guidance of CT or ultrasound [59]. If catheter drainage is unsuccessful, pancreatic necrosectomy has to be performed using a minimally invasive approach [22, 52, 60–64] (LE2). Laparoscopy for necrosectomy is not so widely supported. Most commonly a retroperitoneoscopic route is used [65, 66], taking advantage of the previous percutaneous tract, usually created under CT-guided drainage, or making a first brand new tract, then adding one or two further trocars or, in case of "hybrid" technique, a small—5 to 7 cm—subcostal incision to perform necrosectomy and irrigation. All variants of retroperitoneoscopy are collectively known either as sinus tract endoscopy or video-assisted retroperitoneal debridement (VARD).

There is an increasing strong evidence that endoscopic drainage and necrosectomy using a transgastric or transduodenal approach ensures good results, but these data still require validation [61, 67–70] (LE3). Endoscopic necrosectomy is a form of natural orifice trans-luminal endoscopic surgery (NOTES) and is theoretically the less invasive intervention: it can be performed under conscious sedation without the need for general anesthesia and it can be repeated, but it can only be used when stomach or duodenum is apposed to the area of necrosis, while retroperitoneoscopic approach is effective to access fluid collections close to the lateral abdominal wall, usually in the pancreatic tail or the left paracolic gutter and less frequently for fluid collections of the right paracolic gutter [62] (LE3).

The rationale behind the step-up approach is the aim to control the sepsis, rather than complete removal of the infected necrosis, in a disease which evolves progressively. This reduces the rate of complications and death by minimizing the surgical trauma and the inflammatory response to a surgical intervention in already critically ill patients [20, 63]. Minimally invasive techniques such as percutaneous drainage and video-assisted retroperitoneoscopic debridement reduce complications, whereas open necrosectomy does not maintain abdominal compartmentalization and may therefore cause further intra-abdominal spread of the infection [71].

3.5 Abdominal Compartment Syndrome

Abdominal compartment syndrome (ACS), a life-threatening sustained elevation of the intraabdominal pressure associated with new onset organ failure or acute worsening of existing organ failure [72], is the most lethal complication in the course of severe AP. This syndrome has been described in many severe clinical situations such as abdominal trauma, burns, hemoperitoneum, and in the course of emergency abdominal surgery. Its development in AP is thought to be directly related to the inflammation of the pancreas. Proinflammatory cytokines start a cascade of pancreatic and visceral edema, acute peripancreatic fluid collections, capillary leakage causing ascites, paralytic ileus, and gastric dilatation by upper gastrointestinal tract obstruction leading to an elevated intra-abdominal pressure. It seems that the incidence of ACS has increased, probably as a result of current therapeutic strategy: conservative or a minimally invasive approach and efforts to delay open surgery with massive aggressive fluid resuscitation and prolonged stay in the intensive care unit worsen the evolving visceral edema further increasing the intra-abdominal pressure [73]. This complication leads to reduced perfusion and subsequent ischemia of splanchnic organs followed by further progression of the existing organ failure leading to a potentially lethal downward spiral; also diaphragm motility is compromised, with evolving respiratory failure, and cardiac output is diminished, with lower organ perfusion pressure subject to further decrease due to the intra-abdominal pressure [74, 75].

Nonoperative strategies to prevent and counteract intra-abdominal hypertension are sedation and mechanical ventilation, enteral decompression with nasogastric and rectal tube, prokinetic and diuretic medication, and hemodialysis, but conservative measures can provide only a short period of relief from the increase in abdominal pressure, after that early surgical decompression should be performed. Currently, there is no uniform consensus on the indication and the optimal timing of invasive intervention and which method is most effective. The clinical outcome of patients suffering from ACS is very poor, whatever the adopted technique [76].

Traditional full-thickness midline laparostomy or transverse bilaterally extended incision below the costal margins ensures decompression, but facilitates infection, fistula formation, and incisional hernia [77]. To avoid open abdomen, subcutaneous linea alba fasciotomy was proposed through three short horizontal skin incisions to perform an anterior abdominal midline fasciotomy with the peritoneum left intact [78].

In the recent literature, evidence has grown on vacuum-assisted closure in the management of laparostomy, but very few articles specifically on ACS were published [79]. Regarding minimally invasive procedures, three works about minimally invasive drainage in case of abdominal compartment syndrome were written in the last 5 years, but on low impact factor journals and/or with a low level of evidence [80–82]. A trial named the "DECOMPRESS Study" was designed in 2010 to compare decompressive laparotomy and percutaneous drainage [83], but to date no definitive result has yet been published. The optimal timing and method of minimally invasive interventions, as well as their efficacy, should be further evaluated. Pancreatic necrosectomy is not advised during surgery for decompression and the standard indications for necrosectomy apply [84].

3.6 Acute Pancreatitis and Pregnancy

The most common causes of AP during pregnancy are biliary disease and congenital or acquired hypertriglyceridemia, which can occur during any trimester but over a half comes about in the third one. In case of gallstone-related mild disease, many small series have confirmed the safety of both ERCP and laparoscopic cholecystectomy in any trimester of pregnancy [85, 86], but, despite the lack of significant adverse fetal outcomes in published literature, the uncertainty of long-term effects of radiation on the fetus still poses a significant concern to clinicians [87], suggesting the use of ERCP and endoscopic sphincterotomy without radiation.

The most adopted strategy during the first trimester consists in conservative treatment; antepartum cholecystectomy with correct patient positioning and deep vein thrombosis prophylaxis should be strongly considered in case of gallstone pancreatitis of the second trimester, and not only after failure of a nonoperative approach. Patients treated with nonoperative management are at a significant risk for recurrent symptoms; during the third trimester, if surgery is not performed, antepartum ERCP and endoscopic sphincterotomy appear to be protective with a decrease of symptom recurrence, but early postpartum cholecystectomy is strongly recommended [88–90]. In case of severe AP, most often due to hypertriglyceridemia, and life-threatening for the mother and fetus, a pregnancy interruption is mandatory, as soon as possible, either by abortion or by delivery if possible [91].

References

1. Bradley EL, Dexter ND (2010) Management of severe acute pancreatitis: a surgical odyssey. Ann Surg 251:6–17. doi:10.1097/SLA.0b013e3181c72b79
2. Banks PA, Bollen TL, Dervenis C et al (2013) Classification of acute pancreatitis—2012: revision of the Atlanta classification and definitions by international consensus. Gut 62:102–111
3. Talukdar R, Bhattacharrya A, Rao B et al (2014) Clinical utility of the revised Atlanta classification of acute pancreatitis in a prospective cohort: have all loose ends been tied? Pancreatol Off J Int Assoc Pancreatol IAP Al 14:257–262. doi:10.1016/j.pan.2014.06.003
4. Dellinger EP, Forsmark CE, Layer P et al (2012) Determinant-based classification of acute pancreatitis severity: an international multidisciplinary consultation. Ann Surg 256:875–880
5. Acevedo-Piedra NG, Moya-Hoyo N, Rey-Riveiro M et al (2014) Validation of the determinant-based classification and revision of the Atlanta classification systems for acute pancreatitis. Clin Gastroenterol Hepatol Off Clin Pract J Am Gastroenterol Assoc 12:311–316. doi:10.1016/j.cgh.2013.07.042
6. van Santvoort H, Bakker O, Besselink M et al (2011) Prediction of common bile duct stones in the earliest stages of acute biliary pancreatitis. Endoscopy 43:8–13. doi:10.1055/s-0030-1255866
7. Schepers NJ, Besselink MGH, van Santvoort HC et al (2013) Early management of acute pancreatitis. Best Pract Res Clin Gastroenterol 27:727–743. doi:10.1016/j.bpg.2013.08.007
8. Bollen TL, Singh VK, Maurer R et al (2012) A comparative evaluation of radiologic and clinical scoring systems in the early prediction of severity in acute pancreatitis. Am J Gastroenterol 107:612–619. doi:10.1038/ajg.2011.438
9. Brisinda G, Crocco A, Giustacchini P (2014) Classification of the severity of acute pancreatitis: how much is really needed for a new classification? Ann Surg. doi:10.1097/SLA.0000000000000625
10. Bernardoni L, Frulloni L, Benini L, Gabbrielli A (2014) Aggiornamento delle linee guida della pancreatite acuta. Giorn Ital Endosc Dig 37:25–30
11. Cho JH, Kim TN, Chung HH, Kim KH (2015) Comparison of scoring systems in predicting the severity of acute pancreatitis. World J Gastroenterol 21:2387–2394. doi:10.3748/wjg.v21.i8.2387
12. Bakker OJ, Issa Y, van Santvoort HC et al (2014) Treatment options for acute pancreatitis. Nat Rev Gastroenterol Hepatol 11:462–469. doi:10.1038/nrgastro.2014.39

13. Kuo DC, Rider AC, Estrada P, et al (2015) Acute pancreatitis: what's the score? J Emerg Med. doi:10.1016/j.jemermed.2015.02.018
14. Andersson B, Andrén-Sandberg Å, Nilsson J, Andersson R (2012) Survey of the management of acute pancreatitis in surgical departments in Sweden. Scand J Gastroenterol 47:1064–1070. doi:10.3109/00365521.2012.685752
15. Talukdar R, Rau BM (2015) Determinant-based classification of severity of acute pancreatitis: have we really reached consensus? Ann Surg 261, e22. doi:10.1097/SLA.0000000000000507
16. Petrov MS, Vege SS, Windsor JA (2012) Global survey of controversies in classifying the severity of acute pancreatitis. Eur J Gastroenterol Hepatol 24:715–721. doi:10.1097/MEG.0b013e328351d340
17. (2013) IAP/APA evidence-based guidelines for the management of acute pancreatitis. Pancreatology 13:e1–e15. doi:10.1016/j.pan.2013.07.063
18. Tenner S, Baillie J, DeWitt J, et al (2013) American College of Gastroenterology guideline: management of acute pancreatitis. Am J Gastroenterol 108:1400–1415, 1416. doi:10.1038/ajg.2013.218
19. Yadav D (2014) Acute pancreatitis: too many classifications-what is a clinician or researcher to do? Clin Gastroenterol Hepatol Off Clin Pract J Am Gastroenterol Assoc 12:317–319. doi:10.1016/j.cgh.2013.09.051
20. Kokosis G, Perez A, Pappas TN (2014) Surgical management of necrotizing pancreatitis: an overview. World J Gastroenterol 20:16106–16112. doi:10.3748/wjg.v20.i43.16106
21. Yokoe M, Takada T, Mayumi T et al (2015) Japanese guidelines for the management of acute pancreatitis: Japanese Guidelines 2015. J Hepato-Biliary-Pancreat Sci 22:405–432. doi:10.1002/jhbp.259
22. Italian Association for the Study of the Pancreas (AISP), Pezzilli R, Zerbi A, et al (2015) Consensus guidelines on severe acute pancreatitis. Dig Liver Dis Off J Ital Soc Gastroenterol Ital Assoc Study Liver. doi:10.1016/j.dld.2015.03.022
23. Shen H-N, Wang W-C, Lu C-L, Li C-Y (2013) Effects of gender on severity, management and outcome in acute biliary pancreatitis. PLoS One 8, e57504. doi:10.1371/journal.pone.0057504
24. Yadav D, Lowenfels AB (2013) The epidemiology of pancreatitis and pancreatic cancer. Gastroenterology 144:1252–1261. doi:10.1053/j.gastro.2013.01.068
25. Gurusamy KS, Nagendran M, Davidson BR (2013) Early versus delayed laparoscopic cholecystectomy for acute gallstone pancreatitis. Cochrane Database Syst Rev 9, CD010326
26. Zhao X, Chen D-Z, Lang R et al (2013) Enhanced recovery in the management of mild gallstone pancreatitis: a prospective cohort study. Surg Today 43:643–647. doi:10.1007/s00595-012-0364-9
27. Pérez LJR, Parra JF, Aldana Dimas G (2014) Seguridad de la colecistectomía laparoscópica temprana (<48h) para pacientes con pancreatitis aguda biliar leve: revisión sistemática de la literatura y metaanálisis. Cir Esp 92:107–113. doi:10.1016/j.ciresp.2013.01.024
28. van Baal MC, Besselink MG, Bakker OJ et al (2012) Timing of cholecystectomy after mild biliary pancreatitis: a systematic review. Ann Surg 255:860–866
29. Nguyen GC, Rosenberg M, Chong RY, Chong CA (2012) Early cholecystectomy and ERCP are associated with reduced readmissions for acute biliary pancreatitis: a nationwide, population-based study. Gastrointest Endosc 75:47–55. doi:10.1016/j.gie.2011.08.028
30. Mador BD, Panton ONM, Hameed SM (2014) Early versus delayed cholecystectomy following endoscopic sphincterotomy for mild biliary pancreatitis. Surg Endosc 28:3337–3342. doi:10.1007/s00464-014-3621-8
31. Bakker OJ, van Santvoort HC, Hagenaars JC et al (2011) Timing of cholecystectomy after mild biliary pancreatitis. Br J Surg 98:1446–1454. doi:10.1002/bjs.7587
32. da Costa DW, Bouwense SA, Schepers NJ et al (2015) Same-admission versus interval cholecystectomy for mild gallstone pancreatitis (PONCHO): a multicentre randomised controlled trial. Lancet Lond Engl 386:1261–1268. doi:10.1016/S0140-6736(15)00274-3
33. Bouwense SAW, Bakker OJ, van Santvoort HC et al (2011) Safety of cholecystectomy in the first 48 hours after admission for gallstone pancreatitis not yet proven. Ann Surg 253:1053–1054. doi:10.1097/SLA.0b013e3182172dd7

34. Isogai M, Kaneoka Y, Maeda A (2011) Is early cholecystectomy within 48 hours of admission for mild gallstone pancreatitis classified by ranson score appropriate? Ann Surg 253:1052–1053. doi:10.1097/SLA.0b013e3182172dc4
35. Johnson PM, Walsh MJ (2012) The impact of intraoperative cholangiography on recurrent pancreatitis and biliary complications in patients with gallstone pancreatitis. J Gastrointest Surg 16:2220–2224. doi:10.1007/s11605-012-2041-0
36. Castoldi L, De Rai P, Zerbi A et al (2013) Long term outcome of acute pancreatitis in Italy: results of a multicentre study. Dig Liver Dis 45:827–832. doi:10.1016/j.dld.2013.03.012
37. Johnstone M, Marriott P, Royle TJ et al (2014) The impact of timing of cholecystectomy following gallstone pancreatitis. Surgeon 12:134–140. doi:10.1016/j.surge.2013.07.006
38. Judkins SE, Moore EE, Witt JE et al (2011) Surgeons provide definitive care to patients with gallstone pancreatitis. Am J Surg 202:673–678. doi:10.1016/j.amjsurg.2011.06.031
39. El-Dhuwaib Y, Deakin M, David G et al (2012) Definitive management of gallstone pancreatitis in England. Ann R Coll Surg Engl 94:402–406. doi:10.1308/003588412X13171221591934
40. Hwang SS, Li BH, Haigh PI (2013) Gallstone pancreatitis without cholecystectomy. JAMA Surg 148:867. doi:10.1001/jamasurg.2013.3033
41. Trust MD, Sheffield KM, Boyd CA et al (2011) Gallstone pancreatitis in older patients: are we operating enough? Surgery 150:515–525. doi:10.1016/j.surg.2011.07.072
42. Bencini L (2014) Modern approach to cholecysto-choledocholithiasis. World J Gastrointest Endosc 6:32. doi:10.4253/wjge.v6.i2.32
43. de C Ferreira LEVV, Baron TH (2013) Acute biliary conditions. Best Pract Res Clin Gastroenterol 27:745–756. doi:10.1016/j.bpg.2013.08.008
44. Sandzén B, Haapamäki MM, Nilsson E et al (2012) Treatment of common bile duct stones in Sweden 1989-2006: an observational nationwide study of a paradigm shift. World J Surg 36:2146–2153. doi:10.1007/s00268-012-1648-3
45. Dasari BVM, Tan CJ, Gurusamy KS et al (2013) Surgical versus endoscopic treatment of bile duct stones. Cochrane Database Syst Rev 12, CD003327. doi:10.1002/14651858.CD003327.pub4
46. Baucom RB, Feurer ID, Shelton JS, et al (2015) Surgeons, ERCP, and laparoscopic common bile duct exploration: do we need a standard approach for common bile duct stones? Surg Endosc doi:10.1007/s00464-015-4273-z
47. Tse F, Yuan Y (2012) Early routine endoscopic retrograde cholangiopancreatography strategy versus early conservative management strategy in acute gallstone pancreatitis. Cochrane Database Syst Rev 5, CD009779. doi:10.1002/14651858.CD009779.pub2
48. van Geenen E-JM, van Santvoort HC, Besselink MGH et al (2013) Lack of consensus on the role of endoscopic retrograde cholangiography in acute biliary pancreatitis in published meta-analyses and guidelines: a systematic review. Pancreas 42:774–780. doi:10.1097/MPA.0b013e318287d208
49. Bignell M, Dearing M, Hindmarsh A, Rhodes M (2011) ERCP and endoscopic sphincterotomy (ES): a safe and definitive management of gallstone pancreatitis with the gallbladder left in situ. J Gastrointest Surg Off J Soc Surg Aliment Tract 15:2205–2210. doi:10.1007/s11605-011-1729-x
50. Worhunsky DJ, Visser BC (2013) Gallstone pancreatitis: why not cholecystectomy? JAMA Surg 148:872. doi:10.1001/jamasurg.2013.3063
51. Mustafa A, Begaj I, Deakin M et al (2014) Long-term effectiveness of cholecystectomy and endoscopic sphincterotomy in the management of gallstone pancreatitis. Surg Endosc 28:127–133. doi:10.1007/s00464-013-3138-6
52. van Santvoort HC, Bakker OJ, Bollen TL et al (2011) A conservative and minimally invasive approach to necrotizing pancreatitis improves outcome. Gastroenterology 141:1254–1263. doi:10.1053/j.gastro.2011.06.073
53. Hajjar NA, Iancu C, Bodea R (2012) Modern therapeutic approach of acute severe forms of pancratitis. A review of the literature and experience of Surgical Department No III Cluj. Chir Buchar Rom 1990 107:605–610

54. Phillip V, Steiner JM, Algül H (2014) Early phase of acute pancreatitis: assessment and management. World J Gastrointest Pathophysiol 5:158–168. doi:10.4291/wjgp.v5.i3.158
55. Rodriguez JR, Razo AO, Targarona J et al (2008) Debridement and closed packing for sterile or infected necrotizing pancreatitis: insights into indications and outcomes in 167 patients. Ann Surg 247:294–299. doi:10.1097/SLA.0b013e31815b6976
56. Raraty MGT, Halloran CM, Dodd S et al (2010) Minimal access retroperitoneal pancreatic necrosectomy: improvement in morbidity and mortality with a less invasive approach. Ann Surg 251:787–793. doi:10.1097/SLA.0b013e3181d96c53
57. Sermoneta D, Di Mugno M, Spada PL et al (2010) Intra-abdominal vacuum-assisted closure (VAC) after necrosectomy for acute necrotising pancreatitis: preliminary experience. Int Wound J 7:525–530. doi:10.1111/j.1742-481X.2010.00727.x
58. Besselink MGH, van Santvoort HC, Nieuwenhuijs VB et al (2006) Minimally invasive "step-up approach" versus maximal necrosectomy in patients with acute necrotising pancreatitis (PANTER trial): design and rationale of a randomised controlled multicenter trial [ISRCTN13975868]. BMC Surg 6:6. doi:10.1186/1471-2482-6-6
59. Mamlouk MD, van Sonnenberg E (2011) Interventional radiology for necrotizing pancreatitis. J Gastrointest Surg Off J Soc Surg Aliment Tract 15:1101–1103. doi:10.1007/s11605-011-1507-9
60. Fink D, Soares R, Matthews JB, Alverdy JC (2011) History, goals, and technique of laparoscopic pancreatic necrosectomy. J Gastrointest Surg 15:1092–1097. doi:10.1007/s11605-011-1506-x
61. Bakker OJ, van Santvoort HC, van Brunschot S et al (2012) Endoscopic transgastric vs surgical necrosectomy for infected necrotizing pancreatitis: a randomized trial. JAMA 307:1053. doi:10.1001/jama.2012.276
62. Bausch D, Wellner U, Kahl S et al (2012) Minimally invasive operations for acute necrotizing pancreatitis: comparison of minimally invasive retroperitoneal necrosectomy with endoscopic transgastric necrosectomy. Surgery 152:S128–S134. doi:10.1016/j.surg.2012.05.021
63. Babu RY, Gupta R, Kang M et al (2013) Predictors of surgery in patients with severe acute pancreatitis managed by the step-up approach. Ann Surg 257:737–750. doi:10.1097/SLA.0b013e318269d25d
64. Dupuis CS, Baptista V, Whalen G et al (2013) Diagnosis and management of acute pancreatitis and its complications. Gastrointest Interv 2:36–46. doi:10.1016/j.gii.2013.03.001
65. Tang C, Wang B, Xie B et al (2011) Treatment of severe acute pancreatitis through retroperitoneal laparoscopic drainage. Front Med 5:302–305. doi:10.1007/s11684-011-0145-7
66. Wronski M, Cebulski W, Slodkowski M et al (2012) Retroperitoneal minimally invasive pancreatic necrosectomy using single-port access. Surg Laparosc Endosc Percutan Tech 22:e8–e11. doi:10.1097/SLE.0b013e31823fbec5
67. Fogel EL (2011) Endoscopic pancreatic necrosectomy. J Gastrointest Surg Off J Soc Surg Aliment Tract 15:1098–1100. doi:10.1007/s11605-011-1505-y
68. Worhunsky DJ, Qadan M, Dua MM et al (2014) Laparoscopic transgastric necrosectomy for the management of pancreatic necrosis. J Am Coll Surg 219:735–743. doi:10.1016/j.jamcollsurg.2014.04.012
69. Bang JY, Holt BA, Hawes RH et al (2014) Outcomes after implementing a tailored endoscopic step-up approach to walled-off necrosis in acute pancreatitis. Br J Surg 101:1729–1738. doi:10.1002/bjs.9664
70. Tan V, Charachon A, Lescot T et al (2014) Endoscopic transgastric versus surgical necrosectomy in infected pancreatic necrosis. Clin Res Hepatol Gastroenterol 38:770–776. doi:10.1016/j.clinre.2014.06.016
71. Bausch D, Keck T (2013) Laparoscopic pancreatic resections. Langenbecks Arch Surg 398:939–945. doi:10.1007/s00423-013-1108-z
72. Kirkpatrick AW, Roberts DJ, De Waele J et al (2013) Intra-abdominal hypertension and the abdominal compartment syndrome: updated consensus definitions and clinical practice guidelines from the World Society of the Abdominal Compartment Syndrome. Intensive Care Med 39:1190–1206. doi:10.1007/s00134-013-2906-z

73. Boone B, Zureikat A, Hughes SJ et al (2013) Abdominal compartment syndrome is an early, lethal complication of acute pancreatitis. Am Surg 79:601–607
74. Mentula P, Leppäniemi A (2014) Position paper: timely interventions in severe acute pancreatitis are crucial for survival. World J Emerg Surg 9:15. doi:10.1186/1749-7922-9-15
75. Trikudanathan G, Vege SS (2014) Current concepts of the role of abdominal compartment syndrome in acute pancreatitis – an opportunity or merely an epiphenomenon. Pancreatol Off J Int Assoc Pancreatol IAP Al 14:238–243. doi:10.1016/j.pan.2014.06.002
76. van Brunschot S, Schut AJ, Bouwense SA et al (2014) Abdominal compartment syndrome in acute pancreatitis: a systematic review. Pancreas 43:665–674. doi:10.1097/MPA.0000000000000108
77. Anand RJ, Ivatury RR (2011) Surgical management of intra-abdominal hypertension and abdominal compartment syndrome. Am Surg 77(Suppl 1):S42–S45
78. Leppäniemi A (2009) Surgical management of abdominal compartment syndrome; indications and techniques. Scand J Trauma Resusc Emerg Med 17:17. doi:10.1186/1757-7241-17-17
79. Camps I, Arméstar F, Cuadrado M, Mesalles E (2009) VAC (vacuum-assisted closure) "covered" laparostomy to control abdominal compartmental syndrome in a case of emphysematous pancreatitis. Cir Esp 86:250–251. doi:10.1016/j.ciresp.2009.05.011
80. Hu HK, Du XJ, Li A, et al (2012) A minimally invasive management for abdominal compartment syndrome in severe acute pancreatitis. Pak J Med Sci. doi:10.12669/pjms.291.2721
81. Park S, Lee S, Lee HD et al (2014) Abdominal compartment syndrome in severe acute pancreatitis treated with percutaneous catheter drainage. Clin Endosc 47:469. doi:10.5946/ce.2014.47.5.469
82. Zhu H (2015) Embryonic natural orifice transluminal endoscopic surgery in the treatment of severe acute pancreatitis complicated by abdominal compartment syndrome. World J Emerg Med 6:23. doi:10.5847/wjem.j.1920-8642.2015.01.004
83. Radenkovic DV, Bajec D, Ivancevic N et al (2010) Decompressive laparotomy with temporary abdominal closure versus percutaneous puncture with placement of abdominal catheter in patients with abdominal compartment syndrome during acute pancreatitis: background and design of multicenter, randomised, controlled study. BMC Surg 10:22. doi:10.1186/1471-2482-10-22
84. De Waele JJ, Ejike JC, Leppäniemi A et al (2015) Intra-abdominal hypertension and abdominal compartment syndrome in pancreatitis, paediatrics, and trauma. Anaesthesiol Intensive Ther 47:219–227. doi:10.5603/AIT.a2015.0027
85. Pearl J, Price R, Richardson W, Fanelli R (2011) Guidelines for diagnosis, treatment, and use of laparoscopy for surgical problems during pregnancy. Surg Endosc 25:3479–3492. doi:10.1007/s00464-011-1927-3
86. Polydorou A, Karapanos K, Vezakis A et al (2012) A multimodal approach to acute biliary pancreatitis during pregnancy: a case series. Surg Laparosc Endosc Percutan Tech 22:429–432
87. Chan CHY, Enns RA (2012) ERCP in the management of choledocholithiasis in pregnancy. Curr Gastroenterol Rep 14:504–510. doi:10.1007/s11894-012-0294-0
88. Othman MO, Stone E, Hashimi M, Parasher G (2012) Conservative management of cholelithiasis and its complications in pregnancy is associated with recurrent symptoms and more emergency department visits. Gastrointest Endosc 76:564–569. doi:10.1016/j.gie.2012.04.475
89. Ducarme G, Maire F, Chatel P et al (2013) Acute pancreatitis during pregnancy: a review. J Perinatol 34:87–94
90. Veerappan A, Gawron AJ, Soper NJ, Keswani RN (2013) Delaying cholecystectomy for complicated gallstone disease in pregnancy is associated with recurrent postpartum symptoms. J Gastrointest Surg 17:1953–1959. doi:10.1007/s11605-013-2330-2
91. Qihui C, Xiping Z, Xianfeng D (2012) Clinical study on acute pancreatitis in pregnancy in 26 cases. Gastroenterol Res Pract 2012:1–5. doi:10.1155/2012/271925

Laparoscopic Appendectomy

4

Nereo Vettoretto, Sarah Molfino, Giulia Montori, Fabio Cesare Campanile, and Mauro Zago

4.1 Introduction

Five years after our previous guidelines on laparoscopic surgery in appendicitis [1] technical aspects and outcomes are still debated, despite recent guidelines [2,3]. The publication, in recent years, of many longitudinal or retrospective database studies [4] on large national populations has added more hints to the problem [5] concerning new complications which deserve further confirmation by higher evidence comparative studies to come: wound rupture, negative appendectomy ratio and incidence of small bowel obstruction, intestinal injury, hospital readmission, and urinary infections. The former seem to carry a higher incidence in open appendectomy (OA) series, while the latter have become typical complications of laparoscopic appendectomy (LA). A Swedish national database study [5], including a large cohort of 169,896 patients comparing LA with OA, evidenced a shorter length of hospital stay, a lower frequency of negative appendicectomy (adjusted odds ratio 0.59; $P<0.001$), lower rates of wound infection (adjusted OR 0.54;

N. Vettoretto (✉)
Montichiari Surgery Department, ASST Spedali Civili di Brescia, V.le Ciotti 154, 25018 Montichiari, BS, Italy
e-mail: nereovet@gmail.com

S. Molfino
Surgical Clinic, University of Brescia, P.zza Mercato 15, 25121 Brescia, Italy

G. Montori
Surgical Clinic, University of Parma, Via Gramsci 14, 43100 Parma, Italy

F.C. Campanile
General Surgery Department, Ospedale Andosilla, Via Ferretti 169, 01033 Civita Castellana, VT, Italy

M. Zago
General Surgery Department, Minimally Invasive Surgery Unit, Policlinico San Pietro, Via Forlanini 15, 24036 Ponte San Pietro, BG, Italy

F. Agresta et al. (eds.), *Emergency Laparoscopy*,
DOI 10.1007/978-3-319-29620-3_4

$P=0.004$), and wound rupture (adjusted OR 0.44; $P=0.010$) associated with LA; on the other hand, laparoscopy carries higher rates of previously infrequent complications, like intestinal injuries (adjusted OR 1.32; $P=0.042$), readmission (adjusted OR 1.10; $P<0.001$), postoperative abdominal abscess (adjusted OR 1.58; $P<0.001$), and urinary infection (adjusted OR 1.39; $P=0.020$). Moreover, this paper analyzes small bowel obstructions during the first 2 years after surgery, proving a lower hospitalization in Las, during the first 2 years following operation.

4.2 Preoperative Study

Concerning preoperative study, where possible, ultrasound (US) should be added to clinical examination and computed tomography proves useful, especially in equivocal cases, in order to lower negative appendectomy rate (NAR) and missed perforations. A systematic review of the literature, including a total of 802 patients, showed that an additional radiological imaging was routinely performed in 96.3 % of patients with suspected appendicitis ($n=164$). The use of CT scan was kept to a minimum (17.9 %), due to radiation risk and costs, with a US:CT ratio of approximately 6:1. Different positive and negative predictive values have been referred to clinical examination alone (63 % and 98 %), US (94 % and 97 %), and CT (100 % and 100 %). The negative appendicitis rate was 3.3 %, the perforation rate was 23.5 %, and the missed perforated appendicitis rate was 3.4 %. This meta-analysis supports the hypothesis that the use of preoperative abdominal CT is associated with lower negative appendectomy rates [6].

This is particularly true for obese patients: in these the difference of negative appendectomy rates for overweight patients, obese patients, and morbidly obese patients who underwent preoperative CT, compared with patients in the same BMI category who did not undergo preoperative CT, was statistically significant ($P\leq 0.001$). An analogous significance was found for negative appendectomy rates in favor of preoperative CT scan [7].

Many diagnostic scoring systems have been studied in recent years, in order to stratify patients affected by acute appendicitis. These scores consider clinical history, physical examination, and laboratory values. Popular and validated examples include Alvarado score [8], Pediatric Appendicitis Score (PAS) [9], and RIPASA score [10]. Other scores have been published, including variations on the abovementioned scores. The primary data are derived from retrospective and prospective cross-sectional studies and represent either level 2 or 3 evidence.

The Alvarado score is the most extensively studied score, and its validity has been summarized in a recent meta-analysis [11], including 5960 patients in 29 studies. The score's performance is dependent on the cutoff value: a clinical cutoff score of less than 5 results in a sensitivity of 99 % (95 % CI 97–99 %) and a specificity of 43 % (36–51 %), while a cutoff score of less than 7 results in a sensitivity of 82 % (76–86 %) and a specificity of 81 % (76–85 %).

Alvarado score (with a cut-off of 4) is also useful for the selection of candidates to CT scan [12] (Tables 4.1 and 4.2).

Table 4.1 Characteristics of Alvarado score[a]

Characteristics	Score when present
Migration of pain	1
Anorexia	1
Nausea	1
Tenderness in right lower qua	2
Rebound pain	1
Elevated temperature	1
Leukocytosis	2
Neutrophilia	1
Total (maximum)	10

[a]Modified from Jones RP et al., The Alvarado score as a method for reducing the number of CT studies when appendiceal ultrasound fails to visualize the appendix in adults

Table 4.2 CT scan using Alvarado score[a]

Alvarado score	Pathologically proved appendicitis, evident on CT (%)	Pathologically proved appendicitis (%)	Patients with CT showing neither significant alternative findings nor appendicitis (%)
≤3	0	0	85.7
≥4	15.7	17.1	58.6
P	0.003	0.001	0.002

[a]Modified from Jones RP et al., The Alvarado score as a method for reducing the number of CT studies when appendiceal ultrasound fails to visualize the appendix in adults

In 2014, Shogiley and colleagues published an evidence-based review on diagnosis of acute appendicitis, comprehending studies regarding imaging, Alvarado score, common laboratory markers, and novel markers. They stated that CT is the most accurate mode of imaging for suspected cases of appendicitis but the associated increase in radiation exposure remains an unsolved issue. Alvarado score can help by potentially decreasing the use of CT imaging. Regarding laboratory tests, white blood cell (WBC), C-reactive protein (CRP), granulocyte count, and proportion of polymorphonuclear (PMN) cells are frequently elevated in patients with appendicitis, but are insufficient as isolated tests, for their low specificity. Whenever used in combination, their diagnostic sensitivity is greatly increased [13]. Still, at present, no specific biologic marker has changed the diagnostic or therapeutic management of acute appendicitis.

4.3 Patient Selection

LA is to be considered the gold standard in premenopausal women. A meta-analysis carried out in the Cochrane Library, MEDLINE, EMBASE, LILACS, CNKI, SciSearch, study registries, and the congress proceedings of endoscopic surgical societies and including randomized clinical trials comparing laparoscopic (LA) versus open appendectomy (OA) in adults or children demonstrated as diagnostic laparoscopy reduced the risk of a negative appendectomy, but this effect was stronger in fertile women (RR 0.20; CI 0.11–0.34) as compared to unselected adults (RR 0.37; CI 0.13–1.01). In those clinical settings where surgical expertise and equipment are available and affordable, diagnostic laparoscopy and LA (either in combination or separately) seem to have various advantages over OA. Some of the clinical effects of LA, however, are small and of limited clinical relevance [14].

Regarding the elderly, a recent database study on more than 250,000 patients aged >65 years entails improved clinical outcomes for laparoscopic appendectomy compared with OA in terms of length of stay (LOS, 4.44 days vs. 7.86 days, $P<0.001$), fewer total patient safety indicator events (1.8 % vs. 3.5 %, $P<0.001$), and a decreased mortality rate (0.9 % vs. 2.8 %, $P<0.001$). On multivariate analysis, a decreased probability of patient safety events occurring in LA vs. OA was observed (odds ratio, 0.68) as measured by patient safety indicators [15].

As for obese patients, a meta-analysis of prospective and retrospective comparative series evidences superiority of LA vs. OA also in BMI > 30, with a significantly lower wound infection rate ($P<0.001$) and postoperative complication rate ($P<0.001$). Also, operation time was considered as a hallmark of technical challenge and was diminished in the laparoscopic group ($P=0.018$). Intra-abdominal abscesses formation rate was higher in the open appendectomy group ($P=0.058$), although slightly above the statistical significance threshold [16].

LA is also feasible in men, even if advantages over OA in the latter group are not demonstrated. In fact in a Greek comparative study, 147 men with suspected acute appendicitis were randomized to either OA ($n=75$) or LA ($n=72$). LA took longer operating time (60 min; range, 20–120 min vs. 45 min; range, 20–90 min; $P=0.0027$), and LA did not result in any significant difference for the safety issues, and the length of hospital stay (LOS) did not differ significantly [17].

4.4 Complicated Appendicitis

Complicated appendicitis (defined as abscess, perforation, gangrene, or generalized peritonitis) can be approached laparoscopically in experienced context, with significant advantages, comprehending lower overall complications, readmission rate, SBO rate, infections of the surgical site (minor advantage following Clavien's criteria), and faster recovery [18]. Several database series involving more than 20,000 patients demonstrated that age, comorbidity, and severity of appendicitis were determinants of costs and LOS for both LA and OA. Although the costs and LOS for appendectomy increased with age and number of comorbidities, a sharper increase was noted for OA patients. Laparoscopic appendectomy mildly decreased LOS at the expense of significantly higher costs for young patients, those without comorbidities, and patients with uncomplicated appendicitis. In contrast, compared with OA, LA was associated with comparable costs and reduced LOS for the elderly, patients with comorbidities, and those with complicated appendicitis. In addition,

Table 4.3 Risk of conversion for LA[a]

Author	Risk factors	Definition threshold	Conversion rate (%)	*P* value
X	Abnormal CT findings	Abscess, phlegmon, rupture	17.0	0.001
X	Age	>45 years	9.1	0.006
X	Symptoms duration	>48 h	10.4	0.012
Y	Retrocecal appendix	Yes	15.2	0.016
Y	Gangrenous	Yes	19.4	0.0001
Y	Perforated	Yes	26.3	0.0001
Y	Abscess	Yes	27.7	0.0001
Y	Peritonitis	Diffuse	27.8	0.0001

[a]Modified from Gupta N et al., Identification of preoperative risk factors associated with the conversion of laparoscopic to open appendectomies [X] and Antonacci N et al., Laparoscopic appendectomy: which factors are predictors of conversion? A high-volume prospective cohort study [Y]

hospital mortality and readmission rates for postoperative complications did not differ significantly between LA and OA [19–21].

Conversion to laparotomy is another interesting issue. Two prospective observational cohorts have been analyzed for the detection of factors associated with conversion: higher rates of conversion affect patients with more than 5 days since the onset of symptoms, a WBC count higher than 20,000, males aged more than 45 years, or ruptured appendicitis detected on CT scan; anatomical and pathological intraoperative findings which bring to a higher conversion rate are perforation, retrocecal position, abscess and generalized peritonitis [22, 23] (Table 4.3).

Peritoneal lavage and aspiration have been suggested by a low-powered study to be detrimental [24], but these conclusions are based on low-volume lavage and scarce numbers; a definitive conclusion cannot be drawn even though a study in children [25] has not demonstrated advantages in terms of intra-abdominal abscesses (IAA) of >500 ml, although >6–8 l are needed to lower bacterial charge significantly [26]. Further studies are auspicated as the issue is still controversial and guidelines on behavior are of utmost importance.

Routine drainage has not proven its utility, as established in a case match study in which 130 patients operated for complicated appendicitis with prophylactic intraperitoneal drainage were matched one by one to 130 patients operated without drainage. Drainage is not useful except in generalized peritonitis and seems to cause more complications, LOS, and transit recovery time [27], despite the widespread opinion that aspiration of the residual fluid after peritoneal lavage in the first 24 h postoperatively might lower the incidence of IAA in case of insufficient lavage [28].

The increase in postoperative IAA has been a major issue in favor of OA since the Cochrane meta-analysis by Sauerland [14] which demonstrated a threefold increase in spite of a threefold decrease in superficial wound infections. More recent randomized studies have reappraised the problem, ascribing it to the initial experiences, and not confirming those data [29]. On the contrary, database longitudinal studies still demonstrate a higher incidence in LA although lowered to a twofold increase [30].

Interval appendectomy in adults has been advised in case of appendiceal masses (3.8 % of appendicites) [31], as an initial nonsurgical treatment carries a lower morbidity when compared to immediate surgery; moreover, nonsurgical treatment followed by interval appendectomy has higher morbidity than no appendectomy [32], but controversies over the treatment options are present, since there is a 7.2 % rate of failure of conservative antibiotic treatment, a 7.4 % rate of recurrence of symptoms and disease, and a 1.5 % rate of malignancies in the adult population, which grows in the patients aged over 40 years [32–34].

When indicated, interval appendectomy carries better outcomes if performed by means of laparoscopy [31].

Despite evidence and American guidelines [2], which considers LA safe in pregnancy [35], the choice must be put in each surgeons' hands, as advantages are minor (less pain, less infections, less early deliveries) if compared to the risk of fetal loss; in fact recent data from reviews of comparative studies (599 LA vs. 2816 OA) show an increased fetal loss for LA, without significant advantages [36], while a database study on 859 pregnant women with appendicitis confirms a better outcome for those treated surgically while seeking no difference in maternal complications between LA and OA [37].

Removal of a normal appendix in the presence of other diseases at exploration is not opportune. If no other pathology is encountered while a normal appearing appendix is found, the surgeon is entailed with a therapeutical dilemma. In order to clarify therapeutical options, an English database data on 20,000 patients who underwent either simple exploratory laparoscopy or normal appendectomy suggest a removal to prevent a 32.9 % of readmission for abdominal pain [38]. In support of these conclusions, the data on morbidity of appendectomy do not significantly exceed those of explorative laparoscopy. Thus, if the practice's rate of abscesses is minimal and the surgeon carries a thorough experience in laparoscopic surgery, then appendectomy might be advised in order to prevent recurrent pain and readmission and to gain the "endoappendicites," which accounts for 11–26 % of normal appendices at pathologic examination [39]. Another important hint comes from preoperative findings regarding the presence of fecaliths in the appendix base. If a normal appendix is associated with preoperatory discovery of fecaliths or fecal impaction, then appendectomy is advised. A case series of more than 1000 patients demonstrates an association with recurrence of symptoms and fecaliths' presence also in healthy appendix: the fecalith rate was 13–16 % and the main groups with fecaliths were those with acute/nonperforated appendicitis ($n = 121$, 65.1 %, $P = 0.041$) and those with a pathologically normal appendix ($n = 65$, 34.9 %, $P = 0.003$) [40].

4.5 Technical Notes

Appendiceal stump closure can be performed either with the use of endoloops or with a mechanical suture. Stapler reduces operative time and superficial wound infections [41], but since no significant differences are evidenced in the rate of

IAA [42], higher costs (6- to 12-fold) influence the choice toward loop-closure; nevertheless, attention must be paid to training issues since LA is mostly performed by younger surgeons; hence, an easier and technically standardized closure device might prove advantageous [28].

Trocar size and position are variable in different practices: according to the more often used technique, once pneumoperitoneum is established, another two trocars are required, in order to obtain the proper triangulation: lower left quadrant (LLQ) and suprapubic, LLQ and lower right quadrant (LRQ), suprapubic and LRQ, or both trocars in the suprapubic position (the latter one is particularly appreciated for cosmetic reasons since scars are hidden in pubic hair) [43].

One trocar technique is particularly used in children: the so-called transumbilical laparoscopic-assisted *appendectomy (TULAA)*. There are many advantages in the use of TULAA: excellent diagnostic and therapeutic approach to the acute abdomen, observation of the entire abdominal cavity, high therapeutic reliability, high versatility, optimal cosmetic result, excellent postoperative recovery, and high feasibility, even in obese patients. The current literature does not report real contraindications to the use of this technique apart from those generally indicated for pneumoperitoneum. As for laparoscopy, it is important to remember that insufflation pressure and flow rate must be kept as low as possible, especially in the pediatric age, in order to reduce postoperative pain. Specifically speaking for TULAA, it is necessary to deflate the abdomen before extracting the appendix since this prevents excessive traction on the mesoappendix and facilitates extraction of the appendix through the umbilicus even if a 4.4 % rate of umbilical infections is reported [44].

Needlescopy might be applied only in selected and not complicated cases due to its higher rate of conversions and prolonged OT time [45] and failure to prove any benefit in a recent comparison with standard LA [46].

Single-port appendectomy has proven equivalent in experienced hands, as demonstrated in a recent Italian meta-analysis [47] even with conventional and low-cost devices [48] with benefits in the patient's perceived cosmesis. This technique could be the next step in minimally invasive surgery after conventional laparoscopy, but an economic evaluation of the various techniques for single access must be performed before its widespread clinical introduction. Better-designed randomized controlled trials are necessary to define a population in which single-port appendectomy could have major benefits [49].

Natural orifice translumenal endoscopic surgery (NOTES) appendectomy, principally performed via a transvaginal route (both with flexible operative endoscopes and with hybrid rigid and flexible devices) in women with uncomplicated appendicitis, has seen a growing interest, with more than 100 cases published in a recent systematic review [50], and seems to carry advantages on pain and recovery over LA [51].

Fast-track procedures in the post-op care of LA are studied prevalently in children [52] and 1-day or outpatient surgery is beginning to be studied also for adults. A recent prospective protocol involving more than 300 patients demonstrates that outpatient laparoscopic appendectomy can be performed with a high rate of success, a low morbidity, and a low readmission rate for uncomplicated appendicitis [53].

Costs should not be determining in favoring open or LA, unless there is a routine application of costly technology, as analyzed in an European meta-analysis in which from a health-economic view, laparoscopic and open appendectomies are generally similar with respect to the direct in-patient and indirect costs [54].

References

1. Agresta F, Ansaloni L, Baiocchi GL, Bergamini C, Campanile FC, Carlucci M, Cocorullo G, Corradi A, Franzato B, Lupo M, Mandalà V, Mirabella A, Pernazza G, Piccoli M, Staudacher C, Vettoretto N, Zago M, Lettieri E, Levati A, Pietrini D, Scaglione M, De Masi S, De Placido G, Francucci M, Rasi M, Fingerhut A, Uranüs S, Garattini S (2012) Laparoscopic approach to acute abdomen from the Consensus Development Conference of the Società Italiana di Chirurgia Endoscopica e nuove tecnologie (SICE), Associazione Chirurghi Ospedalieri Italiani (ACOI), Società Italiana di Chirurgia (SIC), Società Italiana di Chirurgia d'Urgenza e del Trauma (SICUT), Società Italiana di Chirurgia nell'Ospedalità Privata (SICOP), and the European Association for Endoscopic Surgery (EAES). Surg Endosc 26(8):2134–2164
2. Korndorffer JR Jr, Fellinger E, Reed W (2010) SAGES guideline for laparoscopic appendectomy. Surg Endosc 24(4):757–761
3. Vettoretto N, Gobbi S, Corradi A, Ricciardelli L, Belli F, Piccolo D, Mannino L (2011) Consensus conference on laparoscopic appendectomy: development of guidelines. Colorectal Dis 13(7):748–754
4. Vettoretto N, Agresta F, Presenti L, Morino M (2013) Evidence-based laparoscopic appendectomy practice requires national database studies. Surg Endosc 27(7):2652–2653
5. Andersson RE (2014) Short-term complications and long-term morbidity of laparoscopic and open appendicectomy in a national cohort. Br J Surg 101(9):1135–1142
6. Toorenvliet BR, Wiersma F, Bakker RFR, Merkus JWS, Breslau PJ, Hamming JF (2010) Routine ultrasound and limited computed tomography for the diagnosis of acute appendicitis. World J Surg 34:2278–2285
7. Coursey CA, Nelson RC, Moreno RD, Patel MB, Beam CA, Vaslef S (2011) Appendicitis, body mass index, and CT: is CT more valuable for obese patients than thin patients? Am Surg 77(4):471–475
8. Alvarado A (1986) A practical score for the early diagnosis of acute appendicitis. Ann Emerg Med 15:557
9. Samuel M (2002) Pediatric appendicitis score. J Ped Surg 37(6):877
10. Chong CF, Adi MIW, Thien A et al (2010) Development of the RIPASA score: a new appendicitis scoring system for the diagnosis of acute appendicitis. Singapore Med J 51:220
11. Ohle R, O'Reilly F, O'Brien KK et al (2011) The Alvarado score for predicting acute appendicitis: a systematic review. BMC Med 9:139
12. Jones RP, Jeffrey RB, Shah BR, Desser TS, Rosenberg J, Olcott EW (2015) Journal Club: The Alvarado score as a method for reducing the number of CT studies when appendiceal ultrasound fails to visualize the appendix in adults. Am J Roentgenol 204(3):519–526
13. Shogilev DJ, Duus N, Odom SR, Shapiro NI (2014) Diagnosing appendicitis: evidence-based review of the diagnostic approach in 2014. West J Emerg Med 15(7):859–871
14. Sauerland S, Jaschinski T, Neugebauer EA (2010) Laparoscopic versus open surgery for suspected appendicitis. Cochrane Database Syst Rev 10, CD001546
15. Ward NT, Ramamoorthy SL, Chang DC, Parsons JK. Laparoscopic appendectomy is safer than open appendectomy in an elderly population. JSLS. 2014 Jul-Sep;18(3). pii: e2014.00322
16. Ciarrocchi A, Amicucci G (2014) Laparoscopic versus open appendectomy in obese patients: a meta-analysis of prospective and retrospective studies. J Minim Access Surg 10(1):4–9

17. Tzovaras G, Baloyiannis I, Kouritas V, Symeonidis D, Spyridakis M, Poultsidi A, Tepetes K, Zacharoulis D (2010) Laparoscopic versus open appendectomy in men: a prospective randomized trial. Surg Endosc 24(12):2987–2992
18. Wang CC, Tu CC, Wang PC, Lin HC, Wei PL (2013) Outcome comparison between laparoscopic and open appendectomy: evidence from a nationwide population-based study. PLoS One 8(7), e68662
19. Yeh CC, Wu SC, Liao CC, Su LT, Hsieh CH, Li TC (2011) Laparoscopic appendectomy for acute appendicitis is more favorable for patients with comorbidities, the elderly, and those with complicated appendicitis: a nationwide population based study. Surg Endosc 25:2932–2942
20. Masoomi H, Mills S, Dolich MO, Ketana N, Carmichael JC, Nguyen NT, Stamos MJ (2011) Comparison of outcomes of laparoscopic versus open appendectomy in adults: data from the Nationwide Inpatient Sample (NIS), 2006-2008. J Gastrointest Surg 15:2226–2231
21. Isaksson K, Montgomery A, Moberg AC, Andersson R, Tingstedt B (2014) Long-term follow-up for adhesive small bowel obstruction after open versus laparoscopic surgery for suspected appendicitis. Ann Surg 259(6):1173–1177
22. Gupta N, Machado-Aranda D, Bennett K, Mittal VK (2013) Identification of preoperative risk factors associated with the conversion of laparoscopic to open appendectomies. Int Surg 98(4):334–339
23. Antonacci N, Ricci C, Taffurelli G, Monari F, Del Governatore M, Caira A, Leone A, Cervellera M, Minni F, Cola B (2015) Laparoscopic appendectomy: which factors are predictors of conversion? A high-volume prospective cohort study. Int J Surg 21:103–107
24. Moore CB, Smith RS, Herbertson R, Toevs C (2011) Does use of intraoperative irrigation with open or laparoscopic appendectomy reduce post-operative intra-abdominal abscess? Am Surg 77(1):78–80
25. St Peter SD, Adibe OO, Iqbal CW, Fike FB, Sharp SW, Juang D, Lanning D, Murphy JP, Andrews WS, Sharp RJ, Snyder CL, Holcomb GW, Ostlie DJ (2012) Irrigation versus suction alone during laparoscopic appendectomy for perforated appendicitis: a prospective randomized trial. Ann Surg 256(4):581–585
26. Ohno Y, Furui J, Kanematsu T (2004) Treatment strategy when using intraoperative peritoneal lavage for perforated appendicitis in children: a preliminary report. Pediatr Surg Int 20:534–537
27. Allemann P, Probst H, Demartines N, Schäfer M (2011) Prevention of infectious complications after laparoscopic appendectomy for complicated acute appendicitis: the role of routine abdominal drainage. Langenbecks Arch Surg 396(1):63–68
28. Lin HF, Lai HS, Lai IR (2014) Laparoscopic treatment of perforated appendicitis. World J Gastroenterol 20(39):14338–14347
29. Kapischke M, Caliebe A, Tepel J, Schulz T, Hedderich J (2006) Open versus laparoscopic appendectomy: a critical review. Surg Endosc 20:1060–1068
30. Tuggle KR, Ortega G, Bolorunduro OB, Oyetunji TA, Alexander R, Turner PL, Chang DC, Cornwell EE III, Fullum TM (2010) Laparoscopic versus open appendectomy in complicated appendicitis: a review of the NSQIP database. J Surg Res 163(2):225–228
31. Rashid A, Nazir S, Kakroo SM, Chalkoo MA, Razvi SA, Wani AA (2013) Laparoscopic interval appendectomy versus open interval appendectomy: a prospective randomized controlled trial. Surg Laparosc Endosc Percutan Tech 23(1):93–96
32. Andersson RE, Petzold MG (2007) Nonsurgical treatment of appendiceal abscess or phlegmon: a systematic review and meta-analysis. Ann Surg 246:741–748
33. Meshikhes AW (2008) Management of appendiceal mass: controversial issues revisited. J Gastrointest Surg 12(4):767–775
34. Carpenter SG, Chapital AB, Merritt MV, Johnson DJ (2012) Increased risk of neoplasm in appendicitis treated with interval appendectomy: single-institution experience and literature review. Am Surg 78(3):339–343
35. Jackson H, Granger S, Price R, Rollins M, Earle D, Richardson W, Fanelli R (2008) Diagnosis and laparoscopic treatment of surgical diseases during pregnancy: an evidence-based review. Surg Endosc 22(9):1917–1927

36. Wilasrusmee C, Sukrat B, McEvoy M, Attia J, Thakkinstian A (2012) Systematic review and meta-analysis of safety of laparoscopic versus open appendicectomy for suspected appendicitis in pregnancy. Br J Surg 99(11):1470–1478
37. Cheng HT, Wang YC, Lo HC, Su LT, Soh KS, Tzeng CW, Wu SC, Sung FC, Hsieh CH (2015) Laparoscopic appendectomy versus open appendectomy in pregnancy: a population-based analysis of maternal outcome. Surg Endosc 29(6):1394–1399
38. Bhangu A, Begaj I, Ray D (2014) Population level analysis of diagnostic laparoscopy versus normal appendicectomy for acute lower abdominal pain. Int J Surg 12(12):1374–1379
39. Garlipp B, Arlt G (2009) Laparoscopy for suspected appendicitis. Should an appendix that appears normal be removed? Chirurg 80(7):615–621
40. Ramdass MJ, Young Sing Q, Milne D, Mooteeram J, Barrow S (2015) Association between the appendix and the fecalith in adults. Can J Surg 58(1):10–14
41. Kazemeier G, in't Hof KH, Saad S, Bonjer HJ, Sauerland S (2006) Securing the appendiceal stump in laparoscopic appendectomy: evidence for routine stapling? Surg Endosc 20:1473–1476
42. Sahm M, Kube R, Schmidt S, Ritter C, Pross M, Lippert H (2011) Current analysis of endoloops in appendiceal stump closure. Surg Endosc 25:124–129
43. Vettoretto N, Agresta F (2011) A brief review of laparoscopic appendectomy: the issues and the evidence. Tech Coloproctol 15:1–6
44. Nicola Z, Gabriella S, Alberto M, Saverio CF (2014) Transumbilical laparoscopic-assisted appendectomy in children: clinical and surgical outcomes. World J Gastrointest Endosc 6(4):101–104
45. Sajid MS, Khan MA, Cheek E, Baig MK (2009) Needlescopic versus laparoscopic appendectomy: a systematic review. Can J Surg 52:129–134
46. Özsan İ, Karabuğa T, Yoldaş Ö, Alpdoğan Ö, Aydın Ü (2014) Laparoscopic appendectomy versus mini-incision appendectomy in patients with lower body mass index and noncomplicated appendicitis. Gastroenterol Res Pract 2014:138648
47. Vettoretto N, Cirocchi R, Randolph J, Morino M (2015) Acute appendicitis can be treated with single-incision laparoscopy: a systematic review of randomized controlled trials. Colorectal Dis 17(4):281–289
48. Lee SE, Choi YS, Kim BG, Cha SJ, Park JM, Chang IT (2014) Single port using glove port and conventional rigid instruments. AnnSurg Treat Res 86(1):35–38
49. SCARLESS Study Group, Ahmed I, Cook JA, Duncan A, Krukowski ZH, Malik M, MacLennan G, McCormack K (2015) Single port/incision laparoscopic surgery compared with standard three-port laparoscopic surgery for appendicectomy: a randomized controlled trial. Surg Endosc 29(1):77–85
50. Yagci MA, Kayaalp C (2014) Transvaginal appendectomy: a systematic review. Minim Invasive Surg 2014:384706
51. Bernhardt J, Steffen H, Schneider-Koriath S, Ludwig K (2015) Clinical NOTES appendectomy study: comparison of transvaginal NOTES appendectomy in hybrid technique with laparoscopic appendectomy. Int J Colorectal Dis 30(2):259–267
52. Lasso Betancor CE, Ruiz Hierro C, Vargas Cruz V, Orti Rodríguez RJ, Vázquez Rueda F, Paredes Esteban RM (2013) Implementation of "fast-track" treatment in paediatric complicated appendicitis. Cir Pediatr 26(2):63–68
53. Frazee RC, Abernathy SW, Davis M, Hendricks JC, Isbell TV, Regner JL, Smith RW (2014) Outpatient laparoscopic appendectomy should be the standard of care for uncomplicated appendicitis. J Trauma Acute Care Surg 76(1):79–82
54. Gorenoi V, Dintsios CM, Schonermark M, Hagen A (2006) Laparoskopische vs. offene Appendektomie. Systematische Ubersicht zur medizinischen Wirksamkeit und gesundheitsokonomische Analyse. HTA-Bericht 148. In: Deutsche Agentur fur Health Technology Assessment des Deutschen Instituts fur Medizinische Dokumentation und Information (DAHTA@DIMDI) (Hrsg) Schriftenreihe Health Technology Assessment (HTA) in der Bundesrepublik Deutschland. DAHTA-Datenbank des DIMDI, Koln

Laparoscopy in Gynecologic Emergencies

5

Federico Coccolini, Giuseppe D'Amico, Giulia Montori, Fausto Catena, Gustavo Fraga, and Luca Ansaloni

5.1 Introduction

An acute abdomen results usually from peritoneal irritation due to inflammation or rupture of an abdominal organ or obstruction of a hollow organ. In hospital practice, patients with acute abdominal pain either go spontaneously to the emergency room or are sent there by their family doctor with a provisional diagnosis, which reportedly has no more than a 50 % chance of being correct [1].

Determining the cause of lower acute abdominal pain is one of the greatest challenges faced by physicians in emergency services. It is a common reason for hospitalization since 67 % of all patients show nonspecific lower acute abdominal pain. Among women, for anatomic, physiological, and pregnancy reasons, it is the most frequent cause of hospitalization [2].

In women, acute pain can be essentially caused by pelvic inflammatory disease (PID), appendicitis, ectopic pregnancy, abortion, torsion of adnexa, endometriosis, and hemorrhagic ovarian cysts.

"Wait and see" has been the most widely used clinical, or paraclinical, method of observation of patients with nontypical clinical signs. The predictive value of clinical diagnosis reached with this method, which varies with the underlying cause, has been estimated between 68 % and 92 %. On the one hand, this method entails

F. Coccolini • G. D'Amico • G. Montori • L. Ansaloni (✉)
Department of General Surgery, Papa Giovanni XXIII Hospital, 24127 Bergamo, Italy
e-mail: lansaloni@hpg23.it

F. Catena
Department of Emergency and Trauma Surgery, University Hospital of Parma, Parma, Italy

G. Fraga
Division of Trauma Surgery, Department of Surgery, School of Medical Sciences, University of Campinas (Unicamp), Campinas, SP, Brazil

F. Agresta et al. (eds.), *Emergency Laparoscopy*,
DOI 10.1007/978-3-319-29620-3_5

risk to patients because of possible complications such as peritonitis, hemorrhage, or infertility; on the other hand, laparotomy might be unnecessarily performed.

Laparoscopy is an alternative way of making an early diagnosis of the cause of pain and treating the underlying disease. The accuracy of laparoscopy in acute pelvic pain varies within a range of 65–97 %. It depends on the complete visualization of the whole abdominal pelvic cavity and the diagnostic standard to which it is compared. However, laparoscopy should not be considered as a routine diagnostic tool for every case of acute abdomen, as it carries its own morbidity and requires a general anesthesia. Although it is incorrect to hypothesize that all patients with acute abdominal pain would benefit from laparoscopic surgery, it is evident that over the years an increasing number of patients have been managed successfully in emergency thanks to the laparoscopic approach [3].

5.2 Clinical Evaluation

In cases of pelvic pain, taking a thorough patient history is mandatory prior to physical examination. The obstetric history is important, particularly if the woman has suffered a late miscarriage, ectopic pregnancy, or undergone a Cesarean section. The number and outcome of all pregnancies should be noted together with eventual complications suffered such as abortion, prenatal and postnatal infections (endometritis), and thromboembolism.

The gynecologic history should focus on conditions such as pelvic inflammatory and infective processes which are relatively common in women of reproductive age. Previous surgical interventions such as laparoscopy, hysteroscopy, and surgical and medical termination of pregnancy, particularly if recent, have to be taken into careful consideration. The patient's menstrual history should be checked completely, gathering information relating to her menarche (first menstruation), menstrual cycle pattern, and menopausal symptoms. The date of her last menstruation should be recorded as well. The surgeon should enquire as to whether the woman has used any contraceptive methods and their nature. A delay in the menstruation should lead the surgeon to suspect an ectopic pregnancy, even when the urine pregnancy test result is negative. In such circumstances, a serum beta-hCG evaluation would confirm or exclude the diagnosis of a pregnancy. An ectopic pregnancy should also be suspected in the presence of a positive pregnancy test where an intrauterine contraceptive device (IUCD) or oral contraception has been used. Other irregularities in the menstrual cycle should be recorded.

Clinical examination can confirm or refute a diagnosis suggested by the patient history. Generally, a painful abdomen with localized or widespread tenderness, rebound tenderness, and reduced bowel movements should be considered a surgical problem. Urgent hematologic and abnormal ultrasound will help to establish the correct diagnosis. The clinical assessment must always be completed by checking for hernias in the groin or in the site of previous surgery. Rectal and vaginal examination should not be unduly painful and the reason for performing it must be explained to the patients. The vaginal examination should be avoided in very young patients and in those with virgo intacta. The physical examination will include palpating the cervix, the uterus, and the adnexa. Local tumor, fluid collection, and signs of pelvic and peritoneal tenderness will be searched for. Signs of tenderness may indicate the presence of inflammations and infections and suggest peritonitis.

Laboratory investigations should include a full blood count. The red blood cell count and hematocrit will give information on possible anemia. Leukocytosis is always present in cases of infections and inflammations such as salpingitis, PID, and pelvic abscesses. It is also often present in the initial stages of an ovarian cyst rupture and in ovarian torsion. Blood cross-matching is advisable before surgery. Likewise, the clotting screen is also necessary in the presence of heavy blood loss or if acute anemia is suspected. The serum human chorionic gonadotropin (beta-hCG) should be urgently tested, particularly in women with irregular menstrual cycles or those using contraception. The serum beta-hCG test should be carried out even when a negative urine pregnancy test result has been obtained, due to a false-negative rate of 5 %. Testing for CA-125 is not required in an emergency setting. However, it is worth knowing that a raised CA-125 is a specific marker of peritoneal reactions. Levels can be elevated up to hundred times in endometriosis and pregnancy and a thousand times in ovarian cancer.

5.3 Most Common Gynecologic Emergencies

The most common gynecologic emergencies causing acute pelvic pain are reported below:

1. Adnexal–ovarian torsion
2. Pelvic inflammatory disease (PID)
3. Ectopic pregnancy
4. Endometriosis
5. Hemorrhagic ovarian cysts

5.3.1 Adnexal Torsion

5.3.1.1 Etiology

The adnexa of the uterus, formed by the ovaries and fallopian tube, are prone to torsion. Ovary and/or fallopian tube torsion happens when the adnexa suffer a complete or partial rotation on its ligamentous support, resulting in compromise of their blood supply and in sudden onset of pelvic pain. Adnexal torsion can be unilateral or bilateral, with the last one being extremely rare. It is the fifth most common gynecological emergency [4], with a reported incidence ranging from 2.7 % to 3.0 % [4, 5]. Adnexal torsion can affect women of all ages 28–31, but it is more frequent among women of reproductive age 26. Most of these women desire future fertility; thus, an accurate diagnosis and prompt treatment are important in an attempt to preserve ovarian function.

The major risk factors for adnexal torsion are an ovarian mass (physiologic cyst or neoplasm) [6], pregnancy and ovarian stimulation [6], previous pelvic surgery, particularly tubal ligation [6], past history of ovarian torsion [7], hypermobile adnexa [8], and an excessive length of the utero-ovarian ligament, particularly in the pediatric population [9].

5.3.1.2 Signs and Symptoms

Patients presenting with adnexal torsion complain of an acute, intermittent, unilateral pelvic pain. This pain may be exacerbated by positional shifts. Approximately, 70 % of patients have associated gastrointestinal complaints including nausea and vomiting, which can lead some providers to include in their differential appendicitis, bowel obstruction, or mesenteric ischemia. The episodes may have intermittently persisted for the past few days to weeks. On physical examination, a tender, unilateral adnexal mass is appreciated in roughly 70 % of patients [10]. This tender mass becomes enlarged because in a partial torsion, there is enough arterial pressure for blood to flow into the adnexa. The venous blood is unable to return, however, because of the pressure dampening of the torsion. If the torsion persists or progresses, then the arterial blood flow is unable to oxygenate the ovary and the tissue begins to undergo necrosis. Many women only develop a fever once necrosis ensues.

5.3.1.3 Diagnosis

Adnexal torsion remains as one as the most challenging conditions to diagnose preoperatively. Traditionally, diagnosis has stood on the clinical and sonography findings. Numerous retrospective analyses were undertaken to evaluate the clinical profile of adnexal torsion. Abdominal pain was the most common symptom (77.8–98 %), followed by nausea and vomiting (46–80.5 %), mass in clinical examination (22.2–72 %), elevated white blood count (22.1–75 %), lower urinary tract symptoms (14.5 %), fever (5.6–7.8 %), and abnormal genital tract bleeding (4 %) [4, 5]. A gynecological ultrasound is usually the first imaging tool used in the approach of pelvic pain. The sonography findings that may be found in adnexal torsion are ovarian enlargement, visualization of a cyst, solid or complex mass at the location of the adnexa, abnormal ovarian position in the pouch of Douglas, thickening of the adnexal wall, peripherally enlarged follicles, cystic hemorrhage, and free pelvic fluid [5]. Lo et al. reported that an adnexal or pelvic mass could be detected using gynecological ultrasound in almost all of the patients (98.3 %) [4]. Oltmann et al. stated that the finding most consistent with torsion on transvaginal ultrasound (TVU) was simply the presence of an enlarged ovary or adnexal mass and confirmed that the sole presence of a mass larger than 5 cm had the best sensitivity for torsion (83 %) [11].

Color doppler ultrasound detects the ovarian blood flow, while spectral Doppler can enable the differentiation between venous and arterial flow in the ovary. These techniques have been suggested as an additional tool to improve the accuracy of diagnosing ovarian torsion. The absence of venous, or arterial and venous flow in an enlarged or cystic ovary on color and spectral doppler studies, is highly predictive of ovarian torsion [12]. Studies reported that, although highly specific, doppler sonography was not sufficiently sensitive. A normal flow by doppler sonography does not rule out ovarian torsion and should not delay surgical exploration if the patient presents with suggestive signs and symptoms.

Computerized tomography scan (CT scan) and magnetic resonance image (MRI) can detect ovarian torsion, but they are not necessary in most cases and should not delay treatment. Moreover, CT scan is contraindicated in pregnant women. Tumor markers, such as beta-human chorionic gonadotropin (β-HCG), alpha-fetoprotein (α-FP), cancer antigen 125 (CA-125), and lactate dehydrogenase (LDH), are not routinely screened in an emergency setting.

At the present time, there is no reliable method enabling the diagnosis of adnexal torsion to be confirmed preoperatively. Studies still report a poor correlation between preoperative diagnosis and surgery findings: Bar-On et al. found that women who underwent laparoscopy for suspected ovarian torsion were correctly diagnosed in only 46.1 % of cases [13]; Cohen et al. stated that among 100 emergency laparoscopies performed due to acute abdomen, ovarian torsion was the most difficult to diagnose preoperatively, with only 44 % of cases being confirmed by laparoscopy [14]; Houry et al. reported that, among women with ovarian torsion, the diagnosis was initially considered in 47 % of patients [6], while White et al. found that it was considered in only 19 % of patients [7]. Thus, diagnostic laparoscopy can reduce the uncertainty of diagnosis in ovarian torsion. Also, it offers a lot of other advantages: enables a rapid and accurate assessment [15], reduces the incidence of negative laparotomies, reduces morbidity and mortality from the underlying disease [16], and, most of all, enables treatment.

5.3.1.4 Treatment

Surgical approach by laparoscopy is the standard of care for adnexal torsion; it allows the physician to diagnose adnexal torsion in a first step and to treat it in a second step. Multiple studies have confirmed the safety and efficacy of the laparoscopic approach for adnexal torsion in children [9, 17] and pregnant patients [18].

Results of Lo et al. show that patients undergoing laparoscopy had a smaller ovarian mass, a shorter hospital stay, and fewer of them suffered from postoperative fever, comparing to patients undergoing laparotomy [4]. Oltmann et al. also reported that a preoperative imaging mass size of less than 5 cm was associated with the use of a laparoscopic approach. They also found that laparoscopy rates increased from 18 % in the 1993–2000 to 42 % in the 2001–2008 period, reflecting the change over time in surgical practice [11]. Laparoscopy approach has demonstrated to be superior to laparotomy as it results in lower rate of febrile morbidity, reduces consumption of analgesic drugs, and shortens hospital stay [19, 20].

Intraoperative management of adnexal torsion has been largely debated. In the past, treatment consisted of radical surgery. An ipsilateral oopherectomy by laparotomy was the standard of care, due to both concerns regarding thromboembolic phenomena and "black-bluish" appearance of twisted adnexa [19]. Nowadays, treatment is rather conservative. It is initiated by untwisting the adnexa, even when it appears necrotic, and completed, as required, by treatment of any cyst present and/or oophoropexy. All these steps are easily accomplished by laparoscopy [21, 22].

In a pregnant patient, there have been successful cases of laparoscopic adnexal torsion reduction. The incidence of adnexal torsion in pregnancy is 1 in 5000 pregnancies. Many authors recommend entering in an open manner as opposed to Verres needle or in a direct approach; however, there has been documentation of complications in all three approaches. In pregnant patients, precautions should be taken as the uterus may be in the abdominal cavity and surgical pneumoperitoneum poses the risk for decreased uterine blood flow secondary to increased intra-abdominal pressure [18, 23]. Fetal cardiac activity should be documented before and after the procedure and the patient should be positioned in the dorsal supine position with left lateral tilt during the operation.

5.3.2 Pelvic Inflammatory Disease

5.3.2.1 Etiology

Pelvic inflammatory disease refers to the acute infection of the upper genital tract in women. It includes any combination of cervicitis, endometritis, salpingitis, tubo-ovarian abscess, and pelvic peritonitis [24]. Originally, PID was associated with *Neisseria gonorrhea* and *Chlamydia trachomatis* infection. Nowadays, it is recognized that these microorganisms cause only two-thirds of cases. *Gardnerella vaginalis*, *Mycoplasma genitalium/hominis*, Ureaplasma spp., Diphtheroids, Prevotella, Bacteroides, other anaerobes, and streptococci may also be involved [24]. It is the most common infectious disease affecting young women, accounting for 94 % of sexually transmitted disease-associated morbidity in well-resourced countries. This condition can cause significant reproductive health sequelae, including tubo-ovarian abscesses, pelvic adhesions, recurrent PID, chronic pelvic pain, infertility due to obstruction of fallopian tubes, and ectopic pregnancy in an increased factor of 7–10 [25]. Such complications are related to disease severity and timing of diagnosis. Prompt investigation is essential in order to attenuate disease impact.

5.3.2.2 Signs and Symptoms

Approximately, 90 % of patients present with the chief complaint of abdominal pain and approximately 75 % of those patients have an elevated white count. Other signs and symptoms can be vaginal discharge, abnormal uterine bleeding, nausea, vomiting, and fever.

5.3.2.3 Diagnosis

The accuracy of different signs and symptoms in predicting the presence of PID has been extensively evaluated using laparoscopy as the gold standard [26, 27]. Currently, the clinical diagnosis of PID is based on recommendations from the Center for Disease Control and Prevention (CDC). Minimum diagnostic criteria (presence of cervical motion, uterine and adnexal tenderness) have been set with a high sensitivity and low specificity, in order to detect as many cases of clinical disease as possible. If all these criteria are present in sexually active young women, empiric treatment should be instituted. The CDC also provides a list of additional criteria that may help to improve diagnostic specificity: elevated oral temperature (>38.3 °C), abnormal cervical or vaginal discharge, elevated erythrocyte sedimentation rate, elevated C-reactive protein concentration, and laboratory documentation of cervical infection with *Neisseria gonorrhoeae* or *Chlamydia trachomatis* [24].

Peipert et al. showed that the clinical finding of adnexal tenderness had a sensitivity of 95.5 %, which was superior to that of the CDC's minimal clinical criteria (83 %) [28].

There is not a pathognomonic laboratory test for upper genital tract infection. Ultrasound examination is able to detect thickening of fallopian tubal walls and tubo-ovarian abscesses and rule out other possible diagnoses like ovarian cysts and ovarian torsion [29]. However, the sensitivity and specificity of ultrasound features is highly dependent on the severity of the disease [29].

Laparoscopic exploration is warranted whenever the diagnosis is unclear and the symptomatology is unremitting, especially in young women for whom the preservation of fertility is important. Laparoscopic visualization of the triad of edema, hyperemia, and a purulent exudate from the ends or surface of the fallopian tube has been considered the gold standard for PID diagnosis [30, 31]. Laparoscopy can be used to directly visualize pelvic anatomy and diagnose PID without aggravating the inflammatory process and exclude other pathologies (which may be present in approximately 20 % of patients) [32]. However, its sensitivity varies depending on the stage of illness, being less sensitive in milder forms where diagnostic criteria are less objective. In cases where there is no visual evidence of salpingitis by laparoscopy, endometrial biopsy is warranted because some women with PID can have endometritis alone.

Gaitán et al. reported that endometrial biopsy showed 75 % of global accuracy, comparing with a global accuracy of 91 % with laparoscopy. Laparoscopy showed an optimum specificity (100 %), proving to be very useful in excluding other causes of abdominal pain in patients presenting with an atypical course [31].

Among these lines, in cases of abdominal pain of unknown cause where there is a suspicion of PID, laparoscopic surgery has become a diagnostic tool that permits not only confirmation of the process but also to take a microbiologic culture from the fallopian tubes to apply specific antibiotic therapy, a classification of the severity of the disease, the evaluation of the future fertility status of the patient, and therapeutic options, such as lysis of adhesions, aspiration of tubo-ovarian abscess, and irrigation of the peritoneal cavity [15, 25].

In patients without PID, laparoscopy permits rapid recognition and treatment of differential pathologies like appendicitis, ovarian cyst, ovarian torsion, and endometriosis, avoiding unnecessary antibiotic therapy. Costs, limited access, surgical risks, and the fact that not all institutions have the facilities or scheduling to submit all patients with acute abdominal pain to diagnostic laparoscopy prevent the universal use of laparoscopy for the diagnosis of PID [16]. However, the costs can be balanced by a shorter hospital stay and a reduction in unnecessary abdominal imaging.

5.3.2.4 Treatment

Tubo-ovarian abscess is not a disease entity, but rather a finding in the spectrum of PID. Treatment includes analgesia, fluids, and intravenous broad-spectrum antibiotics.

Although 60–80 % will resolve without surgical intervention, it is prudent to identify those individuals who require immediate surgical intervention because delay can be fatal [12].

Currently, there are three situations where surgical intervention is recommended: a concern for an alternative surgical emergency, failure of clinical response after 48–72 h of medical therapy, or ruptured tubo-ovarian abscess with generalized peritonitis and septic shock. A review on the management options for tubo-ovarian abscess reported that laparoscopy should be considered in all patients with tubo-ovarian abscess who desire future conception. They reported pregnancy rates ranging from 32 % to 63 % in patients treated with medical therapy followed by immediate laparoscopy drainage within 24 h, comparing to pregnancy rates ranging from 4 % to 15 % in patients treated with medical management alone, both without suspected rupture. They also report the major advantages of an immediate laparoscopy: it allows an accurate diagnosis and effective treatment under magnification with minimal complications and shows faster response rates with shorter hospitalization times and decreased infertility [33]. Surgical procedures can include laparoscopy with drainage of purulent fluid, adhesion lysis, tubal lavage, dissection and excision of necrotic tissue, and thorough irrigation of the peritoneal cavity before completion of the procedure [32, 34]. A particularly simple, safe, and efficacious alternative approach is the use of ultrasound-guided transvaginal drainage of the abscess in combination with antibiotics.

5.3.3 Ectopic Pregnancy

5.3.3.1 Etiology

Ectopic pregnancy occurs when the embryo fails to implant within the uterine cavity. The majority of ectopic pregnancies (95 %) are located in the fallopian tube. The rising incidence of ectopic pregnancy in the past 30 years has been attributed to a number of factors including a greater prevalence of sexually transmitted disease (PID), tubal sterilization and reversal, delayed childbearing, assisted reproductive technologies, and more successful clinical detection [35]. Ectopic pregnancy is the leading cause of maternal mortality during the first trimester of pregnancy [36]. Although spontaneous resolution of ectopic pregnancy can occur, patients are at risk of tubal rupture and catastrophic hemorrhage. Most fatal cases result from delayed diagnosis and inappropriate management. However, recent improvements made in diagnostic techniques have led to a marked reduction in mortality rates.

5.3.3.2 Signs and Symptoms

Patients who have ectopic pregnancies usually show abdominal pain, amenorrhea, and irregular vaginal bleeding. On physical examination, the most common findings include ipsilateral adnexal tenderness, abdominal tenderness, and an adnexal mass [37].

Not all patients who have an ectopic pregnancy, even those who have a hemoperitoneum, have rebound tenderness or peritoneal signs. Also of note, vigorous pressure during bimanual examination can cause a previously unruptured ectopic pregnancy to rupture; therefore, gentle examination is required.

5.3.3.3 Diagnosis

In women of early pregnancy/history of amenorrhea presenting with acute pelvic pain and/or vaginal bleeding, a diagnosis of ectopic pregnancy should always be considered. On physical examination, an adnexal mass may be palpated. The diagnosis of ectopic pregnancy has evolved since the 1980s. Advanced ultrasonography techniques as well as improved β-HCG measurements have largely replaced laparoscopy as primary diagnostic tools. These tests allow us to detect an early ectopic pregnancy before clinical symptoms have the chance to set in [34]. These days, the role of laparoscopy is limited to cases in which the diagnosis is still in doubt. In such cases, a choice must be made between expectant observation and laparoscopic confirmation.

5.3.3.4 Treatment

To date, the management options of tubal ectopic pregnancy are threefold: expectant management, medical treatment, or surgery. These three options have been compared in terms of efficacy, financial costs, and future fertility. The criteria for choosing between therapeutic modalities in ectopic pregnancy remain unsettled. Expectant management has been advocated based on the knowledge that an early ectopic pregnancy can be self-limiting, resulting in tubal abortion or re-absorption. It has been advised in a selective group of patients asymptomatic with serum β-HCG cutoff level relatively low and declining. Medical treatment with methotrexate has been widely used in patients with minimal symptoms, who are hemodynamically stable, have no more than a moderate amount of intra-abdominal free-fluid on TVU scan, and have β-HCG concentrations <3000 IU/L [38]. The major contraindications for medical management are β-HCG level greater than 15,000 IU/L, fetal cardiac activity, and free fluid in the cul-de-sac on TVU. Surgical management is indicated if the patient is not eligible for medical therapy, if medical therapy has failed, or if there are symptoms and signs of tubal rupture [38].

Ectopic pregnancy represents a hallmark in the history of laparoscopic surgery: it was one of the first surgical pathology being treated through a laparoscope [39]. Nowadays, laparoscopy is the accepted approach to perform both a salpingostomy and salpingectomy. Mol et al. reported that although laparoscopic approach was significantly less successful than the open surgical approach in eliminating trophoblastic tissue, it was significantly less costly. The cost savings after laparoscopic surgery resulted from a significantly shorter operation time, less perioperative blood loss, shorter duration of hospital stay, and shorter convalescence time. Laparoscopy was the most cost-effective treatment in women with tubal ectopic pregnancy. The fertility outcome was comparable to laparotomy [40]. Laparoscopy also results in less postoperative adhesion formation and impairment of the pelvic status than laparotomy [35].

Laparoscopic surgery is the gold standard for the treatment of ectopic pregnancy in hemodynamically stable women. However, it is estimated that approximately 15 % of women with ectopic pregnancy experience hypovolemic shock. In these cases, both the volume of hemoperitoneum and the hemodynamic status of the patient have been critical factors in deciding whether to perform a laparoscopy or a laparotomy. Although historically contraindicated, numerous case reports and studies have proven that laparoscopy can be successful in cases of ruptured ectopic pregnancy with hemodynamic instability [41, 42]. Laparoscopy has also been contraindicated in certain situations such as interstitial and cornual pregnancy and severe adhesions. The improvement of surgeons' skills and instrumentation has made these contraindications obsolete. Laparoscopy efficacy has been reported in interstitial and cornual pregnancies in various case reports [43, 44]. Thus, laparoscopy leaves little space for laparotomy in ectopic pregnancy management.

There is a controversy on whether to perform a conservative treatment (salpingostomy) or a radical treatment (salpingectomy) in ectopic pregnancy. The possible advantage of radical approach would be to eliminate the possibility of recurrence, but with lower rates of fertility (66 %). In conservative approach, rates of 8 % of persistent ectopic pregnancy have been reported, but with higher rates of fertility (89 %). So the conservative approach should be preferred whenever future fertility is required. Most authors agree that salpingectomy should only be performed in women with uncontrolled bleeding, recurrent ectopic pregnancy in the same tube, a severely damaged tube, or a tubal gestational sac greater than 5 cm in diameter [36].

5.3.4 Endometriosis

5.3.4.1 Etiology

Endometriosis, the presence of endometrial glands and stroma outside of the endometrial cavity, represents one of the most challenging gynecologic conditions to manage given its insidious onset, surgical diagnosis, association with pelvic pain and infertility, and often progressive nature.

The cause of endometriosis is unclear. There are several theories postulated to explain its pathogenesis. These include retrograde menstruation and implantation, the metaplasia theory, lymphatic and vascular spreading, and genetic predisposition [45, 46].

Endometriosis is a chronic disease affecting at least 10 % of reproductive-aged women, but is found in approximately 40 % of infertile women and up to 90 % of women with pelvic pain [47]. Risk factors include family history, low body mass index, alcohol use, smoking, particularly in the setting of infertility, Caucasian race, prolonged estrogen exposure as with early menarche or late menopause, and nutritional/environmental factors.

5.3.4.2 Signs and Symptoms

During menstruation these ectopic tissue areas undergo changes such as edema and bleeding, causing symptoms like acute pelvic pain, dysmenorrhea, dyspareunia, signs of peritoneal irritation, dyschezia, rectal pain and bleeding, each being dependent upon the location of endometriosis. Chronic symptoms with acute bouts of pain are characteristics of endometriosis affecting the ovaries with bleeding, torsion, or rupture of an endometrioma.

5.3.4.3 Diagnosis

Apart from the clinical evaluation, diagnosis is helped by transvaginal or transabdominal US and by MRI. Laparoscopy is the gold standard to evaluate pelvic endometriosis as it allows the collection of histologic specimens needed to confirm diagnosis. Deep infiltrating or subperitoneal endometriosis is not always visible at laparoscopy and MRI can therefore be helpful in such conditions. Laboratory investigations are restricted to serum CA-125 which usually increases to values of up to 100–200 IU/mL, but is not useful for the diagnosis. The role of CA-125 is limited to the follow-up of recurrences.

5.3.4.4 Treatment

Medical treatment with NSAIDs reduces the production of local prostaglandin, therefore reducing inflammation but more importantly reducing the pain. The medical treatment of endometriosis consists of ceasing ovarian estrogen production. Estroprogestinic preparations are the most useful drugs as they can be used for months if common contraindications such as obesity, breast cancer, smoking, and high blood pressure do not exist.

Medical treatment by danazol or a GnRH analog are also very effective as a means of stopping ovarian function and estrogen production, but are associated, due to hypo-estrogenization, with undesired side effects including osteoporosis, vaginal dryness, hot flushes, and other vasomotor symptoms. The use of danazol or a GnRH analog if protracted for more than 6 months should be associated with an estroprogestinic preparation to reduce the menopausal symptoms, osteoporosis, and fracture risk. The medical treatment is only effective in minimal endometriosis, while moderate and severe forms need to be treated by surgery [48].

Surgical treatment consists of trying to remove as much endometriotic tissue as possible. It is rare to perform emergency surgery for pelvic pain exclusively due to endometriosis, unless it is secondary to an operation performed for hemoperitoneum due to an ovarian cyst rupture (endometriomas) or for suspected appendicitis. At surgery the removal of endometriosis requires careful manipulation of the organs involved. A careful approach needs to be applied during surgery for endometriosis infiltrating the serosa of the bowel, above the urethra and bladder and above major blood vessels [49].

Laparoscopy allows a mapping of the disease and the collection of material for histology that will eventually confirm the diagnosis. Surgical staging of endometriosis consists of a scoring to be attributed to each site, localization, and extension of the lesion. The most commonly used scoring system suggested by the American Fertility Society helps in the evaluation of patient fertility prognosis [50].

In young women, surgical treatment of ovarian endometriosis must not compromise the reproductive function of the ovary and electrosurgery should be minimally used. The laparoscopic approach is favored compared to open surgery as it allows clearer visibility and access to the pelvic cavity and reduces the postoperative morbidity and hospital stay. Moreover, laparoscopy may increase chances of future pregnancy and live birth [51, 52].

It is important to remember that the endometriotic tissue has the capacity to implant and therefore careful peritoneal cavity washing and adequate removal of the surgical specimens should be performed to reduce the risk of distal implant on scars and trocar access points.

5.3.5 Hemorrhagic Ovarian Cysts

5.3.5.1 Etiology

Approximately 2–4 days after ovulation, the ovary becomes increasingly vascular. With neovascularization, blood from the vascular theca zone often fills the cavity of the cyst. Often, the cyst reabsorbs the blood; however, if the amount of bleeding is large or a cyst ruptures the bleeding may continue, producing a hemoperitoneum. Increased caution should be taken in patients who are anticoagulated.

5.3.5.2 Signs and Symptoms

Pertinent history should include when the patient's last menstrual period took place. Pain can occur with ovulation of a follicular cyst, otherwise known as Mittelschmerz syndrome. Enlarging ovarian follicles often produce a colicky or dull unilateral tenderness in the lower abdomen or pelvic region. Rarely, patients may present with hypovolemia and hemodynamic instability. Nausea and/or vomiting are associated as nonspecific symptoms. A bimanual examination should be performed to evaluate the size of the cyst and tenderness. On physical examination, a corpus luteal cyst can mimic an ectopic pregnancy. Originally described by Halban, a triad of symptoms includes a delay in menses, followed by spotting, unilateral pelvic pain, and a small, tender, adnexal mass [53].

5.3.5.3 Diagnosis

Diagnosis of a hemorrhagic or ruptured cyst is often made by narrowing the differential. Transvaginal ultrasound often demonstrates an adnexal mass; however, the ovary may be normal in size if rupture has decompressed any cysts. In these cases, a large amount of pelvic fluid is usually noted [54]. A quantitative pregnancy test can rule out an ectopic pregnancy. A CBC should be taken to assess the current blood count. An elevated white count is rarely seen in a ruptured luteal cyst. Once

Table 5.1 Indications for different surgical approaches

Laparotomy
High suspicion for malignancy
Large cysts
History of or risk factors for abdominopelvic adhesions
Hemodynamically unstable patient—hypovolemia
Significant cardiopulmonary disease
Obesity
Laparoscopy
Minimizing the risks of subsequent infertility resulting from pelvic adhesions
Every effort should be made to conserve ovarian tissue

pregnancy is ruled out, an abdominal/pelvic CT with contrast can further assist in evaluating other potential causes, including acute appendicitis.

5.3.5.4 Treatment

Initial management of a suspected follicular or hemorrhagic cyst is supportive management and continued observation with a repeat pelvic ultrasound in approximately 4–6 weeks to document resolution. Oral contraceptive medication can be started in patients to halt further ovulation.

Indications for immediate operative intervention include a large amount of peritoneal fluid found on a transvaginal ultrasound, hemodynamic instability, and severe pain. Delayed operative management is indicated for patients in whom pain is not improving with conservative management or for persistent tumors to rule out a neoplastic process. A cystectomy is recommended as opposed to a unilateral salpingo-oophorectomy in reproductive-aged women. Laparoscopic evaluation is usually feasible; however, if cancer is suspected, laparotomy may be necessary to ensure intact removal and for staging purposes [53]. The indications for laparotomy or laparoscopy are summarized in Table 5.1. Intraoperative spillage of a malignant tumor does not necessarily worsen prognosis, but it does necessitate adjuvant chemotherapy. If the cyst is benign, a ruptured cyst may still cause postoperative abdominal pain secondary to chemical peritonitis.

5.4 Discussion and Conclusion

Anteby et al. highlighted the value of laparoscopy in the evaluation of acute pelvic pain in 1974. Since then, great advances in anesthesia care and cardiovascular monitoring, together with the development of a great number of devices and different techniques, have made possible the use of diagnostic and therapeutic laparoscopy procedures for gynecologic emergencies.

Nowadays, early diagnostic laparoscopy in the emergency setting improves diagnostic rates and reduces hospital stays and costs, when compared to other diagnostic modalities. Still, laparoscopy is an invasive technique and it should only be used after a first-line investigation combining clinical and sonography examination.

Therapeutic laparoscopy procedures in gynecology emergencies are now universal practice. The efficacy and safety are comparable to laparotomy procedures but with several additional advantages: shorter operation times, impairment of pelvic status with less postoperative adhesions; few postoperative pain, fever, and blood loss; reduction on consumption of analgesic drugs; fast recovery rates; shorter hospital stays; better cosmetics outcomes; and lower costs. However, the safest approach should always be the one that the surgeon feels more comfortable with, and this should always be a factor regarding the type of intervention.

In a pregnant woman laparoscopy and laparotomy may increase the possibility of spontaneous abortion in the first trimester and premature delivery in the last trimester of pregnancy, respectively. It is, however, a common opinion that the use of laparoscopy is preferable to laparotomy. In this regard, the advantages of laparoscopy over open surgery are represented by a reduced administration of anesthetic drugs, a reduced need for postoperative analgesia, a low incidence of infective complications, and a faster recovery. Major risks of surgery in pregnant women include uterine injuries due to the increased uterine size, with or without rupture of the amniotic membrane, bleeding, and gaseous embolism, as well as technical difficulties related to the limited working space [55]. Therefore, when operating on a pregnant woman, all the necessary precautions must be taken prior to the use of laparoscopy including a low intra-abdominal pressure and deep vein thrombosis prophylactic measures even for minor procedures.

In conclusion, it is important to remember that the multidisciplinary approach to the patient is essential for establishing the correct diagnosis and treatment in the shortest time. The use of modern laboratory and radiologic resources associated with the progress in endoscopic surgical techniques provides both general surgeons and gynecologists with all the means necessary to ensure the best surgical result.

References

1. Jones PF (1987) Emergency abdominal surgery. Blackwell Science, Oxford
2. Sheridan WG, White AT, Havard T, Crosby DL (1992) Non-specific abdominal pain: the resource implications. Ann R Coll Surg Engl 74:181–185
3. Sauerland S, Agresta F, Bergamaschi R, Borzellino G, Budzynski A, Champault G et al (2006) Laparoscopy for abdominal emergencies: evidence-based guidelines of the European Association for Endoscopic Surgery. Surg Endosc 20:14–29
4. Lo LM, Chang SD, Horng SG, Yang TY, Lee CL, Liang CC (2008) Laparoscopy versus laparotomy for surgical intervention of ovarian torsion. J Obstet Gynaecol Res 34:1020–1025
5. Vijayalakshmi K, Reddy GM, Subbiah VN, Sathiya S, Arjun B (2014) Clinico-pathological profile of adnexal torsion cases: a retrospective analysis from a tertiary care teaching hospital. J Clin Diagn Res 8:OC04–OC07
6. Houry D, Abbott JT (2001) Ovarian torsion: a fifteen-year review. Ann Emerg Med 38:156–159

7. White M, Stella J (2005) Ovarian torsion: 10-year perspective. Emerg Med Australas 17:231–237
8. Peña JE, Ufberg D, Cooney N, Denis AL (2000) Usefulness of Doppler sonography in the diagnosis of ovarian torsion. Fertil Steril 73:1047–1050
9. Spinelli C, Buti I, Pucci V, Liserre J, Alberti E, Nencini L et al (2013) Adnexal torsion in children and adolescents: new trends to conservative surgical approach – our experience and review of literature. Gynecol Endocrinol 29:54–58
10. Kardakis S, Barranca A, Vitelli A, Amore I, Trento F, Caccia G (2013) Isolated fallopian tube torsion. Case Rep Obstet Gynecol 2013:479698
11. Oltmann SC, Fischer A, Barber R, Huang R, Hicks B, Garcia N (2009) Cannot exclude torsion–a 15-year review. J Pediatr Surg 44:1212–1216, discussion 1217
12. Ramphal SR, Moodley J (2006) Emergency gynaecology. Best Pract Res Clin Obstet Gynaecol 20:729–750
13. Bar-On S, Mashiach R, Stockheim D, Soriano D, Goldenberg M, Schiff E et al (2010) Emergency laparoscopy for suspected ovarian torsion: are we too hasty to operate? Fertil Steril 93:2012–2015
14. Cohen SB, Weisz B, Seidman DS, Mashiach S, Lidor AL, Goldenberg M (2001) Accuracy of the preoperative diagnosis in 100 emergency laparoscopies performed due to acute abdomen in nonpregnant women. J Am Assoc Gynecol Laparosc 8:92–94
15. Aulestia SN, Cantele H, Leyba JL, Navarrete M, Llopla SN (2003) Laparoscopic diagnosis and treatment in gynecologic emergencies. JSLS 7:239–242
16. Golash V, Willson PD (2005) Early laparoscopy as a routine procedure in the management of acute abdominal pain: a review of 1,320 patients. Surg Endosc 19:882–885
17. Kao JK, Chiu CC, Wang PY, Yu MK (2012) Pediatric ovarian torsion in a medical center in Taiwan: case analysis. Pediatr Neonatol 53:55–59
18. Koo YJ, Lee JE, Lim KT, Shim JU, Mok JE, Kim TJ (2011) A 10-year experience of laparoscopic surgery for adnexal masses during pregnancy. Int J Gynaecol Obstet 113:36–39
19. Cohen SB, Wattiez A, Seidman DS, Goldenberg M, Admon D, Mashiach S et al (2003) Laparoscopy versus laparotomy for detorsion and sparing of twisted ischemic adnexa. JSLS 7:295–299
20. Oelsner G, Cohen SB, Soriano D, Admon D, Mashiach S, Carp H (2003) Minimal surgery for the twisted ischaemic adnexa can preserve ovarian function. Hum Reprod 18:2599–2602
21. Huchon C, Fauconnier A (2010) Adnexal torsion: a literature review. Eur J Obstet Gynecol Reprod Biol 150:8–12
22. Fujishita A, Araki H, Yoshida S, Hamaguchi D, Nakayama D, Tsuda N et al (2015) Outcome of conservative laparoscopic surgery for adnexal torsion through one-stage or two-stage operation. J Obstet Gynaecol Res 41:411–417
23. Bouet PE, Fressard S, Combaud V, Descamps P, Sentilhes L (2013) Laparoscopic management of recurrent adnexal torsion in the second and third trimesters of pregnancy. Eur J Obstet Gynecol Reprod Biol 170:294–295
24. Workowski KA, Bolan GA, C. f. D. C. a. Prevention (2015) Sexually transmitted diseases treatment guidelines, 2015. MMWR Recomm Rep 64:1–137
25. Schindlbeck C, Dziura D, Mylonas I (2014) Diagnosis of pelvic inflammatory disease (PID): intra-operative findings and comparison of vaginal and intra-abdominal cultures. Arch Gynecol Obstet 289:1263–1269
26. Munday PE (2000) Pelvic inflammatory disease–an evidence-based approach to diagnosis. J Infect 40:31–41
27. Simms I, Warburton F, Weström L (2003) Diagnosis of pelvic inflammatory disease: time for a rethink. Sex Transm Infect 79:491–494
28. Peipert JF, Ness RB, Blume J, Soper DE, Holley R, Randall H et al (2001) Clinical predictors of endometritis in women with symptoms and signs of pelvic inflammatory disease. Am J Obstet Gynecol 184:856–863, discussion 863–864

29. Romosan G, Valentin L (2014) The sensitivity and specificity of transvaginal ultrasound with regard to acute pelvic inflammatory disease: a review of the literature. Arch Gynecol Obstet 289:705–714
30. Mitchell C, Prabhu M (2013) Pelvic inflammatory disease: current concepts in pathogenesis, diagnosis and treatment. Infect Dis Clin N Am 27:793–809
31. Gaitán H, Angel E, Diaz R, Parada A, Sanchez L, Vargas C (2002) Accuracy of five different diagnostic techniques in mild-to-moderate pelvic inflammatory disease. Infect Dis Obstet Gynecol 10:171–180
32. Agresta F, Ansaloni L, Baiocchi GL, Bergamini C, Campanile FC, Carlucci M et al (2012) Laparoscopic approach to acute abdomen from the Consensus Development Conference of the Società Italiana di Chirurgia Endoscopica e nuove tecnologie (SICE), Associazione Chirurghi Ospedalieri Italiani (ACOI), Società Italiana di Chirurgia (SIC), Società Italiana di Chirurgia d'Urgenza e del Trauma (SICUT), Società Italiana di Chirurgia nell'Ospedalità Privata (SICOP), and the European Association for Endoscopic Surgery (EAES). Surg Endosc 26(8):2134–2164
33. Rosen M, Breitkopf D, Waud K (2009) Tubo-ovarian abscess management options for women who desire fertility. Obstet Gynecol Surv 64:681–689
34. Porpora MG, Gomel V (1997) The role of laparoscopy in the management of pelvic pain in women of reproductive age. Fertil Steril 68:765–779
35. Luciano AA, Roy G, Solima E (2001) Ectopic pregnancy from surgical emergency to medical management. Ann NY Acad Sci 943:235–254
36. Murray H, Baakdah H, Bardell T, Tulandi T (2005) Diagnosis and treatment of ectopic pregnancy. CMAJ 173:905–912
37. Hughes GJ (1979) The early diagnosis of ectopic pregnancy. Br J Surg 66:789–792
38. Westaby DT, Wu O, Duncan WC, Critchley HO, Tong S, Horne AW (2012) Has increased clinical experience with methotrexate reduced the direct costs of medical management of ectopic pregnancy compared to surgery? BMC Pregnancy Childbirth 12:98
39. Bruhat MA, Manhes H, Mage G, Pouly JL (1980) Treatment of ectopic pregnancy by means of laparoscopy. Fertil Steril 33:411–414
40. Mol F, Mol BW, Ankum WM, van der Veen F, Hajenius PJ (2008) Current evidence on surgery, systemic methotrexate and expectant management in the treatment of tubal ectopic pregnancy: a systematic review and meta-analysis. Hum Reprod Update 14:309–319
41. Cohen A, Almog B, Satel A, Lessing JB, Tsafrir Z, Levin I (2013) Laparoscopy versus laparotomy in the management of ectopic pregnancy with massive hemoperitoneum. Int J Gynaecol Obstet 123:139–141
42. Sagiv R, Debby A, Sadan O, Malinger G, Glezerman M, Golan A (2001) Laparoscopic surgery for extrauterine pregnancy in hemodynamically unstable patients. J Am Assoc Gynecol Laparosc 8:529–532
43. Woh L, Koh PR, Wong CN, Sun YL, Lin ET, Huang MH (2007) Laparoscopic management of a large viable cornual pregnancy. JSLS 11:506–508
44. Moawad NS, Dayaratna S, Mahajan ST (2009) Mini-cornual excision: a simple stepwise laparoscopic technique for the treatment of cornual pregnancy. JSLS 13:87–91
45. Sampson JA (1927) Metastatic or embolic endometriosis, due to the menstrual dissemination of endometrial tissue into the venous circulation. Am J Pathol 3:93–110.43
46. Matsuura K, Ohtake H, Katabuchi H, Okamura H (1999) Coelomic metaplasia theory of endometriosis: evidence from in vivo studies and an in vitro experimental model. Gynecol Obstet Invest 47(Suppl 1):18–20, discussion 20–22
47. Farquhar C (2007) Endometriosis. BMJ 334:249–253
48. Hughes E, Brown J, Collins JJ, Farquhar C, Fedorkow DM, Vandekerckhove P (2007) Ovulation suppression for endometriosis. Cochrane Database Syst Rev (3):CD000155
49. Kodaman PH (2015) Current strategies for endometriosis management. Obstet Gynecol Clin N Am 42:87–101

50. Lin SY, Lee RK, Hwu YM, Lin MH (1998) Reproducibility of the revised American Fertility Society classification of endometriosis using laparoscopy or laparotomy. Int J Gynaecol Obstet 60:265–269
51. Jin X, Ruiz Beguerie J (2014) Laparoscopic surgery for subfertility related to endometriosis: a meta-analysis. Taiwan J Obstet Gynecol 53:303–308
52. Duffy JM, Arambage K, Correa FJ, Olive D, Farquhar C, Garry R et al (2014) Laparoscopic surgery for endometriosis. Cochrane Database Syst Rev 4, CD011031
53. McWilliams GD, Hill MJ, Dietrich CS (2008) Gynecologic emergencies. Surg Clin N Am 88:265–283, vi
54. Ding Z, Zhang D, Ying W, Wang J (2010) Sonographic value in diagnosis of hemorrhagic ovarian cysts. Eur J Gynaecol Oncol 31:87–89
55. Barnett MB, Liu DT (1974) Letter: Complication of laparoscopy during early pregnancy. Br Med J 1:328

Nonspecific Abdominal Pain

6

Michele Carlucci, Aldo Alberto Beneduce, Guido Fiorentini, and Giovanni Burtulo

6.1 Introduction

Five to ten percent of all admissions to the emergency department (ED) are due to acute abdominal pain. Within this patient population, up to a third of all patients will leave the hospital without a clear and unambiguous diagnosis explaining the cause of their abdominal pain, despite a mean hospital stay of up to 6 days. Acute nonspecific abdominal pain (NSAP) is defined as acute abdominal pain less than 1 week in duration, for which there is no diagnosis despite investigations and comprises a spectrum of undiagnosed conditions, both somatic and functional, and remains a "diagnosis of exclusion." Depending on the severity of the symptoms, some patients are admitted to the hospital for repeated active clinical observation, classically known as the "wait and see" approach, resulting in a substantial use of financial and human resources [1].

Although attempts have been made toward developing consensus guidelines and diagnostic algorithms, no prospective evidence-based clinical guidelines for the exclusion of NSAP have been developed or validated to date [2, 3]. The necessity to achieve a correct diagnosis and a systematic approach to NSAP should be useful in order to reduce the admission rate for NSAP because of the costs and morbidity associated with this condition in terms of excessive hospital stay, multiple investigations, and unnecessary surgical explorations [3–5].

Systematic baseline character examination, abdominal ultrasound (US) [6], abdominal computed tomography (CT) [7], and early laparoscopy (EL) [8–13] have all been described as potential methods for improving the diagnostic accuracy in the emergency setting.

M. Carlucci (✉) • A.A. Beneduce • G. Fiorentini • G. Burtulo
IRCCS Ospedale San Raffaele, Milan, Italy
e-mail: carlucci.michele@hsr.it

F. Agresta et al. (eds.), *Emergency Laparoscopy*,
DOI 10.1007/978-3-319-29620-3_6

Nevertheless, the most important part of the evaluation remains a thorough history and a careful physical examination given the wide variety of disorders which may cause abdominal pain. The physician is called to establish a differential diagnosis, plan appropriate imaging studies, and determine whether surgery is necessary.

In conclusion, the management of acute NSAP can be divided into three stages. The first stage is the initial history, physical examination, baseline investigations, and formulation of a working and differential diagnosis. The second stage involves the judicious use of radiologic techniques.

The third stage should be represented by diagnostic laparoscopy [12].

6.2 Baseline Investigation

Although standing as the bedrock of medical practice, the physical examination often is both insensitive and nonspecific in the diagnosis of NSAP. Likewise, diagnostic adjuncts such as laboratory studies and plain abdominal radiographs have played fundamental yet controversial roles in the assessment of NSAP. When combined with a plain chest radiograph, the upright and supine plain abdominal radiographs compose the acute abdominal series (AAS) in many institutions. This series is ordered frequently for the evaluation of abdominal pain; however, its low sensitivity and specificity limit utility. Some authors suggest a systematic collection of baseline data (Table 6.1) with the end-point of discriminate, among patients with NSAP, patients who need urgent procedure or further diagnostic procedure [3].

However, history and clinical examination with the addition of laboratory tests and abdominal radiographs do not reach a sufficient level of sensitivity and specificity to lead to a proper management of NSAP (56 % and 81 %, respectively) [3–5]. An early use of CT in the diagnostic workup of acute abdominal pain has led to a correct diagnosis in 96.8 % of cases [14].

6.3 Imaging Studies

Several studies designed to identify the most effective diagnostic strategy for patients with acute abdominal pain have demonstrated that the highest sensitivity for detecting urgent diagnoses is achieved when ultrasonography is performed in all patients and a CT only in the event of inconclusive or negative ultrasonography [3, 15, 16]. Using this strategy, CT is only needed when conventional radiology or US does not achieve diagnosis.

Even though CT exposes patients to a higher radiation dose, it still remains the preferred standard diagnostic modality if ultrasound fails to diagnose the cause

Table 6.1 Baseline Data Collection

Age	Does examination change during ED visit?
Sex	Does pain resolve during ED visit?
Pulse rate initial	Does patient vomit during ED visit?
Systolic blood pressure initial	Urinalysis, leukocyte esterase positive?
Respiratory rate initial	Urinalysis nitrite positive?
Temperature initial	Urinalysis ketones positive?
Pain diffuse\localized	Urinalysis leukocytes present?
Pain localization (if localized)	Urinalysis erythrocytes present?
Pain onset (sudden/gradual)	Venous pH
Does pain radiate?	Venous base excess
Nausea in past 24 hours?	Complete blood count, leukocyte count
Vomiting in past 24 hours?	Amylase, serum
Anorexia in past 24 hours?	Lipase, serum
Diarrhea in past 24 hours?	AST, serum
Flatus in past 24 hours?	ALT, serum
Melena in past 24 hours?	ALP, serum
Hematochezia in past 24 hours?	Total bilirubin, serum
Hematemesis in past 24 hours?	Direct bilirubin, serum
Bowel sounds present?	Glucose, serum
Rebound tenderness?	Serum urea nitrogen
McBurney point tenderness?	Creatinine, serum
Murphy sign present?	AAS predicts UI required?
Rovsing sign present?	
Costovertebral angle tenderness present?	
Stool grossy bloody?	
Stool heme positive?	

of acute abdominal pain correctly. Plain radiography demonstrates low sensitivity and accuracy and is, therefore, generally unhelpful; because of its low sensitivity and negative predictive value, it can also be misleading in the workup of acute abdominal pain. Although the radiation dose is lower than that of CT, the mediocre test characteristics of plain radiography may delay appropriate treatment and are therefore detrimental.

Moreover, CT is increasingly being used as a first-line investigation in abdominal pain because it is not only good at determining the correct diagnosis but also the severity of the disease and its potential complications. It can also accurately demonstrate clinically relevant unexpected and important second abnormalities, which may be critical to patient management [16].

Except certain patients, such as children or pregnant women, in which US or MRI should be considered the method of choice because of concerns about radiation dose, a CT should be considered to guide treatment and avoid harmful delays [17, 18]. Therefore, if the diagnosis is still uncertain or CT is not accessible, the next stage of the management of NSAP should be diagnostic laparoscopy.

6.4 The Role of Diagnostic Laparoscopy: When and Always?

Several studies have documented the feasibility and safety of diagnostic laparoscopy (DL) using general anesthesia for patients with acute abdominal pain [19, 20]. The diagnostic accuracy of the procedure is high, ranging between 90 and 100 %, and prevents unnecessary laparotomies in 36–95 % of patients in the published series [21]. Open access or the Veress technique has been used for initial access without reported untoward events. Overall morbidity, also in ICU patients, has been reported between 0 % and 8 % in expert hands and no mortality directly associated with the procedure has been described [22, 23]. Contraindications for DL do not differ from contraindications to exploratory laparotomy, except for patients unable to tolerate pneumoperitoneum and those with a tense and distended abdomen (i.e., clinically suspected abdominal compartment syndrome) [21]. The role of early laparoscopy compared with the traditional "wait and see" in the management of NSAP in patients with unclear diagnosis after baseline examinations and tests has been evaluated by randomized controlled trials [9, 10, 12] with controversial results due to poor sample size or no long-term follow-up. DL seems to drive to an improved diagnosis (81–97 % vs. 28–36 % in observational group) and subsequent treatment of patients with NSAP leading to save costs for hospitalization and reduced hospital stay but seems unuseful in prevention of recurrence of symptoms [12, 14–24]. In conclusion, DL is technically feasible and can be applied safely by surgeons with appropriate training and expertise for selected patients with acute nonspecific abdominal pain after baseline examination. The results of our systematic review suggest that there is insufficient evidence at present to justify routine use of early laparoscopy in patients with undifferentiated acute abdominal pain. Conversely, there is no evidence of harm. Cost-effectiveness data are lacking and there have been no comparisons with alternative strategies, particularly early cross-sectional imaging. There is a need for robust large-scale randomized controlled trials to clarify the role of this technique.

The timing and the real necessity of laparoscopy should be evaluated on the basis of patients' course and observation.

6.5 Conclusions

Despite their initial presentation of NSAP, approximately 13 % of our subject sample required UI within 24 hours of ED presentation, and an additional 34 % of subjects underwent elective interventions that likely mitigated morbidity and mortality, approximating proportions reported in larger retrospective studies [25, 26].

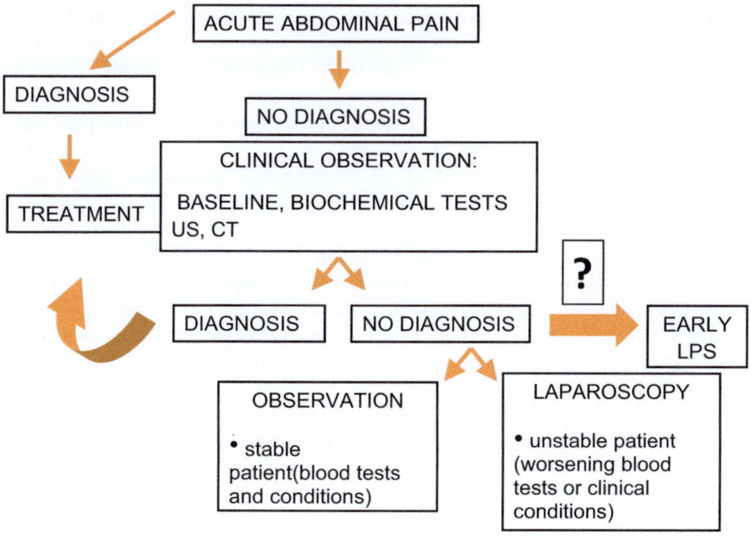

Fig. 6.1 Algorithm for approach to NSAP

Enhanced or non-enhanced computed tomography of the abdomen and pelvis is a crucial step, after baseline examination and before invasive diagnostic methods such as diagnostic laparoscopy.

Diagnostic laparoscopy is helpful in the treatment of patients with NSAP because it improves the achievement of correct diagnosis and reduces hospital stay and per-patient costs but seems to be unuseful in prevention of recurrence of symptoms. The available literature has a number of limitations including the lack of homogeneity in the reported patient populations and the frequent absence of high-quality preoperative imaging studies which may have provided the diagnosis without the need for an invasive procedure.

The results of our systematic review suggest that there is insufficient evidence at present to justify routine use of early laparoscopy in patients with undifferentiated acute abdominal pain. For this reason, laparoscopy should be reserved for patients with worsening course or when urgency is reasonably suspected after baseline.

However, on the basis of the literature selected, we tried to design an algorithm (Fig. 6.1) for the systematic approach to NSAP.

References

1. Society of American Gastrointestinal and Endoscopic Surgeons (SAGES) (2007) Guidelines for diagnostic laparoscopy practice/clinical guidelines
2. American College of Emergency Physicians (2000) Clinical policy: critical issues for the initial evaluation and management of patients presenting with a chief complaint of nontraumatic acute abdominal pain. Am Emerg Med 36:406–415

3. Gerhardt RT et al (2005) Derivation of clinical guidelines for the assessment of nonspecific abdominal pain in the ED Setting (GAPEDS) Phase 1 Study. Am J Emerg Med 23:709–717
4. Wilson DH, Wilson PD, Walmsley RG et al (1977) Diagnosis of acute abdominal pain in the accident and emergency department. Br J Surg 64:250–254
5. Sheridan WG, White AT, Havard T et al (1992) Non-specific abdominal pain: the resource implications. Ann R Coll Surg Engl 74:181–185
6. Raheja SK, McDonald PJ, Taylor I (1990) Non-specific abdominal pain—an expensive mystery. J R Soc Med 83:10–11
7. Allemann F, Cassina P, Röthlin M et al (1999) Ultrasound scans done by surgeons for patients with acute abdominal pain: a prospective study. Eur J Surg 165:966–970
8. Rao PM, Rhea JT, Novelline RA et al (1998) Effect of computed tomography of the appendix on treatment of patients and use of hospital resources. N Engl J Med 338:141–146
9. Champault G, Rizk N, Lauroy J et al (1993) Right iliac fossa pain in women. Conventional diagnostic approach versus primary laparoscopy. A controlled study (65 cases). Ann Chir 7:316–319
10. Decadt B, Sussman L, Lewis MP et al (1999) Randomized clinical trial of early laparoscopy in the management of acute non-specific abdominal pain. Br J Surg 86:1383–1386
11. Gaitán H, Angel E, Sánchez J et al (2002) Laparoscopic diagnosis of acute lower abdominal pain in women of reproductive age. Int J Gynaecol Obstet 76:149–158
12. Morino M, Pellegrino L, Castagna E et al (2006) Acute nonspecific abdominal pain: a randomized, controlled trial comparing early laparoscopy versus clinical observation. Ann Surg 244:881–886
13. Schietroma M, Carlei F, Cappelli S et al (2007) "Acute abdomen": early laparoscopy or active laparotomic-laparoscopic observation. Hepatogastroenterology 54:1137–1141
14. Strömberg C, Johansson G, Adolfsson A (2007) Acute abdominal pain: diagnostic impact of immediate CT scanning. World J Surg 31:2347–2354
15. Agresta F, Mazzarolo G, Ciardo LF et al (2008) The laparoscopic approach in abdominal emergencies: has the attitude changed: a single-center review of a 15-year experience. Surg Endosc 22:1255–1262
16. Gans SL, Stoker J et al (2012) Plain abdominal radiography in acute abdominal pain: past present and future. Int J Gen Med 5:525–533
17. Butala P, Greenstein AJ, Sur MD et al (2010) Surgical management of acute right lower-quadrant pain in pregnancy: a prospective cohort study. J Am Coll Surg 211:490–494
18. Chen MM, Coakley FV, Kaimal A et al (2008) Guidelines for computed tomography and magnetic resonance imaging use during pregnancy and lactation. Obstet Gynecol 112:333–340
19. Sozuer EM, Bedirli A, Ulusal M et al (2000) Laparoscopy for diagnosis and treatment of acute abdominal pain. J Laparoendosc Adv Surg Tech A 10:203–207
20. Poulin EC, Schlachta CM, Mamazza J (2000) Early laparoscopy to help diagnose acute nonspecific abdominal pain. Lancet 355:861–863
21. Stefanidis D, Richardson WS et al (2009) The role of diagnostic laparoscopy for acute abdominal conditions: an evidence based review. Surg Endosc 23:16–23
22. Gagne DJ, Malay MB et al (2002) Bedside diagnostic minilaparoscopy in the intensive care patients. Surgery 131(5):491–496
23. Pecoraro AP, Cacchione R et al (2001) The routine use of diagnostic laparoscopy in the intensive care unit. Surg Endosc 15(7):638–641
24. Maggio AQ, Reece-Smith AM et al (2008) Early laparoscopy versus active observation in acute abdominal pain: systematic review and meta-analysis. Int J Surg 6:400–403
25. Irvin TT (1989) Abdominal pain: a surgical audit of 1190 emergency admissions. Br J Surg 76(11):1121–1125
26. Brewer RJ, Golden GT, Hitch DC et al (1976) Abdominal pain—an analysis of 1000 consecutive cases in a university hospital emergency room. Am J Surg 131:219–223

Perforated Gastroduodenal Ulcer

7

Antonino Mirabella, Massimo Lupo, Ferdinando Agresta,
Stefano Mandalà, Gabriele Anania, Mario Campli, and Kjetil Soreide

7.1 Introduction

The complications to perforated ulcers remain one of the most frequent causes of death and disability worldwide. While the incidence and mortality of bleeding ulcers have decreased and its management—mainly guided by endoscopy and interventional radiology—has largely made surgery obsolete, the rates and incidence of perforated peptic ulcers have largely been unchanged in the past decades.

The use of more tolerable drugs able to control hyperacidity (H2 antagonists, proton pump inhibitors) and the radical treatment of HP made possible by antibiotics

A. Mirabella, MD (✉) • M. Lupo, MD
General and Emergency Surgery, Villa Sofia – Cervello Hospital, Piazza Salerno 1, Palermo 90146, Italy
e-mail: antoninomirabella@gmail.com; antonellomirabella@libero.it; massimolupo60@gmail.com

F. Agresta
Department of General Surgery, Azienda ULSS19 del Veneto, Adria (RO), Italy

S. Mandalà
General Surgery, Clinica Noto Hospital, Via Dante, Palermo, Italy
e-mail: stefano.mandala@gmail.com

G. Anania
Department of Morfology, Surgery and Experimental Medicine, School of Medicine, University of Ferrara, Ferrara, Italy

M. Campli
Division of Surgery, "Nuova Itor" Private Health Facility, Rome, Italy

K. Soreide, MD, PhD
Department of Clinical Medicine, University of Bergen, Bergen, Norway

Department of Gastrointestinal Surgery, Stavanger University Hospital, POB 8100, 4068 Stavanger, Norway
e-mail: ksoreide@mac.com

F. Agresta et al. (eds.), *Emergency Laparoscopy*,
DOI 10.1007/978-3-319-29620-3_7

have led to reduced need for acid-reductive surgery (vagotomy, gastric resection) and a reduction of ulcerative recurrence (and so the need for re-intervention surgery) [1, 2].

By contrast, the number of patients requiring surgical intervention for complications, such as perforations, remains relatively unchanged and the peptic ulcer remains the most common cause of gastroduodenal perforation with incidence ranging from 2 % to 10 % of the patients with a peptic ulcer [3]. This is attributed to the increasingly widespread use of anti-inflammatory drugs (NSAIDs), especially in the elderly with considerable comorbidity, where a high mortality rate (up to 25 %) and a morbidity rate of up to 50 % have been reported, even in recent studies. Almost 70 % of deaths from peptic ulcer disease are the result of perforation [4]. Consequently, the treatment of perforated peptic ulcer (PPU) remains today the most frequent indication for gastric emergency surgery [5].

Considering these conditions, the mini-invasive technique, as in other fields, has been adopted to treat a PPU, because it allows the advantages of laparoscopic surgery (better tolerability for the patients) and the definitive treatment of the disease, with a simple surgical procedure. After the first report published in 1990 by Mouret [6] that described the closure of the PPU through an omental patch maintained in situ by fibrin glue, in the same year Nathanson [7] reported the first laparoscopy for PPU by direct suturing.

However, even today, some concerns on the use of laparoscopy in the PPU, especially with regard to the real advantages that the technique would have compared to traditional treatment, have partially limited the spread, at least in terms predictable after the initial experiences. However, in most centers the rate of laparoscopy is gradually increasing [8].

In January 2010, the SICE (Italian Society of Endoscopic Surgery), under the auspices of the EAES, decided to revisit the clinical recommendations for the role of laparoscopy in abdominal emergencies in adults, with the primary intent being to update the 2006 EAES indications [9, 10].

The papers were selected and classified based on highest evidence design of the study (following Oxford's hierarchy of March 2009). The results of Consensus, published in 2012, showed, surprisingly for PPU, that "previous strong recommendations have to be challenged after review of recent research," so as to advise some caution in the use of laparoscopy in the PPU, waiting for new and more reliable publications (Figs. 7.1 and 7.2; Table 7.1).

Gastroduodenal ulcer

If symptoms and diagnostic findings are suggestive of perforated peptic ulcer, diagnostic laparoscopy and laparoscopic repair are recommended (GoR A).

Fig. 7.1 From evidence based guidelines of the European Association for Endoscopic Surgery. Surg Endosc 2006 [9]

Fig. 7.2 From laparoscopic approach to acute abdomen—Consensus Development Conference, Surg Endosc 2012 [10]

Perforated peptic ulcer

Laparoscopy is a useful diagnostic tool when preoperative findings are not conclusive, especially if a laparoscopic treatment is likely (GoR A). Laparoscopy is a possible alternative to open surgery in the treatment of perforated peptic ulcer (GoR B).

Table 7.1 EAES 2006 and 2012 Guidelines "evidence" of the effectiveness of laparoscopy in acute abdomen

	2006 consensus	2011 consensus
Perforated gastroduodenal ulcer	+++	++
Acute cholecystitis	+++	++
Acute pancreatitis	+	++
Acute appendicitis	+++	+++
Acute diverticulitis	–?	+
Small bowel obstruction	+?	+
Incarcerated hernia	+?	+
Ventral hernias		+
Mesenteric ischemia	–?	–
Gynecologic disorders	+++	+++
Nonspecific abdominal pain	+++	+++
Abdominal trauma	+?/–?	+

+, effectiveness from strongest (+++) to weakest (+); –, no effectiveness; ?, doubtful effectiveness

In this study, the results of the Consensus of 2012, which we consider a sort of milestones about emergency laparoscopy, will be reconsidered, first of all in light of the new classification Oxford of 2011. These results will also reevaluated based on the experiences published in the last 4 years (after Consensus), for any confirmations or criticisms. We also would like to refer to our monograph on the use of laparoscopy in emergency, published by Springer in 2011 [11].

7.2 Radiological Imaging and Diagnostic Laparoscopy

The diagnosis of perforated peptic ulcer (PPU) is based on patient history (history of ulcer disease, taking NSAIDs), clinical examination (absence or reduction of hepatic obtuse area on physical examination), and imaging studies.

Sometimes the clinical examination may not be decisive, especially when the leakage from the gastric cavity and the spread of free air in the peritoneum are contained. Generally, laboratory tests are of little use in the acute phase and nonspecific, even if the association of leukocytosis, metabolic acidosis, and hyperamylasemia may be present in case of PPU [12].

The finding of sickle air at the base of the right hemi-diaphragm on the radiograph (plain abdomen and chest bases Rx), associated with a history of peptic ulcer and a history and peritonitis on examination, is an indication of surgery [13]. Although the first instrumental investigation used, radiological examination has, however, a limited sensitivity (50–70 %) for the detection of pneumoperitoneum [14–16]. Current practice is to perform a CT scan in the stable patient and avoid upright chest X-ray or plain radiographs due to the lower sensitivity and potential added delay in diagnosis.

The CT is the most reliable survey not only in the diagnosis of perforation. However, few studies have evaluated the reliability of CT to specify the location of perforation.

The Consensus of 2012 has considered two prospective studies. Hainaux et al. prospectively studied 85 consecutive patients with extraluminal air on MDCT who had surgically proven gastrointestinal tract perforations. Two experienced radiologists, blinded to the surgical diagnosis, reached a consensus on prediction of the site of the perforation. Analysis of MDCT images was predictive of the site of gastrointestinal tract perforation in 73 (86 %) of 85 patients [17].

Earls et al. examined 27 CT scans and 27 abdominal radiographs in 17 patients after uncomplicated abdominal surgery. Fifteen patients were examined 3 days after surgery and 12 were examined 6 days after surgery. The studies were evaluated in a blinded fashion for the presence, location, and volume of free air. The results of this study showed that CT is significantly more sensitive than plain radiography for detecting small amounts of free intraperitoneal air in postoperative patients [18].

Chen et al. in a retrospective study of 14 patients with PPU reported a 100 % reliability of a CT scan to determine a pneumoperitoneum, but only 36 % in determining the perforation site [19].

The Consensus concluded, based on two prospective studies, that "A CT scan of the abdomen is the most reliable exam, not only for the diagnosis of perforation (sensibility nearly 100 % for the detection of pneumo-peritoneum), but also to identify the perforation site (specificity approximately 86 %)."

In the review of Bertleff [20] of 54 articles published on the subject in the last two decades, the diagnosis of perforation with the presence of free air in the abdomen was possible in 85 % of cases. Moreover, as can be seen from RCT of the same authors, in 8 of 109 patients examined (7 %) intraoperative diagnosis was different from that of a PPU undertaken prior to the operation [21]. This underlines the importance of the role of laparoscopy to confirm the diagnosis and to define the location, size, and nature of the perforation (differential diagnosis with other diseases which can cause perforation of the visceral cavity), when the preoperative imaging studies are inconclusive.

The Consensus 2012 that refers to two randomized controlled trials [21, 22], a systematic review [23] and a meta-analysis [24], concludes "A DL is possible when preoperative exams are not sufficiently clear for definitive diagnosis" and "However, failing to identify a PPU represents one of the most frequent causes of conversion to laparotomy."

7.3 Selection of Patients/Prognostic Factors

From the data obtained from the literature, it is evident that laparoscopic technique cannot be used in all patients with PPU. In an attempt to select preoperatively the patients with objective criteria undergoing minimally invasive surgery, several clinical parameters have been defined.

A number of risk scores are utilized and reported in PPU, as reviewed extensively by Thorsen et al. [8].

Boey already in 1987 had established a scale of surgical risk, from 0 to 3, in the treatment of perforated peptic ulcer, according to the presence of three parameters: state of shock on admission (SBP < 90 mmHg), ASA III–V (presence of severe comorbidities), and duration of symptoms (>24 h) [25]. The laparoscopic treatment is preferred as a safe option for the classes 0 and 1 and should be avoided in those capable of higher degree. For patients in extremis, a "damage control" approach should be considered to minimize the insult on physiology and get early control on sepsis.

The conclusions of Lau's meta-analysis [24] are favorable to the use of laparoscopy in the PPU in patients without risk factors (Boey score = 0). In higher risk classes, the conversion rate and mortality are significantly higher. This fact is evident especially in some limited experiences where there was a high proportion of patients at risk: Katkhouda [26] presents 10 patients in shock (22 % of the total); Robertson [27] contains 17 subjects (47 % of cases) with ASA III–IV, of which 11 underwent laparoscopy.

Studies by Bertleff et al. [20, 21] have shown that the risk classification according to the Boey score is highly reliable to decide the choice of best technique. However, the limited number of patients with advanced Boey score (2–3) in the study, especially of those who underwent laparoscopic treatment, makes it difficult to find a definitive confirmation of this statement.

Overall, the use of clinical risk scores is difficult and not reliable; valid score exists with a high predictive value and wide generalizability. The investigations of scores have proved difficult, likely due to the complexity and heterogeneity of the disease.

The systematic review by Lunevicius and Morkevicius reached the same conclusion that the laparoscopic approach, which involves an extended operating time compared to the open technique, is not recommended in patients with higher risk factors [23]. The authors include among the risk factors of laparoscopic surgery the advanced Boey score, patients over 70 years, the APACHE II = 5, and lastly the surgeon's skill in laparoscopic surgery (this parameter is not simple evaluation). Even these authors underline that a conclusive opinion on the matter cannot be given yet, because of the lack of sufficient quantitative data, concerning the high-risk patients who undergo laparoscopic surgery.

Notashi et al. [28] have demonstrated the reliability of MPI (Mannheim Peritonitis Index) score as a prognostic factor in patients with peritonitis: when the score is lower than 21 the mortality rate varies from 0 to 2.3 %; for higher values the mortality rate is close to 100 %.

In other experiences [29], the APACHE II score has been used to identify patients at risk. The latter is not widely used because it is considered not easily applicable.

The problem of the duration of symptoms and then the diagnostic delay is set in correlation to the possibility that the PPU may become an unrecognized peritonitis, which is responsible for a generalized sepsis. In this eventuality, laparoscopy could play an important role in favoring, thanks to the action of CO_2, the bacterial translocation, as demonstrated in animal models [27]. These experimental results, however, have not been confirmed by clinical experience. The RCT by Lau et al. of 20 patients, which examined possible effects on the acute phase response and the presence of endo-toxemia, found no difference between laparoscopy and open repair [30]. A study by Waidya [31] suggests that the mini-invasive treatment is safe even in patients with peritonitis and a delayed diagnosis: no mortality was recorded on 31 patients treated by laparoscopy for peritonitis caused by PPU and with symptoms for more than 24 h. These findings are confirmed by recent study of Schietroma et al. [32] that showed, in case of peritonitis after PPU, increased incidence of bacteremia, endo-toxemia, and systemic inflammation after open ulcer repair compared with laparoscopy.

The Danish Clinical Register of Emergency Surgery [33], including 2668 patients treated for PPU, however, reports the limits of surgical delay, in a cohort study. A total of 708 patients (26.5 %) died within 30 days of surgery and it was showed that every hour of delay from admission to surgery is associated with an adjusted 2–4 % decreased probability of survival, compared with the previous hour. The authors conclude that prompt surgery for the control of sepsis is of paramount importance in treating patients with PPU.

In 2013, Thorsen et al. [8] compared 11 different scores used to predict outcome in PPU patients, of which the Boey score, the Hacettepe score, the Jabalpur score, the peptic ulcer perforation (PULP) score, the ASA score, the Charlson comorbidity index, the Mannheim Peritonitis Index (MPI), the Acute Physiology and Chronic Health Evaluation II (APACHE II), the simplified acute physiology score II (SAPS II), the Mortality probability models II (MPM II), and the Physiological and Operative Severity Score for the enumeration of Mortality and Morbidity physical subscore (POSSUM-phys score). Only four of the scores were specifically constructed for PPU patients. Considerable variation in performance both between different scores and between different studies was found. The authors concluded that the Boey and ASA scores are most commonly used to predict outcome for PPU patients, while other scoring systems are hampered by a lack of validation or by their complexity, which precludes routine clinical use. The PULP score (Presentation $\geq$ or <24 h; presence of preoperative shock; ASA score, presence of aids, active malignancy, liver failure; serum creatinine >130 mmol/L) seems promising, but it needs external validation before widespread use.

The Consensus 2012 concludes: "Several studies suggest that Boey's shock score on admission [blood pressure (BP)\90 mmHg)], ASA III–V (severe comorbidities), and duration of symptomatology (>24 h) are the most reliable parameters for selecting patients." "The laparoscopic approach is safe in patients with no risk factors (Boey score = 0)." "Other principles of selection have been considered: Mannheim Peritonitis Index (MPI), age >70 years, APACHE II and surgeon's skill in mini-invasive surgery."

However, to date, there is no unanimous agreement about which group of patients might benefit from a laparoscopic approach of PPU and sufficient information regarding the laparoscopic repair in high-risk surgical patients.

Teoh et al. [34], in a retrospective study published in 2015, concluded the adoption of laparoscopy-first approach in patients suffering from PPU was associated with acceptable rates of mortality and morbidity. The approach could also be selectively adopted in patients hemodynamically stable with Boey score ≥ 2 and low ASA grading.

7.4 Surgical Technique/Closure of the Perforation

Placing the patient in the Trendelenburg position at 15–20° is usually recommended. The operator can position between the legs of the patient or at the patient's side. From the review of Bertleff [20], it has been shown that 44 % of the surgeons prefer positioned between the legs of the patient (even in our experience this is a privileged position), 33 % carry out the intervention from the left side, 16 % either between the legs or the side left, and 6 % from the patient's right side. The assistants are positioned each at one side of the patient. The number, location, and the section of the trocars may differ according to the habits and experience of the surgeon, and in relationship to the patient's build. Generally, the first optical trocar, 12 mm, is placed between or over the umbilical area using open technique. Once the pneumoperitoneum has been insufflated (alternatively the Verres needle can be used), the whole abdominal cavity is explored using a 30° optic. Then the other trocars (usually in number of 3) are positioned under visual control. One 5 mm trocar is placed in the epigastric for the lift of the liver and if necessary of the gallbladder. The other two trocars are usually positioned, respectively, in the left abdominal quadrant, on the mild-clavicular line, above the umbilical transverse line (12 mm), and on the right side (5 mm). The position is diametrically opposite on the projection plane of the abdominal wall of the trans-pyloric region. There are other variations in the positioning of trocars, but the one described seems to respond better to the needs of ergonomics and "triangulation" between optics and trocars for the uneventful outcome of a laparoscopy (Fig. 7.3).

Usually, it is easy to identify PPU, but if the perforation is located in a "difficult" site (lateral wall of the descending duodenum, posterior gastric wall) some additional maneuvers need to be performed, i.e., the mobilization of duodenum or the section of the gastrocolic ligament to access to the retro-cavity of great omentum. In case of missed site perforation, despite these maneuvers, the conversion may be necessary. Conversion should not be considered a failure, as the detection and safe closure of the perforation takes precedence over choice of surgical access. The gain

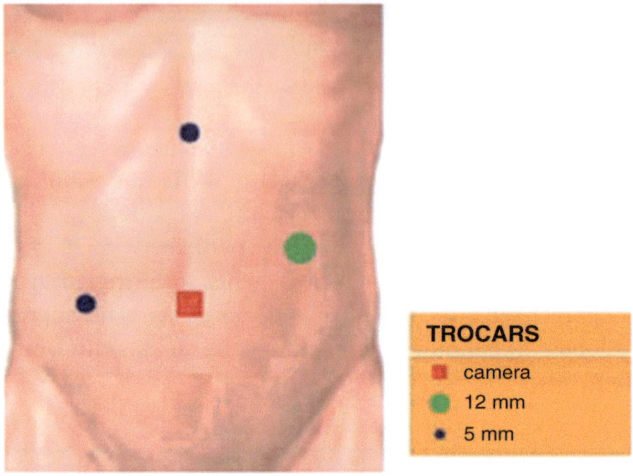

Fig. 7.3 The position of the optical and operating ports on the abdominal wall used to repair perforated peptic ulcer

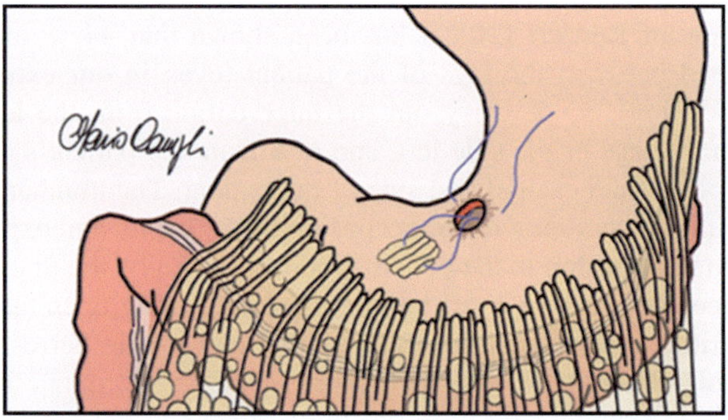

Fig. 7.4 Graham omentoplasty: a free graft of epiploon is used to repair the perforation

of laparoscopy may be lost if the complexity exceeds the level of technical ability or diminish the performance of a safe procedure.

The closure of perforation, probably, represents the most demanding moment of surgery and together with the subsequent extensive washing of the abdominal cavity is responsible for the increase of the operative time of laparoscopy compared to the traditional technique.

The choice of the method of closure depends fundamentally on the characteristics of the lesion: if the margins are infiltrated, friable, and less mobile, the repair must be performed only by applying an omental patch; for easily joined margins without any tension, just a simple suture with an omental flap is sufficient. In the latter 2–3 stitches are suggested to close the lesion to which in the second moment an omental patch is secured. Figs. 7.4, 7.5, and 7.6 show the techniques of laparoscopic closure of PPU [35].

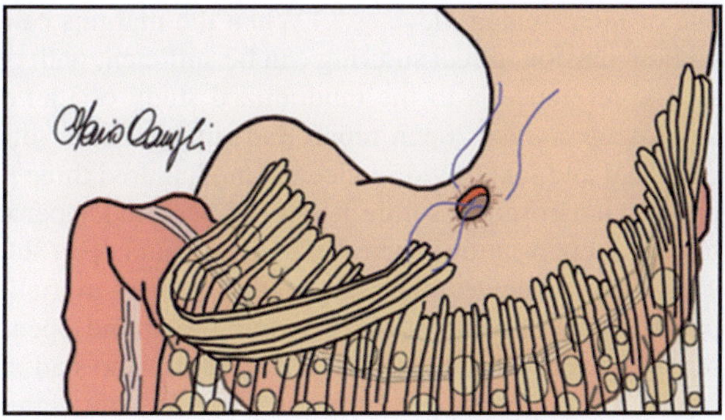

Fig. 7.5 Cellan-Jones repair: a strand of omentum is drawn over the perforation and held in place by full thickness sutures placed on either side of the perforation

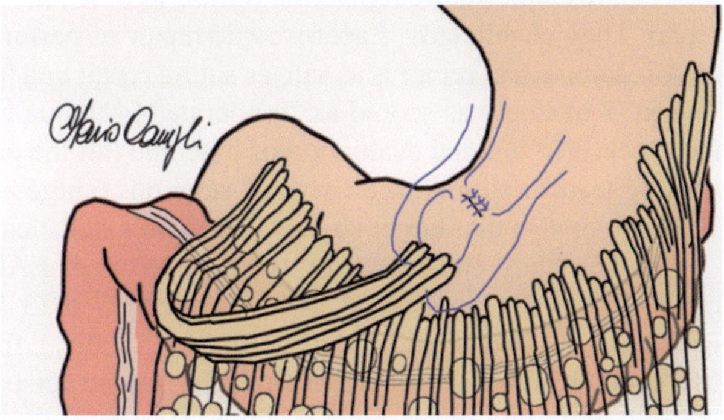

Fig. 7.6 Primary suture of the perforation overlapped by a pedicle omentum flap

As an alternative to classical suturing, several changes have been proposed to simplify the method: "single-stitch laparoscopic repair" [22]; use of a clip to tighten the suture (avoid a knot in the suture) [2]; use of clips full thickness self-locking [36]; use of staplers ("stapled omental patch repair") [37]; and use of combined laparoscopic–endoscopic technique ("gastroscopy-aided repair") [38].

In order to make the repair of the PPU less complex and, consequently, reduce operating time, techniques have been proposed so-called suture-less, which avoids the suture of the perforation (particularly laborious in the case of the edge of the friable and edematous perforation) [39]. The lesion can be repaired by means of an omental flap secured in situ by the affixing of fibrin glue (as in the first case described by laparoscopic Mouret in 1990) [6], or by using a plug to close the perforation, dimensioned on the size of the lesion [39, 40]. Nevertheless, there is still an open question whether the reduction of operating time made possible by simpler procedures does not reduce the safety of the laparoscopic technique at the expense of the patient, favoring a higher incidence of postoperative sequelae (in particular leakage) [5, 24].

The Consensus 2012 states: "The choice of perforation closure technique depends on lesion characteristics: if margins are edematous, friable, and/or difficult to mobilize, repair can be limited to an omental patch, eventually associated with one or more sealant devices." "When the margins can be easily brought together, without tension, direct suturing can be sufficient with or without omentoplasty."

The reference is to the randomized study of Lau et al. [39], which compared laparoscopic versus open repair and suture versus suture-less repair of perforated duodenal and juxta-pyloric ulcers. One hundred three patients were randomly allocated to laparoscopic suture repair (26 patients), laparoscopic suture-less repair (26 patients), open suture repair (25 patients), and open suture-less repair (26 patients). The authors showed that the morbidity and mortality were the same between patients who underwent laparoscopic repair and open repair. Similarly, there was no significant difference between patients who had suture repair and suture-less repair. The laparoscopic suture-less repair took significantly less operation time than laparoscopic suture repair, but it took significantly longer than open suture-less repair. They concluded, "Laparoscopic repair of perforated peptic ulcer is a viable option. Suture-less repair is as safe as suture repair and it takes less time to perform." The RCT of Lau was scored as "moderate" [41], due to some bias present such as the absence of blinded evaluation of outcome (all the patients were assessed by the treating team) and learning curve of surgeons (surgeon's experience was similar). To consider also that larger studies with better statistical power are needed.

Another study considered by the Consensus of EAES is the systematic review conducted by Sanabria et al. [42], updated to 2013 [43]. It involves only three RCTs [21, 22, 39] (evaluated of acceptable quality), for a small diversified of just 315 patients. The authors examined laparoscopic versus open surgery correction of the PPU with any mechanical method (primary suture, omentum patch, synthetic material patch, or resection), with or without insufflation. The suture dehiscence, one of the primary outcomes measured, in order to define the most reliable technique, was reported in four patients in the laparoscopy group (2.4 %) versus two patients in the open group (1.3 %), but any conclusion was not possible, because of few events examined.

7.5 Drainage/Lavage

The withdrawal of intra-abdominal collections, in particular septic fluids, is more frequent when the perforation is not recent, and peritoneal irrigation should reduce the incidence of dangerous postoperative intra-abdominal infections, which are often responsible for re-intervention. It is reasonable to perform irrigation only if necessary and, however, proportional to the quantity and quality (presence of food) of the fluids found in the peritoneal cavity. Saline solution (2–6 L) is generally recommended, but others recommend using greater quantities, up to 30 L. [20, 24].

In this way, laparoscopic technique compared to the traditional technique offers the advantage of easier access to various intra-peritoneal recesses (spaces above and below liver, pericolic areas, left diaphragmatic region, pelvic cavity) without the need to perform extensive and destructive laparotomies.

A single drainage is generally used for prophylactic purposes by the majority of the authors [44, 45], positioned in the hepatic region or closer to the lesion. Only a minority of authors consider it unnecessary [22, 46], considering it as a possible source of contamination of the peritoneal cavity [47].

Consensus 2012 states: "Decontamination of the peritoneal cavity by washing after treatment of PPU is a fundamental step in the surgical procedure."

7.6 Conversion

It has an extreme variable percentage in the different case studies (from 0 to 29 %) [20, 24], probably in relation to the different degrees of experience reached by the various surgical teams involved in the studies. The LAMA randomized multicenter trial, conducted by Bertleff et al. in 2009 [21], shows a conversion rate of only 8 %. This result is due, according to the authors, to good laparoscopic experience gained by the nine centers involved (at least 50 previous laparoscopic procedures) and confirms that this type of surgery should only be undertaken by surgeons with sufficient experience in the field of mini-invasive surgery.

The most common causes of intraoperative conversion are the size of the perforation (for some authors >6 mm, for others >10 mm) [22, 26], the missed diagnosis, the friable margins of the lesion, the gastric non-juxta-pyloric site, and the severity of peritonitis. Moreover, in 2010, Bertleff et al. [20] performed a review including 2788 patients. They stress that, even if a perforation >10 mm should be considered a contraindication to laparoscopy, the size of perforation might not necessarily have to be a reason anymore to convert, using an omental patch.

The presence of those factors considered predictive of conversion can be useful to prevent this eventuality, preferring to the traditional open treatment. Those conditions include the state of shock at admission, risk of conversion up to 50 % vs. 8 % in patients without shock, as well as the time between the beginning of perforation and diagnosis >24 h, rate conversion up to 33 % vs. 0 % of patients without diagnostic delay [6, 26].

The study of Katkhouda [26] was taken into account by Consensus of 2012. The study, despite the limitation, nonrandomized controlled trial, as well as small sample size, only 30 patients underwent laparoscopy using the classic Graham patch technique for PPU), shows that the laparoscopy in PPU is safe and feasible. Two clinical parameters, however, may preclude the results: shock at the admission, defined as a systolic blood pressure less than 80 mmHg, and symptom duration more than 24 h. Patients who presented with evidence of shock and were treated laparoscopically had a high conversion rate and a significantly worse postoperative course than patients without shock on admission. In this clinical situation, a laparoscopic approach that has a high likelihood of failure should not be attempted, and the patient should have an expeditious open repair.

Consensus 2012 states: "Predictive factors of conversion are shock on admittance and the free interval between the beginning of perforation and the diagnosis >24 h)."

In 2015, in a nationwide real-life data on laparoscopic vs. open surgery from Denmark [48], the authors showed the results of 726 patients of whom 238 (32.8 %) were treated laparoscopically and 178 (24.5 %) had a laparoscopic procedure converted to laparotomy. The most frequent causes were a persistent leak and wound dehiscence occurred in 5.9 % and 4.7 % of cases, respectively.

A special condition of conversion can be the suspicion of malignant perforated ulcer. The perforation of a gastric cancer is a rare event (1 % of gastric cancers and about 10–16 % of gastric perforations [49] should be suspected in patients over 65) which is diagnosed intraoperatively in only about 30 % of cases and often is indistinguishable from a benign ulcer, unless a biopsy of the lesion is performed. This is recommended as routine by some authors for all gastric perforations during the same laparoscopic repair [50, 51].

The few studies available are of limited number of cases and limited to open treatment and significant results on the treatment of this disease in emergency surgery cannot be obtained.

According to some authors, a resective surgery (with or without conversion to open?) in case of a perforated gastric cancer can be justified by clinical and oncological criteria. Several studies concluded that the 5-year survival in patients with a perforated gastric cancer is the same as a non-complicated gastric cancer [51, 52].

A multivariate analysis has shown that the degree of lymph node invasion is the only factor related to long-term survival of patients with perforated gastric cancer [53].

In 2000, Lehnert et al. [52] proposed a two-stage treatment: the first, a simple repair of the perforation and the second a radical gastrectomy. This approach would fully meet two fundamental requirements: avoid major surgical procedures in a frail patient because of peritonitis and cancer; improve the patient's clinical condition and after appropriate cancer staging perform the correct oncologic procedure.

7.7 Re-intervention

In a systematic review of seven studies examined, Lunevicius and Mokevicius [23] report no statistically significant difference between the incidence of reoperation between laparoscopic technique and the open approach, although the incidence is almost double after laparoscopy (5.3 % vs. 2.1 %). Even in the meta-analysis of Lau [24], the incidence of reoperation is significantly higher after laparoscopy (3.7 %) compared to traditional surgery (1.6 %). The complication that causes, most frequently, reoperation is represented by the leakage of the suture (seven cases).

Lee has identified APACHE II (>5 points) and the diameter of the ulcer (>10 mm) as independent factors of the risk of postoperative leakage in patients undergoing suture-less laparoscopic repair (plug with fibrin glue) of PPU [29]. The importance of the laparoscopic skill was underlined in this experience. This factor is also confirmed in a study of Lunevicius and Morkevicius: all cases of leakage are reported when the intervention is performed by surgeons with limited learning curve (less than 10 laparoscopic sutures) [54].

Consensus 2012 states: "In Lau's meta-analysis [24], the reoperation rate was higher after the laparoscopic approach (3.7 %) than after conventional surgery

(1.6 %). Suture site leakage represents the most important cause of reoperation" and "APACHE II (5 points) and ulcer size (>10 mm) are independent risk factors for postoperative leak after laparoscopic suture-less fibrin glue repair."

Wilhemsen et al. [48], already mentioned above, showed that 17.1 % of patients needed a re-intervention. The crude risk of re-operative surgery was higher in patients who underwent laparotomy and those with procedures converted to open surgery than in patients who had laparoscopic repair: OR 1.98 (95 % C.I. 1.19–3.27) and 2.36 (1.37–4.08), respectively. The mortality was higher in this group, with crude and adjusted OR 1.53 (1.00–2.34) and 1.06 (0.65–1.72), respectively. They concluded that reoperation was necessary in almost one in every five patients operated on for PPU. Laparoscopy was associated with lower risk of reoperation than laparotomy or a converted procedure. However, there was a risk of bias, including confounding by indication.

7.8 Results

The first RCT that compared the surgical techniques for PPU, open vs. laparoscopic and sutures vs. sutureless repair, was published by Lau et al. in Hong Kong [39] and included 103 procedures. The study showed that the total operative time for laparoscopic repair was significantly increased but resulted in a reduced requirement for postoperative analgesia.

In the same study there was no significant difference found in NG tube drainage, intravenous fluid usage, hospital stay, and return to normal diet. There was also no statistically significant difference between the different techniques, in terms of mortality and morbidity.

Similarly, a second small randomized trial of 20 patients, which examined possible effects on the acute phase response and the presence of endo-toxemia, found no difference between laparoscopy and open repair [30].

A further RCT, from Hong Kong, that included 130 patients reported in 2002 [22], and the only European study (the Dutch LAMA trial [21]) reported in 2009, confirmed these findings. All three RCTs favored laparoscopic repair, as being at least not inferior to open surgery for PPU.

However, a subsequent meta-analysis of Sanabria [43] has provided inconclusive results. From the information provided by the clinical trials included in this review, outcomes from laparoscopic surgery for perforated peptic ulcers were not different from those of open surgery. The authors conclude that laparoscopic surgery could be the first therapeutic after considering other variables such as experience, costs, and availability. However, it is necessary to have randomized controlled trials with large sample sizes, better outcomes assessments, and in different populations. Besides, variables that measure the experience of surgeons with laparoscopic repair must be introduced and assessed. Data for cost and resources consumption variables are also needed.

We will compare the main results obtained by the two approaches, open and laparoscopic.

7.9 Postoperative Pain

In the meta-analysis conducted by Lau in 2004 [24], the first on this topic, which included 13 trials (with 2 RCTs [22, 39]), in 8 was demonstrated a significant reduction in the dose of analgesics in the patients who underwent laparoscopy and in three studies [22, 39, 52] VAS pain score was significantly decreased after laparoscopy.

In contrast, in the RCT of Lau et al. [39] in the earlier measurements (first 24 h postoperative), the VAS pain score was comparable in the two techniques.

According to the authors, there are three possibilities for these apparently inconsistent results. First, laparoscopic surgery was as painful as open surgery, and the less demand in the postoperative analgesic was due to the influence of the psychological impact of minimally invasive surgery and the medical and nursing staffs' positive attitudes toward the procedure. This explanation is difficult to prove or disprove because it is difficult to perform a double-blind study to eliminate these biases. Second, laparoscopic repair actually was less painful than open repair, but it was difficult for the patients to differentiate between pain due to the peritonitis and postoperative pain within 24 h of surgery. Third, there was an actual difference in the postoperative VAS pain score between laparoscopic and open repair, but the difference was too small to be detected by the small number of patients studied (type II statistical error).

Differences regarding postoperative pain in favor of the laparoscopic procedure were confirmed later in the only European study (the Dutch LAMA trial [21]) reported in 2009, which showed a VAS score on postoperative days 1, 3, and 7 significantly lower in the laparoscopic group.

Consensus 2012 concludes: "One of the advantages of laparoscopic surgery is less postoperative pain, but earlier data about pain (within 24 h postoperatively) do not show any difference, probably because of peritoneal inflammation."

7.10 Operating Time

In the meta-analysis of 2004, Lau [24] showed that operative time was significantly higher for laparoscopy in five trials. In further five studies there was no difference between laparoscopy and open treatment. Only in the RCT of Siu the operating time was lower, 42 min for laparoscopy vs. 52.3 min for open treatment [22]. This result in favor of laparoscopy is attributed to the particular technique used: a "single-stitch laparoscopic repair" for the closure of the perforation and the subsequent omental patch.

Contrasting results have been reported in the other two RCTs of Lau [39] and LAMA trial of Bertleff [21], where the results are more favorable for the open surgery. The variability of these results is attributable mainly to the different levels of experience and organization achieved by the surgical teams involved in the study, as well as the technological improvement, in particular the laparoscopic irrigation/drainage system, as also emphasized in the systematic review of Lunevicius and Morkevicius [23].

Consensus 2012 states: "The operative times are longer for laparoscopy (except one study); however, a progressive and constant reduction of operative times over the past 10 years has been seen, probably due to an improvement in the surgeon's skill, better technology, and better organization of the surgical teams."

7.11 Complications

In the evaluation of postoperative morbidity, the parameters most frequently considered are represented by septic sequelae (sepsis, infection of the wall, intra-abdominal abscesses, lung infections), complications of perforated lesion perforation (suture dehiscence, hemorrhage, recurrence of ulcer), systemic complications (e.g., cardiovascular), or other conditions, such as prolonged dynamic ileus.

The first RCT about the use of laparoscopy in PPU performed by Lau, in 1996, showed that there were no statistically significant differences between the two techniques, mini-invasive and traditional, in terms of mortality and morbidity [39].

These results were confirmed later by the other two RCTs of Bertleff [21] and Siu [23], which reaffirmed the excellence of the laparoscopic option in terms of safety and feasibility.

Recent studies, such as the review of Bertleff published in 2010, confirm previous data equivalence in terms of rate of complications between the two techniques and lower incidence of mortality after laparoscopy: 14.3 % and 3.6 % vs. 26.9 % and 6.4 %, respectively, after laparoscopy and open surgery [20]. Even the review of Sanabria [43] (updated to 2013) is indicative of a trend toward a decrease in some complications, such as wall abdominal infections, postoperative ileus, pulmonary infections, as well as the mortality rate, after laparoscopic surgery, although none of these results are statistically significant. In contrast, although not statistically significant, the incidence of intra-abdominal abscesses and re-intervention in comparison with traditional surgery has increased. Lastly, no conclusion has been reached with regard to other complications, such as the incidence of suture dehiscence or the risk of incisional hernia [43].

Antoniou et al. [55], in meta-analysis published in 2013, conclude that laparoscopic surgery could be the first therapeutic after considering other variables such as surgeon's experience, costs, and availability, however, it is necessary to have RCT with large sample sizes, better outcome assessments, and in different populations. They stress the same conclusions of previous work [43, 55].

7.12 Hospitalization

The three most important systemic reviews [23, 24, 43] report favorable results to laparoscopy in terms of time of postoperative hospital stay or at least not worse than those obtained from conventional surgery.

This is highlighted in the RCT by Siu et al. [22], which showed a reduction in hospitalization (6 vs. 7 days) and a significantly earlier shorter return to normal activities (10.4 vs. 26.1 days; $p = 0.001$), in patients treated laparoscopically than those treated traditionally.

In contrast, in the RCTs of Lau [39] and Bertleff [21] the hospital stay was comparable between laparoscopy and open surgery: median, respectively, of 5 vs. 6 days and 6.5 vs. 8.0 days, in the two studies.

Lunevicius and Morkevicius [23] stress that these aspects are also linked to factors outside the medical fields, like the cultural habits of the patients and the different health policies followed by the various surgical centers involved.

Consensus 2012 concludes: "The hospital stay has been shown to be more favorable for the laparoscopic approach compared to traditional surgery in Siu et al., but not in Lau and Bertleff et al."

7.13 Non-operative Management (NOM)

Studies by Taylor, in the first half of the twentieth century, have shown that the positive effects of the adjacent organs buffer at least half of the patients with PPU, in particular by the greater omentum [56]. This has tended to suggest that nonoperative management (NOM) is a possible valid alternative to surgery for PPU in selected cases. Conservative treatment known as the "Taylor method" consists of positioning of nasogastric tube aspiration, administration of parenteral therapy, antibiotics, and proton pump inhibitor (PPI) therapy. Croft et al. conducted a prospective randomized trial comparing the outcome of nonoperative treatment with that of emergency surgery in patients with a clinical diagnosis of PPU [57]. Of the 83 patients entered in the study over a 13-month period, 40 were randomly assigned to conservative treatment. The other 43 patients were assigned to immediate laparotomy and repair of the perforation. Eleven of 40 patients (28 %) who underwent NOM had no clinical improvement after 12 h and required an operation. The overall mortality rates in the two groups were similar (two deaths in each, 5 %) and did not differ significantly in the morbidity rates (40 % in surgical group and 50 % in nonsurgical group). The authors concluded that in patients with perforated peptic ulcer, an initial period of conservative treatment with careful observation may be safely allowed except in patients over 70 years old (where a high failure rate was noted), because such an observation period can avoid the need for emergency surgery in more than 70 % of patients. This is the only RCT on conservative treatment performed thus far. Notably, this was performed before the PPI era, and ranitidine was used as acid suppressant.

Bucher et al. performed NOM on inoperable patients because of their poor clinical condition [49]. The authors pointed out that the eradication of HP and especially the introduction of PPI drugs can positively influence the results of conservative treatment, mortality of 64 % in the group of patients with H2-blockers, compared to 11 % of patients in therapy with PPI. On the other hand, shock is the greatest predictive criterion for the failure of NOM, while no influence would be given to the advanced age of the patient. Thus, hemodynamically unstable patients should be candidates for surgery immediately.

Songne B et al. in 2004 conducted a prospective trial of 82 consecutive patients, with diagnosis of PPU, initially treated with NOM [58]. Clinical improvement was obtained in 44 patients (54 %) with a mortality rate of 1 %. Significant predictive factors of failure of nonoperative treatment were size of pneumoperitoneum, heart beat > 94 bpm, pain at digital rectal exam, age > 59 years, and abdominal meteorism. These results suggested that more than 50 % of patients with perforated peptic ulcer respond to conservative treatment without surgery and that the association of few clinical criteria required emergency surgery.

As confirmed by the recent review of the WSES [59], in the 2013, the most important factor regarding the likely success of NOM of PPU is whether the ulcer has sealed. This can be shown by gastrografin contrast study: if there is free leak of contrast from the ulcer, then surgery is needed; if the ulcer has sealed itself by adherent omentum, etc., then NOM is indicated, provided the patient does not have peritonitis or severe sepsis.

NOM management should be carefully considered in selected patients, knowing that evidence is weak for its efficacy and risk may be high if disease symptoms do not resolve.

7.14 Future Developments

7.14.1 Natural Orifice Transluminal Endoscopic Surgery

A Natural Orifice Transluminal Endoscopic Surgery (NOTES) approach may reduce the physiologic impact of therapeutic intervention after peptic ulcer perforation and provide a technically less challenging procedure. This is especially important in elderly and/or immunocompromised patients.

A retrospective review of Bonin et al. suggested that up to 50 % of patients presenting with perforated ulcer might be candidates for a NOTES repair [60].

Bingener et al. present a pilot clinical study evaluating the feasibility of endoscopic transluminal omental-patch closure for perforated peptic ulcers [61]. Of seven patients (mean age 79, range 64–89) who consented to the study, three underwent the study procedure. All patients had multiple comorbidities. Two patients presented with 4–6 mm perforated peptic ulcers and underwent successful laparoscopic-assisted NOTES omental and falciform ligament patch closure, respectively. Postoperative radiographic contrast studies showed no leak and patients were discharged home on postoperative days 3 and 4. The third patient had undergone enterocutaneous fistula repair with herniorrhaphy 6 weeks prior; a transluminal endoscopic approach was feasible; however, the omentum was under too much tension to be secured. This procedure was converted to an open omental-patch repair.

After induction of general anesthesia, pneumoperitoneum (12–14 cm H_2O) has been established using a periumbilical trocar in Hasson technique. This served to confirm the diagnosis of ulcer perforation and for surveillance of the endoscopic procedure. A standard diagnostic upper endoscope with CO_2 insufflation has been introduced through the oro-pharynx into the stomach and duodenum. The site of perforation was identified and measured. The endoscope was carefully advanced through the perforation when possible. Once in the peritoneal cavity, the endoscopist proceeded with inspection and irrigation. A viable mobile piece of omentum was identified and pulled intraluminally through the site of perforation. The omentum was then fixed to the mucosa of the luminal wall with several endoscopic clips (Figs. 7.7 and 7.8).

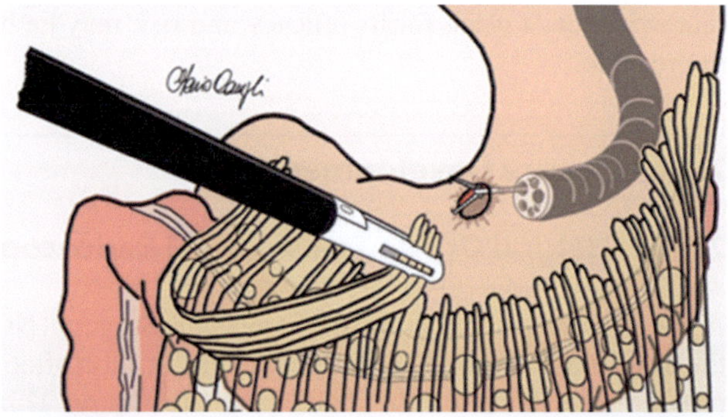

Fig. 7.7 A viable mobile piece of omentum pulled intraluminally through the site of perforation

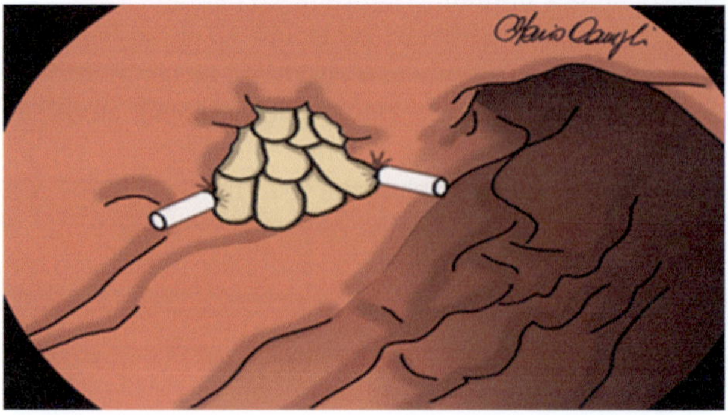

Fig. 7.8 The omentum is fixed to the mucosa of the luminal wall with several endoscopic clips

The falciform ligament was used if a suitable omental patch was not available. Following repair, the stomach or duodenum was insufflated to test for air leak. If the NOTES procedure was unsuccessful, either a laparoscopic or open omental patch repair was considered by the acute care surgical team.

Initial results from a laparoscopic-assisted NOTES approach for closure of perforated peptic ulcers appear promising and enable swift recovery in selected patients. This is especially important in elderly and/or immunocompromised patients.

7.14.2 Stem Cells

In future, development takes place in the Stem Cell Technology. In the literature, among several preclinic studies on stem cells, there is a Chinese experimental study [62] published in 2015 on the effect of local injection of mesenchymal stem cells (MSC) on healing of sutured gastric perforation (GP). Its results were very encouraging. The local injection of adipose tissue-derived MSC significantly promoted the healing of GP, with the highest pneumatic bursting pressure, minimal wound adhesions, and lowest incidence of wound dehiscence and abdominal abscess. The injected MSC favored a reduction of inflammation and an increase of granulation and re-epithelization. The authors concluded that local injection of MSC enhanced the healing of sutured GP by anti-inflammatory process and improved cellular proliferation and earlier onset of granulation. The use of this technology represents the new frontier, for instance, for secure gastrotomy closure after notes, as advocated by the authors.

Thus, in the future, surgeons may take advantage of stem cell technology for enhanced healing of wounds after closure, based on experimental studies. This has yet to be confirmed in a clinical trial.

7.14.3 Other Techniques

Aside from the novel techniques previously described, there are some applications very interesting. Søreide [63] enunciates these techniques superbly in an article published in 2015, such as *Over-the-scope-clip (OTSC), the OverStitch Endoscopic Suturing System, Self-expanding metal stents (SEMS), Nitinol U-clips, Plug with acellular matrix, a biodegradable patch, a patch coated with fibrinogen and thrombin.* Some of these are in an experimental phase.

7.15 Conclusions

After the laparoscopic repair of PPU was first reported in 1990 by Mouret, an increasing numbers of combined meta-analyses of RCTs, prospective observations, and retrospective cohorts have yielded more favorable advantages for laparoscopy, as being at least not inferior to open surgery for PPU. Collective reviews also favor a laparoscopic approach, but most of these were conducted before the advent of guidelines for systematic reviews and have the inherent risk of publication bias. Thus, the current state of evidence remains poor for choosing laparoscopy over laparotomy for PPU and there are inconclusive results owing to the small sample sizes for each outcome measured, between two techniques, open and laparoscopic. Therefore, such data, far from being able to be considered as definitive, deserve further evaluation and, especially, require wider and more numerous trials of quality (randomized prospective studies). In contrast, the literature review has retrieved a decreasing number of published prospective trials from 1996 to date. This trend was also confirmed in the last 5 years.

The best defined prognostic criteria, able to identify patients at higher risk for laparoscopic surgery, and the determination of predictors of laparoscopic to open conversion, are some of priority objectives to be pursued. Especially, the experiences about the use of laparoscopy in higher risk patients are still limited and do not allow definitive conclusions.

The degree of experience achieved by surgical teams in the laparoscopic technique is one of the factors prognostically more relevant to the final result, although it is, at present, extremely difficult to determine. Some data, such as the progressive reduction of operating time and conversion rates, along with the increase in the number of patients undergoing laparoscopy for PPU can be considered indicative of the parameters for the evaluation of the level achieved by the operators in this type of surgery.

There is some variability of the techniques used in laparoscopic repair of the PPU and the ideal technique should respond to some basic requirements, such as the relative easy of implementation with reduced operating times and reliability, in terms of reduced morbidity (in particular of reducing the risk of leakage). The criteria to choose the method of closure basically depend on the characteristics of the lesion: in case of ulcer edges easily closed without tension, just the simple suture with any omentum plastic is enough; instead, if the margins are edematous or little sliding, the repair will be done by affixing omental patch.

There is no reference in the literature to the costs of the laparoscopic technique. However, it seems reasonable to assume that the contraction of the operative time, linked to the more experienced and better organizational skills of the surgical team, as well as advances in technology, may create in the near future a decline in costs directly related to the intervention. However, an overall estimate of costs, also including those relating to the length of postoperative hospital stay and the time required to return to work or normal daily activities, appears complex. The progressive increase in the elderly population suffering from PPU, often in the presence of a clinical picture of frank peritonitis, may represent, in fact, an obstacle to a more rapid discharge and, consequently, to an immediate resumption of normal activities by the patient.

References

1. Pappas TN, Lagoo SA (2002) Laparoscopic repair for perforated peptic ulcer. Ann Surg 235(3):320–321
2. Matsuda M, Nishiyama M, Hanai T, Saeki S, Watanabe T (1995) Laparoscopic omental patch repair for perforated peptic ulcer. Ann Surg 221(3):236–240
3. Lui FY, Davis KA (2010) Gastroduodenal perforation: maximal or minimal intervention? Scand J Surg 99:73–77
4. Bertleff MJ, Lange JF (2010) Perforated peptic ulcer disease: a review of history and treatment. Dig Surg 27:161–169
5. Lagoo S, Mc Mahon RL, Kalkharu M, Pappas TN, Eubanks S (2002) The sixth decision regarding perforated duodenal ulcer. JSLS 6:359–368
6. Mouret J, Francois Y, Vignal J et al (1990) Laparoscopic treatment of perforated duodenal ulcer. Br J Surg 77:1006
7. Nathanson LK, Easter DW, Cuschieri A (1990) Laparoscopic repair peritoneal toilette of perforated duodenal ulcer. Surg Endosc 4:232–233
8. Thorsen K, Søreide JA, Søreide K (2013) Scoring systems for outcome prediction in patients with perforated peptic ulcer. Scand J Trauma Resusc Emerg Med 21:25
9. Sauerland S, Agresta F, Bergamaschi R, Borzellino G, Budzynsky A, Champault G, Fingerhut A, Isla A, Johansson M, Lundorff P, Navez B, Saad S, Neugebauer EA (2006) Laparoscopy for abdominal emergencies: evidence based guidelines of the European Association for Endoscopic Surgery. Surg Endosc 20(1):14–29
10. Agresta F, Ansaloni L, Baiocchi GL, Bergamini C, Campanile FC, Carlucci M, Cocorullo G, Corradi A, Franzato B, Lupo M, Mandalà V, Mirabella A, Pernazza G, Piccoli M, Staudacher C, Vettoretto N, Zago M, Lettieri E, Levati A, Pietrini D, Scaglione M, De Masi S, De Placido G, Francucci M, Rasi M, Fingerhut A, Uranüs S, Garattini S (2012) Laparoscopic approach to acute abdomen from the Consensus Development Conference of the Società Italiana di Chirurgia Endoscopica e nuove tecnologie (SICE), Associazione Chirurghi Ospedalieri Italiani (ACOI), Società Italiana di Chirurgia (SIC), Società Italiana di Chirurgia d'Urgenza e del Trauma (SICUT), Società Italiana di Chirurgia nell'Ospedalità Privata (SICOP), and the European Association for Endoscopic Surgery (EAES). Surg Endosc 26(8):2134–2164. doi:10.1007/s00464-012-2331-3
11. Mandala V, Mirabella A, Lupo M (2012) The role of laparoscopy in emergency abdominal surgery. Springer, Italia
12. Kakhry S, Watts D, Daley B et al (2001) Current diagnostic approach lack sensitivity in the diagnosis of perforating blunt small bowel injury (SBI): findings from a large multi-institutional trial. J Trauma 51:1232
13. Schein M (2005) Perforated peptic ulcer. In: Schein's common sense emergency abdominal surgery. Springer, Berlin, p 143–150
14. Miller RE, Nelson SW (1971) The roentgenologic demonstration of tyni amounts of free intraperitoneal gas: experimental and clinical studies. AJR Am J Roentgenol 112:574–585
15. Chen SC, Wang HP, Chen WJ (2002) Selective use of ultrasonography for the detection of pneumoperitoneum. Acad Emerg Med 9:643–645
16. Phatak MG, Frank SJ, Ellis JJ (1984) Computed tomography of bowel perforation. Gastrointest Radiol 9:133–135
17. Hainaux B, Agneessen E, Bertinotti R, De Maertelaer V, Rubesova E, Capelluto E, Moschopoulos C (2006) Accuracy of MDCT in predicting site of gastrointestinal tract perforation. AJR Am J Roentgenol 187:1179–1183
18. Earls JP, Dachman AH, Colon E, Garrett MG, Molloy M (1993) Prevalence and duration of postoperative pneumoperitoneum: sensitivity of CT vs left lateral decubitus radiography. AJR Am J Roentgenol 161:781–785
19. Chen CH, Huang HS, Yang CC, Yeh YH (2001) Features of perforated peptic ulcers in conventional computed tomography. Hepatogastroenterology 48:1393–1396

20. Bertleff M, Lange JF (2010) Laparoscopic correction of perforated peptic ulcer: first choice? A review of literature. Surg Endosc 24:1231–1239
21. Bertleff M et al (2009) Randomized Clinical trial of laparoscopic versus open repair of the perforated peptic ulcer: the LAMA trial. World J Surg 33:1368–1373
22. Siu WT, Leong HT, Law BKB et al (2002) Laparoscopic repair for perforated peptic ulcer: a randomized controlled trial. Ann Surg 235:313–319
23. Lunevicius R, Morkevicius M (2005) Systemic review comparing laparoscopic and open repair for perforated peptic ulcer. Br J Surg 92:1195–1207
24. Lau H (2004) Laparoscopic repair of perforated peptic ulcer. A meta-analysis. Surg Endosc 18:1013–1021
25. Boey J, Wong J (1987) Perforated duodenal ulcers. World J Surg 11:319–324
26. Katkhouda N, Mavor E, Mason RJ et al (1999) Laparoscopic repair of perforated duodenal ulcers: outcome and efficacy in 30 consecutive patients. Arch Surg 134:845–850
27. Robertson GS, Wemyss-Holden SA, Maddern GJ (2000) Laparoscopic repair of perforated duodenal ulcers. The role of laparoscopy in generalized peritonitis. Ann R Coll Surg Engl 82:6–10
28. Notashi AY, Salimi J, Rahimian H, Fersharaki MH, Abbassi A (2005) Evaluation of Mannheim Peritonitis Index and multiple failure score in patients with peritonitis. Ind J Gastroenterol 24:197–200
29. Lee FY, Leung KL, Lai BS et al (2001) Predicting mortality and morbility of patients operated on for perforated peptic ulcers. Arch Surg 136:90–94
30. Lau JY, Lo SY, Ng EK, Lee DW, Lam YH, Chung SC (1998) A randomized comparison of acute phase response and endotoxemia in patients with perforated peptic ulcers receiving laparoscopic or open patch repair. Am J Surg 175:325–327
31. Vaidya BB, Garg CP et al (2009) Laparoscopic repair of perforated peptic ulcer with delayed presentation. J Laparoendosc Adv Surg Tech A 19(2):153–156
32. Schietroma M, Piccione F, Carlei F, Sista F, Cecilia EM, Amicucci G (2013) Peritonitis from perforated peptic ulcer and immune response. J Invest Surg 26:294–304
33. Buck DL, Vester-Andersen M, Moller MH (2013) Danish clinical register of emergency surgery surgical delay is a critical determinant of survival in perforated peptic ulcer. Br J Surg 100(8):1045–1049
34. Teoh AYB, Chiu PWY, Kok ASY, Wong SKH, Ng EKW (2015) The selective use of laparoscopic repair is safe in high-risk patients suffering from perforated peptic ulcer. World J Surg 39:740–745
35. Søreide K, Thorsen K, Søreide JA (2014) Strategies to improve the outcome of emergency surgery for perforated peptic ulcer. Br J Surg 101(1):e51–e64
36. Guglielminotti P, Bini R, Fontana D, Leli R (2009) Laparoscopic repair for perforated peptic ulcers with U-CLIP. World J Emerg Surg 4:28
37. Darzi A, Chesire NJ, Somers SS (1993) Laparoscopic omental patch repair with an automated stapler. Br J Surg 80:1552
38. Costalat G, Alquier Y (1995) Combined laparoscopic and endoscopic treatment of perforated gastroduodenal ulcers using the ligamentum teres hepatis. Surg Endosc 9:677–679
39. Lau WY, Leung KL, Kwong KH, Davey C, Robertson C, Dawson JJ, Chung SC, Li AK (1996) A randomized study comparing laparoscopic versus open repair of perforated peptic ulcer using suture or sutureless technique. Ann Surg 224(2):131–138
40. Tate JJT, Dawson JW, Lau WY et al (1993) Sutureless laparoscopic treatment of perforated duodenal ulcer. Br J Surg 80:235
41. Jackson N, Waters E (2005) Criteria for the systematic review of health promotion and public health interventions. Health Promotion Int 20:367–374
42. Sanabria AE, Morales CH, Villegas MI (2005) Laparoscopic repair for perforated peptic ulcer disease. Cochrane Database Syst Rev (4):CD004778
43. Sanabria AE, Morales CH, Villegas MI (2005) Laparoscopic repair for perforated peptic ulcer disease. The Cochrane Library, Issue 4, Updated 2013

44. Druart ML, Van Hee R, Etienne J et al (1997) Laparoscopic repair of perforated duodenal ulcer. A prospective multicenter clinical trial. Surg Endosc 11(10):1017–1020
45. Siu WT, Chau CH, Law BKB, Tang CN, Ha PY, Li MKW (2004) Routine use of laparoscopic repair for perforated peptic ulcer. Br J Surg 91:481–484
46. Cellan-Jones CJ (1929) A rapid method of treatment in perforated duodenal ulcer. BMJ 1:1076–1077
47. Petrowsky H, Demartines N, Rousson V, Clavien PA (2004) Evidence-based value of prophylactic drainage in gastrointestinal surgery. A systematic review and meta-analyses. Ann Surg 240:1074–1085
48. Wilhelmsen M, Møller MH, Rosenstock S (2015) Surgical complications after open and laparoscopic surgery for perforated peptic ulcer in a nationwide cohort. Br J Surg 102(4):382–387. doi:10.1002/bjs.9753, Epub 2015 Jan 21
49. Bucher P, Oulbaci W, Morel P, Ris F, Huber O (2007) Results of conservative treatment for perforated gastroduodenal ulcer in patients not eligible for surgical repair. Swiss Med Wkly 137:337–340
50. Adachi Y, Mori M, Maehara Y, Matsumata T, Okudaira Y, Sugimachi K (1997) Surgical results of perforated gastric carcinoma: an analysis of 155 Japanese patients. Am J Gastroenterol 92(3):516–518
51. Roviello F, Rossi S, Marrelli D, De Manzoni G, Pedrazzani C, Morgagni P, Corso G, Pinto E (2006) Perforated gastric carcinoma: a report of 10 cases and review of the literature. World J Surg Oncol 4:19
52. Lehnert T, Buhl K, Dueck M, Hinz U, Herfart C (2000) Two-staged radical gastrectomy for perforated gastric cancer. Eur J Surg Oncol 26:780–784
53. Gertsch P, Yip SK, Chow LW, Launder IJ (1995) Free perforation of gastric carcinoma. Arch Surg 130:177–181
54. Lunevicius R, Morkevicius M (2005) Comparison of laparoscopic versus open repair for perforated duodenal ulcers. Surg Endosc 19:1565–1571
55. Antoniou SA, Antoniou GA, Koch OO, Pointner R, Granderath FA (2013) Meta-analysis of laparoscopic versus open repair of perforated peptic ulcer. JSLS 17(1):15–22
56. Taylor H (1957) The non-surgical treatment of perforated peptic ulcer. Gastroenterology 33:353–368
57. Crofts TJ, Park KG, Steele RJ, Chung SS, Li AK (1989) A randomized trial of nonoperative treatment for perforated peptic ulcer. N Engl J Med 320(15):970–973
58. Songne B, Jean F, Foulatier O, Khalil H, Scottè M (2004) Non operative treatment for perforated peptic ulcer: result of a prospective study. Ann Chir 129(10):578–582
59. Di Saverio S, Bassi M, Smerieri N, Masetti M, Ferrara F, Fabbri C, Ansaloni L, Ghersi S, Serenari M, Coccolini F, Naidoo N, Sartelli M, Tugnoli G, Catena F, Cennamo V, Jovine E (2014) Diagnosis and treatment of perforated or bleeding peptic ulcers: 2013 WSES position paper. World J Emerg Surg 9:45
60. Bonin EA, Moran E, Gostout CJ, McConico AL, Zielinski M, Bingener J (2012) Natural orifice transluminal endoscopic surgery for patients with perforated peptic ulcer. Surg Endosc 26:1534–1538
61. Bingener J, Loomis EA, Gostout J, Zielinski MD, Buttar NS, Song LM, Baron TH, Ghahfarokhi LS, Rajan E (2013) Feasibility of NOTES omental plug repair of perforated peptic ulcers: results from a clinical pilot trial. Surg Endosc 27(6):2201–2208
62. Liu L, Chiu PW, Lam PK, Poon CC, Lam CC, Ng EK, Lai PB (2015) Effect of local injection of mesenchymal stem cells on healing of sutured gastric perforation in an experimental model. Br J Surg 102(2):e158–e168
63. Søreide K, Thorsen K, Harrison EM, Bingener J, Møller MH, Ohene-Yeboah M, Søreide JA (2015) Perforated peptic ulcer. Lancet 386(10000):1288–1298

8 Emergency Lapararoscopy for Colon Obstruction and Acute Diverticulitis

Alberto Arezzo, Marco E. Allaix, Mario Campli, Carlo Bergamini, and Ferdinando Agresta

8.1 Acute Colon Obstruction

8.1.1 Introduction

About 30 % of patients with colorectal cancer present with acute colon obstruction requiring an emergent treatment [1]. There are several surgical options and the choice among these options depends on several factors: tumor location, clinical condition, surgeon expertise, and intraoperative surgical findings.

The different surgical options include:

1. *Colon resection and end colostomy (so-called Hartmann procedure).* This approach is most frequently performed for obstructive left-sided colon cancers, although colostomy reversal is performed in much less than 50 % of patients [2];
2. *Subtotal colectomy and primary ileorectal anastomosis.* It is the alternative to the Hartmann procedure avoiding the need for a loop oostomy and treating in one stage possible synchronous cancers [3];
3. *Loop oostomy followed by colorectal resection.* Currently, this two- or three-staged strategy is reserved to obstructive extraperitoneal rectal cancers to allow neoadjuvant chemoradiation therapy before resection [4];

A. Arezzo, MD, PhD (✉) • M.E. Allaix, MD
Department of Surgical Sciences, University of Torino, Torino, Italy
e-mail: alberto.arezzo@gmail.com; alberto.arezzo@unito.it

M. Campli, MD
Division of Surgery, "Nuova Itor" Private Health Facility, Roma, Italy

C. Bergamini, MD
General, Emergency and Mini-invasive Surgery, Careggi Hospital, Firenze, Italy

F. Agresta, MD
Department of General Surgery, Azienda ULSS19 del Veneto, Adria (RO), Italy

F. Agresta et al. (eds.), *Emergency Laparoscopy*,
DOI 10.1007/978-3-319-29620-3_8

4. *Colon resection with intraoperative washout and primary anastomosis.* This strategy is still quite common in the USA despite it is still missing evidence that intraoperative lavage significantly reduces the risk of postoperative anastomotic leakage [5].

Acute colon obstruction is considered by many an absolute contraindication to the laparoscopic approach. As a consequence, this surgery is mainly performed by an open approach and is associated with significant perioperative mortality, postoperative morbidity, and impaired quality of life [6].

However, the progressive diffusion of the laparoscopic approach to both benign and malignant colorectal diseases and the development of endoluminal stenting is challenging this practice.

8.1.2 Laparoscopic Right Hemicolectomy

Surgery is the standard of care for the treatment of right-sided obstructive colon cancer as this is achieved in a single-stage procedure with no need of protective ileostomy in the vast majority of cases. Elective laparoscopic right hemicolectomy is a well-established procedure for the treatment of right colon cancer, with significantly reduced early postoperative morbidity and mortality. Arezzo [7] has recently published the results of a systematic review and meta-analysis of studies comparing elective laparoscopic and open right hemicolectomy having as primary endpoints 30-day mortality and overall morbidity. Twenty-seven studies were included, representing 3049 patients although only 2 were randomized controlled trials (RCTs) for a total of 211 patients. Mortality was significantly lower after laparoscopic surgery (1.2 % vs. 3.4 %, $p = 0.031$) as well as the raw incidence of overall complications (16.8 % vs. 24.2 %; $p = 0.007$).

Data about emergent laparoscopic right hemicolectomy for obstructing right-sided colon cancer are lacking. The only study published in the literature is the one by Ng [8]. This is a retrospective study comparing 14 patients who underwent emergency laparoscopic-assisted right hemicolectomy and 29 treated by open right hemicolectomy for obstructing right-sided colon cancer. Both groups were similar in terms of age, gender, comorbidities, duration of symptoms, tumor size, and pathological staging. Laparoscopic resection was associated with prolonged operative time (187.5 min vs. 145 min; $p = 0.034$) and reduced intraoperative blood losses (20 vs. 100 ml; $p = 0.020$) when compared to open surgery. Full patients' mobilization occurred 2 days earlier after laparoscopic right hemicolectomy (4 vs. 6 days, $p = 0.016$). No differences were observed in time to resumption of normal diet, time to return to gastrointestinal functions, and length of hospital stay. A higher morbidity rate was observed after open surgery, but the difference despite consistent did not reach statistical significance (55.2 % vs. 28.6 %, $p = 0.119$). The interpretation of the results of this study is limited by the retrospective nature, the small sample size, and the lack of long-term oncologic outcomes. Larger and RCTs are needed to investigate the role of laparoscopic surgery in the emergent treatment of obstructing right-sided colon cancers.

8.1.3 Laparoscopic Left Hemicolectomy

Emergent open Hartmann procedure, subtotal colectomy, and colon resection with intraoperative washout and primary anastomosis are all procedures proposed for the treatment of left-sided obstructive colon cancer, but burdened by high postoperative morbidity and mortality rates and concerns for quality of life and often need of loop oostomy [6].

The insertion of a self-expandable metallic stent (SEMS) has been proposed for the relief of colon obstruction in 1990 by Dohmoto [9], initially with palliative intent in patients with unresectable locally advanced tumor, metastatic disease, or at high operative risk, aiming to avoid an emergent operation and the surgery-related morbidity.

Consequently, this approach has been proposed as a "bridge to surgery" strategy in patients with resectable but obstructing colon cancer [10], the insertion of SEMS allowing for postponed elective surgery and its benefits [11, 12]. There is actually no more controversial topic than this with two RCTs [13, 14] stopped for evidence of superiority of emergency surgery and one [15] stopped vice versa for evidence of superiority of the SEMS bridge to surgery strategy. Still, a temptative meta-analysis by Huang [16] showed despite high heterogeneity that SEMS insertion followed by elective surgery improves the rates of one-stage surgery, increases the rates of primary anastomosis, and reduces the rates of stoma creation and wound infections, while overall short-term mortality and morbidity, anastomotic leakage rates, and intra-abdominal complication rates do not significantly vary between groups. These data, although limited by the heterogeneity of the RCTs published in the literature, show that SEMS placement is a safe and effective procedure in the "bridge to surgery" strategy. In addition, it seems to be associated with earlier adjuvant chemotherapy administration [17, 18]. To explain why so different results were achieved by the various different studies it has to be noticed that the expertise of endoscopists and their case load in those studies that were stopped for advantage of emergency surgery were critical and possibly criticized. At the same time in those studies in which Hartmann's procedure was usually performed in the emergency surgery group, not always Hartmann's reversal procedure was considered when considering complications of surgery. On the other side, the considerably low rate of reversal procedures allows us to say that Hartmann's procedure and SEMS insertion as bridge to surgery have different objectives.

After the first report of laparoscopic-assisted colectomy in 1991 [19], many studies have shown the short-term benefits of laparoscopic resection when compared with open resection for uncomplicated colon cancer, including reduced intraoperative blood loss and postoperative pain, lower complication rates, shorter length of hospital stay, and reduced costs [20–23]. Based on this high-quality evidence, the use of laparoscopy has been proposed in the early 2000s as the second step of the "bridge to surgery" strategy. The SEMS placement relieves bowel distension, thus allowing to create the working space for the laparoscopic procedure and minimizing the risk of intestinal injury that is increased in the presence of dilated and fragile bowel. For instance, Morino [24] reported in 2002 the short-term outcomes in four patients with colon obstruction secondary to left-sided colon cancer. Laparoscopic colon resection was performed 4–5 days after the SEMS placement. No patient experienced postoperative complications and all patients were discharged 5–7 days after laparoscopic resection.

More recently, few studies (Table 8.1) have shown the advantages of combining these two minimally invasive procedures. Balagué [25] described the outcomes in six patients undergoing SEMS insertion followed by laparoscopic colon resection. Conversion to open surgery was necessary in one patient due to adhesions, while conversion to hand-assisted surgery was necessary in one case for challenging dissection of the tumor and the mobilization of the splenic flexure. Median interval between SEMS placement and surgery was 8 days (range 5–14). Postoperative morbidity rate was 16.7 %, including a perianastomotic collection that required a percutaneous drainage. Similarly, Dulucq [26] reported, in 2006, the results in 10 patients diagnosed with acute colon obstruction and treated with SEMS followed by laparoscopic surgery: they observed one case (10 %) of anastomotic leakage that was treated by laparoscopic drainage and loop ileostomy. Chung [27] analyzed 17 patients. All procedures were completed laparoscopically: an Hartmann procedure was performed in two cases (11.8 %), while a diverting ileostomy was created in a patient undergoing anterior resection. Postoperative morbidity rate was 11.8 %. Similar results were obtained by others [18, 28].

A word of caution comes from a recent comparative study on long-term oncologic outcomes. Sabbagh [29] has retrospectively analyzed survival in 48 patients undergoing SEMS and 39 patients treated by emergency surgery. Five-year overall survival and 5-year cancer-specific mortality were significantly worse in the SEMS group, even though a higher number of lymph nodes were harvested in the SEMS group and these patients had a better access to adjuvant chemotherapy. No significant differences between the two groups were observed in 5-year disease-free survival, recurrence rate, and mean time to recurrence. In the multivariable analysis, SEMS insertion was independently correlated with overall survival. The analysis of patients with no metastasis and no colon perforation showed similar worse oncologic outcomes in the SEMS patients compared to the patients undergoing emergency surgery. To justify this, a possible mechanism of cancer cell spreading was advocated [30]. This confirms in a way the hypothesis of Kim [31] who showed in a case-matched study that SEMS insertion had an adverse effect on the 5-year overall survival rate (38.4 % vs. 65.6 %; $p = 0.025$) and the 5-year disease-free survival rate (48.3 % vs. 75.5 %; $p = 0.024$). Nevertheless, it is unclear what magnitude of this effect is related to the underlying obstruction rather than to the SEMS. No other report of long-term results is present in the literature, although necessary to clarify the crucial aspect of oncologic adequacy.

Table 8.1 SEMS and laparoscopic colon resection: data from the literature

Author	Typeof study	*n*	Interval between SEMS and surgery (days)	Stoma (%)	Conversion to open surgery (%)	Early postoperative morbidity (%)	Hospital stay (days)
Morino [24]	R	4	5 (4–5)	0	0	0	7 (5–7)
Balagué [25]	R	6	8 (5–14)	0	16.7 open	16.7	6.5 (5–12)
					16.7 hand-assisted		
Dulucq [26]	P	14	6.5 ± 2	0	0	10	16.4 ± 5[a]
Chung [27]	R	17	7 (2–11)	17.6	0	11.8	9 (7–49)
Stipa [28]	R	6	16.5 (6–18)	0	0	0	7
Lujan [18]	R	12	19 (4–60)	8.3	0	NA	NA

R retrospective, *P* prospective, *NA* not available
[a]Total hospital stay between admission and discharge

8.1.4 Conclusions

The current evidence shows that elective laparoscopic colon resection could be safely performed in patients who had previous successful SEMS insertion, with negligible intraoperative complications, very low stoma rates, and limited postoperative morbidity. However, further larger RCTs including long-term oncologic results are needed to confirm these data and to verify oncologic adequacy.

Based on the little evidence currently available, the European Society for Gastrointestinal Endoscopy has recently published new guidelines for the use of SEMS for obstructing colonic and extracolonic cancer [32, 33] that can be summarized in the following four recommendations:

- Prophylactic colonic metal stent placement is not recommended and should be reserved for symptomatic patients with imaging evidence of obstruction
- Colonic metal stent placement as a bridge to elective surgery is not recommended.
- Colonic metal stent placement is an alternative to emergency surgery only in case of increased risk of postoperative mortality.
- Colonic metal stent placement is recommended as the preferred treatment for palliation.

This seems supported by very weak data and should be applied with caution.

The results of two ongoing RCTs comparing SEMS as "bridge to surgery" and emergency surgery for left-sided colonic malignant obstruction are expected to better clarify the oncologic impact of this minimally invasive strategy: the Colorectal Stent Trial (CreST) [34] and the ESCO trial [35]. Both studies have closed recruitment recently and publication of results is now awaited.

8.2 Acute Diverticulitis

8.2.1 Introduction

The Hinchey classification is the most common grading system used for the classification and treatment of complicated diverticulitis [36]. While Hinchey grade I and II patients are successfully managed in most cases by conservative treatment, surgery is needed in the presence of peritonitis secondary to perforated diverticulitis (grades III and IV according to Hinchey classification).

The traditional surgical treatment of Hinchey III and IV patients includes open sigmoid colon resection with end colostomy and left hemicolectomy with primary anastomosis with or without diverting stoma. Early postoperative mortality rate is about 10–20 % after both sigmoid resection and end colostomy and resection and primary anastomosis. In addition, up to 70 % of patients undergoing nonrestorative resection do not have their colostomy reversed and the anastomotic leakage rate reported in the literature after primary anastomosis is as high as 14 % [37, 38].

In 1996, a minimally invasive approach to patients with Hinchey III diverticulitis based on intravenous antibiotics and laparoscopic peritoneal lavage was proposed to avoid urgent resective surgery, and stoma creation including their high morbidity and mortality [39]. Since then, several studies have challenged both indications and outcomes of the laparoscopic peritoneal lavage in Hinchey III patients [40–57].

8.2.2 Laparoscopic Peritoneal Lavage

This minimally invasive approach to perforated diverticulitis was first proposed by O'Sullivan [39] in 1996. The rationale was that "*in the vast majority of patients with generalized peritonitis secondary to perforated diverticular disease, there is no evidence of fecal contamination, and the perforation is already sealed or cannot be found at surgery*" [58]. They retrospectively reviewed the outcomes in eight patients with generalized peritonitis secondary to perforated diverticular disease of the left colon that was diagnosed laparoscopically and treated by laparoscopic peritoneal lavage and administration of parenteral fluids and antibiotics. All patients had diffuse purulent peritonitis with no fecal contamination. No patients developed postoperative surgical complications. Full normal diet was resumed in all patients within 5–8 days. Mean postoperative hospital stay was 10 days (range, 7–17). Two patients were readmitted to the hospital at 4 and 8 months after the laparoscopic peritoneal lavage with lower quadrant abdominal pain; both patients were treated conservatively. No surgical intervention was required during the follow-up, ranging from 12 to 48 months. Similar results were reported by other small retrospective studies [40, 42].

The first large multicenter prospective study was published by Myers in 2008 [47]. They included 100 patients preoperatively diagnosed with generalized peritonitis undergoing attempted laparoscopic peritoneal lavage. Primary endpoints were operative success and resolution of symptoms. Eight patients with Hinchey IV diverticulitis had conversion to open Hartmann's procedure. The remaining 92 patients underwent laparoscopic peritoneal lavage. The postoperative medical complication rate was 4 % (lower respiratory tract infection, acute myocardial infarction, and pulmonary embolism). Pelvic abscesses occurred in two patients: one patient underwent radiological percutaneous drainage, while the other required an open Hartmann's procedure. The postoperative mortality rate was 3 %, including multiorgan failure in two patients and pulmonary embolism in one. During a median follow-up of 36 (range 12–84) months, two patients were readmitted with acute diverticulitis treated by intravenous antibiotics. No patient required reintervention. The authors concluded that laparoscopic management of perforated diverticulitis with generalized peritonitis is an alternative to open surgery, with low postoperative morbidity and low risk of recurrence in the short term.

Since 2008, several papers have been published on the feasibility and efficacy of laparoscopic peritoneal lavage for the treatment of diffuse peritonitis secondary to perforated diverticulitis. Cirocchi [59] recently published a systematic review of those studies aiming to evaluate the outcomes of this minimally invasive strategy, having as primary outcome for this systematic review the success rate of laparoscopic peritoneal lavage. This was defined as the rate of patients alive without surgical treatment for a recurrent episode of diverticulitis or complication from diverticular disease. Of the 19 articles published between 1996 and 2013, 10 were cohort studies, 8 case series, and 1 controlled clinical trial for a total of 871 patients analyzed with up to 96 months of follow-up. The success rate of laparoscopic peritoneal lavage was 24.3 %. The overall conversion rate for Hinchey III and Hinchey IV patients was 1 % and 45 %, respectively. The 30-day postoperative mortality rate was 2.9 % as a result of multiple organ failure for sepsis and pulmonary embolism. The 30-day postoperative reintervention (surgery or percutaneous drainage) rate was 3.8 %: most common causes were sepsis from generalized peritonitis or intra-abdominal abscess and colonic fistula The hospital readmission rate after the laparoscopic peritoneal lavage was 3.4 %: main reasons were recurrent diverticular phlegmon, generalized peritonitis, colo-vesical fistula, missing colon cancer, inflammatory colonic stenosis, and pelvic abscess. A reintervention (colon resection or percutaneous drainage) was necessary in 19 (63.3 %) of the 30 patients readmitted to the hospital. Elective laparoscopic sigmoid resection was performed in 35.8 % of patients. The timing of the laparoscopic procedure varied greatly, ranging from 2 weeks to 21 months from the laparoscopic peritoneal lavage. In this group of patients, the conversion rate to open surgery was 4.2 %. It has to be pointed out that the technique of laparoscopic lavage is not yet standardized so that there was a vast heterogeneity among the included studies, even in considering the criteria for a further routine sigmoidectomy after resolution of the acute phase.

Four RCTs have been initiated to better define the role of laparoscopic peritoneal lavage in patients with purulent peritonitis secondary to perforated diverticulitis. A few months ago, short-term results of the DILALA trial were published showing feasibility and safety of laparoscopic lavage as treatment for patients with Hinchey III diverticulitis [60]. A total of 83 patients with purulent peritonitis were randomized. Some 39 patients undergoing laparoscopic peritoneal lavage and 36 treated by an Hartmann procedure were available for analysis. Similar early postoperative morbidity and mortality rates were found in the two groups. Patients undergoing laparoscopic lavage had a shorter operative time and shorter hospital stay. On the other side, concerns have been risen about the use of laparoscopic lavage even in selected patients after results of the LADIES trial and SCANDIV trial were presented. The LADIES trial was the largest study on peritoneal lavage designed. Patients with purulent peritonitis were randomized to laparoscopic lavage and drainage, sigmoidectomy with primary anastomosis, and sigmoidectomy with end colostomy in a 2:1:1 ratio. Recruitment was stopped early for the laparoscopic lavage and drainage arm due to safety issues, while the two other arms are still continuing the recruitment [61, 62].

The SCANDIV trial [63] is a multicenter, randomized clinical superiority trial comparing the outcomes in patients undergoing laparoscopic lavage (101) or colon resection (98) for perforated diverticulitis. Ninety-day severe postoperative complication rates (Clavien Dindo > IIIa) were similar in the laparoscopic lavage and colon resection groups (30.7 % vs. 26 %, $p = 0.53$). Ninety-day mortality rates did not significantly differ between the two groups (12.9 % vs. 11.5 %, $p = 0.67$). The reoperation rate was significantly higher after the laparoscopic lavage (20.3 %) than after colon resection (5.7 %) ($p = 0.01$). Operative time was significantly shorter in the laparoscopic lavage group; length of postoperative hospital stay and quality of life did not differ significantly between groups. Four sigmoid cancers were missed with laparoscopic lavage. The results of this study do not support the use of laparoscopic lavage for the treatment of perforated diverticulitis since it is not associated with better postoperative outcomes than colon resection.

The long-term results of the DILALA trials and the results of the other ongoing randomized controlled trial (LAPLAND [64] trial) are needed to more clearly establish the role of laparoscopic peritoneal lavage in the treatment of patients with purulent peritonitis secondary to acute perforated diverticulitis.

8.2.3 Conclusions

According to the evidence currently available in the literature, laparoscopic peritoneal lavage should be considered an option for the treatment of purulent peritonitis secondary to perforated diverticulitis. In addition, the laparoscopic exploration of the peritoneal cavity helps to categorize the patients and better plan the surgical approach. However, the quality of evidence is still quite low; therefore, despite promising results, it seems too early to recommend the routine use of laparoscopic peritoneal lavage in clinical practice. As stated by the American Society of Colon and Rectal Surgeons (ASCRS) [65], *"the poor quality of the existing literature on peritoneal lavage in aggregate and the inherent selection bias in the literature are major obstacles in advocating the widespread adoption of the laparoscopic lavage; the safety of lavage for purulent or fecal peritonitis has not been proven or disproven by the published studies to date."*

Conflict of Interest The authors have no conflicts of interest to declare.

References

1. Landis SH, Murray T, Bolden S, Wingo PA (1998) Cancer statistics, 1998. CA Cancer J Clin 48(1):6–29
2. van de Wall BJ, Draaisma WA, Schouten ES, Broeders IA, Consten EC (2010) Conventional and laparoscopic reversal of the Hartmann procedure: a review of literature. J Gastrointest Surg 14(4):743–752
3. The SCOTIA Study Group (1995) Single-stage treatment for malignant left-sided colonic obstruction: a prospective randomized clinical trial comparing subtotal colectomy with segmental resection following intraoperative irrigation. Br J Surg 82:1622–1627

4. Frago R, Ramirez E, Millan M, Kreisler E, del Valle E, Biondo S (2014) Current management of acute malignant large bowel obstruction: a systematic review. Am J Surg 207:127–138
5. Ortiz H, Biondo S, Ciga MA, Kreisler E, Oteiza F, Fraccalvieri D (2009) Comparative study to determine the need for intraoperative colonic irrigation for primary anastomosis in left-sided colonic emergencies. Colorectal Dis 11:648–652
6. De Salvo GL, Gava C, Pucciarelli S, Lise M (2004) Curative surgery for obstruction from primary left colorectal carcinoma: primary or staged resection? Cochrane Database Syst Rev 2, CD002101
7. Arezzo A, Passera R, Ferri V, Gonella F, Cirocchi R, Morino M (2015) Laparoscopic right colectomy reduces short-term mortality and morbidity. Results of a systematic review and meta-analysis. Int J Colorectal Dis 30(11):1457–1472
8. Ng SS, Lee JF, Yiu RY, Li JC, Leung WW, Leung KL (2008) Emergency laparoscopic-assisted versus open right hemicolectomy for obstructing right-sided colonic carcinoma: a comparative study of short-term clinical outcomes. World J Surg 32(3):454–458
9. Dohmoto M, Rupp KD, Hohlbach G (1990) Endoscopically-implanted prosthesis in rectal carcinoma (article in German). Dtsch Med Wochenschr 15:915
10. Tejero E, Mainar A, Fernández L, Tobío R, De Gregorio MA (1994) New procedure for the treatment of colorectal neoplastic obstructions. Dis Colon Rectum 37(11):1158–1159
11. Baron TH, Dean PA, Yates MR III, Canon C, Koehler RE (1998) Expandable metal stents for the treatment of colonic obstruction: techniques and outcomes. Gastrointest Endosc 47:277–286
12. Mainar A, De Gregorio Ariza MA, Tejero E, Tobio R, Alfonso E, Pinto I, Herrera M, Fernández JA (1999) Acute colorectal obstruction: treatment with self-expandable metallic stents before scheduled surgery—results of a multicenter study. Radiology 210:65–69
13. van Hooft JE, Bemelman WA, Oldenburg B, Marinelli AW, Lutke Holzik MF, Grubben MJ, Sprangers MA, Dijkgraaf MG, Fockens P, Collaborative Dutch Stent-in study group (2011) Colonic stenting versus emergency surgery for acute left-sided malignant colonic obstruction: a multicentre randomised trial. Lancet Oncol 12:344–352
14. Pirlet A, Slim K, Kwiatkowski F, Michot F, Millat BL (2011) Emergency preoperative stenting versus surgery for acute left-sided malignant colonic obstruction: a multicenter randomized controlled trial. Surg Endosc 25:1814–1821
15. Alcántara M, Serra-Aracil X, Falcó J, Mora L, Bombardó J, Navarro S (2011) Prospective, controlled, randomized study of intraoperative colonic lavage versus stent placement in obstructive left-sided colonic cancer. World J Surg 35:1904–1910
16. Huang X, Lv B, Zhang S, Meng L (2014) Preoperative colonic stents versus emergency surgery for acute left-sided malignant colonic obstruction: a meta-analysis. J Gastrointest Surg 18:584–591
17. Karoui M, Charachon A, Delbaldo C, Karoui M, Charachon A, Delbaldo C, Loriau J, Laurent A, Sobhani I, Tran Van Nhieu J, Delchier JC, Fagniez PL, Piedbois P, Cherqui D (2007) Stents for palliation of obstructive metastatic colon cancer: impact on management and chemotherapy administration. Arch Surg 142:619–623
18. Lujan HJ, Barbosa G, Zeichen MS, Mata WN, Maciel V, Plasencia G, Hartmann RF, Viamonte M III, Fogel R (2013) Self-expanding metallic stents for palliation and as a bridge to minimally invasive surgery in colorectal obstruction. JSLS 17:204–211
19. Jacobs M, Verdeja JC, Goldstein HS (1991) Minimally invasive colon resection (laparoscopic colectomy). Surg Laparosc Endosc 1:144–150
20. Lacy AM, Garcia-Valdecasas JC, Delgado S, Castells A, Taurá P, Piqu JM, Visa J (2002) Laparoscopy-assisted colectomy versus open colectomy for treatment of non-metastatic colon cancer: a randomised trial. Lancet 359:2224–2229
21. Clinical Outcomes of Surgical Therapy Study Group (2004) A comparison of laparoscopically assisted and open colectomy for colon cancer. N Engl J Med 350:2050–2059

22. Guillou PJ, Quirke P, Thorpe H, Walker J, Jayne DG, Smith AM, Heath RM, Brown JM, MRC CLASICC trial group (2005) Short-term endpoints of conventional versus laparoscopic-assisted surgery in patients with colorectal cancer (MRC CLASICC trial): multicentre, randomised controlled trial. Lancet 365:1718–1726
23. Veldkamp R, Kuhry E, Hop WC, Jeekel J, Kazemier G, Bonjer HJ, Haglind E, Påhlman L, Cuesta MA, Msika S, Morino M, Lacy AM, COlon cancer Laparoscopic or Open Resection Study Group(COLOR) (2005) Laparoscopic surgery versus open surgery for colon cancer: short-term outcomes of a randomised trial. Lancet Oncol 6:477–484
24. Morino M, Bertello A, Garbarini A, Rozzio G, Repici A (2002) Malignant colonic obstruction managed by endoscopic stent decompression followed by laparoscopic resection. Surg Endosc 16:1483–1487
25. Balagué C, Targarona EM, Sainz S, Montero O, Bendahat G, Kobus C, Garriga J, Gonzalez D, Pujol J, Trias M (2004) Minimally invasive treatment for obstructive tumors of the left colon: endoluminal self-expanding metal stent and laparoscopic colectomy. Preliminary results. Dig Surg 21:282–286
26. Dulucq JL, Wintringer P, Beyssac R, Barberis C, Talbi P, Mahajna A (2006) One-stage laparoscopic colorectal resection after placement of self-expanding metallic stents for colorectal obstruction. Dig Dis Sci 51:2365–2371
27. Chung TS, Lim SB, Sohn DK, Hong CW, Han KS, Choi HS, Jeong SY (2008) Feasibility of single-stage laparoscopic resection after placement of a self-expandable metallic stent for obstructive left colorectal cancer. World J Surg 32:2275–2280
28. Stipa F, Pigazzi A, Bascone B, Cimitan A, Villotti G, Burza A, Vitale A (2008) Management of obstructive colorectal cancer with endoscopic stenting followed by single-stage surgery: open or laparoscopic resection? Surg Endosc 22:1477–1481
29. Sabbagh C, Browet F, Diouf M, Cosse C, Brehant O, Bartoli E, Mauvais F, Chauffert B, Dupas JL, Nguyen-Khac E, Regimbeau JM (2013) Is stenting as "a bridge to surgery" an oncologically safe strategy for the management of acute, left-sided, malignant, colonic obstruction? A comparative study with a propensity score analysis. Ann Surg 258(1):107–115
30. Maruthachalam K, Lash GE, Shenton BK, Horgan AF (2007) Tumour cell dissemination following endoscopic stent insertion. Br J Surg 94(9):1151–1154
31. Kim JS, Hur H, Min BS, Sohn SK, Cho CH, Kim NK (2009) Oncologic outcomes of self-expanding metallic stent insertion as a bridge to surgery in the management of left-sided colon cancer obstruction: comparison with non-obstructing elective surgery. World J Surg 33:1281–1286
32. van Hooft JE, van Halsema EE, Vanbiervliet G, Beets-Tan RG, DeWitt JM, Donnellan F, Dumonceau JM, Glynne-Jones RG, Hassan C, Jiménez-Perez J, Meisner S, Muthusamy VR, Parker MC, Regimbeau JM, Sabbagh C, Sagar J, Tanis PJ, Vandervoort J, Webster GJ, Manes G, Barthet MA, Repici A, European Society of Gastrointestinal Endoscopy (2014) Self-expandable metal stents for obstructing colonic and extracolonic cancer: European Society of Gastrointestinal Endoscopy (ESGE) Clinical Guideline. Endoscopy 46(11):990–1053
33. van Hooft JE, van Halsema EE, Vanbiervliet G, Beets-Tan RG, DeWitt JM, Donnellan F, Dumonceau JM, Glynne-Jones RG, Hassan C, Jiménez-Perez J, Meisner S, Muthusamy VR, Parker MC, Regimbeau JM, Sabbagh C, Sagar J, Tanis PJ, Vandervoort J, Webster GJ, Manes G, Barthet MA, Repici A, European Society of Gastrointestinal Endoscopy (ESGE) (2014) Self-expandable metal stents for obstructing colonic and extracolonic cancer: European Society of Gastrointestinal Endoscopy (ESGE) Clinical Guideline. Gastrointest Endosc 80(5):747–761.e1–75
34. Group CCCS (2009) The role of endoluminal stenting in the acute management of obstructing colorectal cancer. Available from: http://www.birmingham.ac.uk/Documents/college-mds/trials/bctu/crest/CReSTProtocolv2116072009.pdf
35. Enteral Stents for Colonic Obstruction (ESCO). Available from: http://clinicaltrials.gov/ct2/show/NCT00591695
36. Hinchey EJ, Schaal PG, Richards GK (1978) Treatment of perforated diverticular disease of the colon. Adv Surg 12:85–109

37. Toorenvliet BR, Swank H, Schoones JW, Hamming JF, Bemelman WA (2010) Laparoscopic peritoneal lavage for perforated colonic diverticulitis: a systematic review. Colorectal Dis 12:862–867
38. Salem L, Flum DR (2004) Primary anastomosis or Hartmann's procedure for patients with diverticular peritonitis? A systematic review. Dis Colon Rectum 47:1953–1964
39. O'Sullivan GC, Murphy D, O'Brien MG, Ireland A (1996) Laparoscopic management of generalized peritonitis due to perforated colonic diverticula. Am J Surg 171:432–434
40. Faranda C, Barrat C, Catheline JM, Champault GG (2000) Two-stages laparoscopic management of generalized peritonitis due to perforated sigmoid diverticula: eighteen cases. Surg Laparosc Endosc Percutan Tech 10:135–138
41. Da Rold AR, Guerriero S, Fiamingo P, Pariset S, Veroux M, Pilon F, Tosato S, Ruffolo C, Tedeschi U (2004) Laparoscopic colorrhaphy, irrigation and drainage in the treatment of complicated acute diverticulitis: initial experience. Chir Ital 56:95–98
42. Taylor CJ, Layani L, Ghusn MA, White SI (2006) Perforated diverticulitis managed by laparoscopic lavage. ANZ J Surg 76:962–965
43. Mutter D, Bouras G, Forgione A, Vix M, Leroy J, Marescaux J (2006) Two-stage totally minimally invasive approach for acute complicated diverticulitis. Colorectal Dis 8:501–505
44. Galleano R, Di Giorgi S, Franceschi A, Falchero F (2007) Two-stage laparoscopic management of complicated acute diverticulitis. Initial experience. Ann Ital Chir 78:61–64
45. Bretagnol F, Pautrat K, Mor C, Benchellal Z, Huten N, de Calan L (2008) Emergency laparoscopic management of perforated sigmoid diverticulitis: a promising alternative to more radical procedures. J Am Coll Surg 206:654–657
46. Franklin ME Jr, Portillo G, Trevino JM, Gonzalez JJ, Glass JL (2008) Long-term experience with the laparoscopic approach to perforated diverticulitis plus generalized peritonitis. World J Surg 32:1507–1511
47. Myers E, Hurley M, O'Sullivan GC, Kavanagh D, Wilson I, Winter DC (2008) Laparoscopic peritoneal lavage for generalized peritonitis due to perforated diverticulitis. Br J Surg 95:97–101
48. Karoui M, Champault A, Pautrat K, Valleur P, Cherqui D, Champault G (2009) Laparoscopic peritoneal lavage or primary anastomosis with defunctioning stoma for Hinchey 3 complicated diverticulitis: results of a comparative study. Dis Colon Rectum 52:609–615
49. Favuzza J, Friel JC, Kelly JJ, Perugini R, Counihan TC (2009) Benefits of laparoscopic peritoneal lavage for complicated sigmoid diverticulitis. Int J Colorectal Dis 24:797–801
50. Mazza D, Chio F, Khoury-Helou A (2009) Conservative laparoscopic treatment of diverticular peritonitis. J Chir (Paris) 146:265–269
51. Lam HD, Tinton N, Cambier E, Navez B (2009) Laparoscopic treatment in acute complicated diverticulitis: a review of 11 cases. Acta Chir Belg 109:56–60
52. Lippi CE, Beatini L, Cervia S, Fabbricotti A, Miaruelli PA, Spessa E, Sturlese I, Braini A (2009) Laparoscopic lavage and drainage in the surgical treatment of diverticular disease complicated by peritonitis. Chir Ital 61:467–474
53. White SI, Frenkiel B, Martin PJ (2010) A ten-year audit of perforated sigmoid diverticulitis: highlighting the outcomes of laparoscopic lavage. Dis Colon Rectum 53:1537–1541
54. Rogers AC, Collins D, O'Sullivan GC, Winter DC (2012) Laparoscopic lavage for perforated diverticulitis: a population analysis. Dis Colon Rectum 55:932–938
55. Liang S, Russek K, Franklin ME Jr (2012) Damage control strategy for the management of perforated diverticulitis with generalized peritonitis: laparoscopic lavage and drainage vs. laparoscopic Hartmann's procedure. Surg Endosc 26:2835–2842
56. Swank HA, Mulder IM, Hoofwijk AG, Nienhuijs SW, Lange JF, Bemelman WA, Dutch Diverticular Disease Collaborative Study Group (2013) Early experience with laparoscopic lavage for perforated diverticulitis. Br J Surg 100:704–710
57. Edeiken SM, Maxwell RA, Dart BW IV, Mejia VA (2013) Preliminary experience with laparoscopic peritoneal lavage for complicated diverticulitis: a new algorithm for treatment? Am Surg 79:819–825
58. Krukowski ZH, Matheson NA (1988) Acute diverticulitis. Rec Adv Surg 13:125–141

59. Cirocchi R, Trastulli S, Vettoretto N, Milani D, Cavaliere D, Renzi C, Adamenko O, Desiderio J, Burattini MF, Parisi A, Arezzo A, Fingerhut A (2015) Laparoscopic peritoneal lavage: a definitive treatment for diverticular peritonitis or a "bridge" to elective laparoscopic sigmoidectomy? A systematic review. Medicine (Baltimore) 94(1), e334
60. Angenete E, Thornell A, Burcharth J, Pommergaard HC, Skullman S, Bisgaard T, Jess P, Läckberg Z, Matthiessen P, Heath J, Rosenberg J, Haglind E (2016) Laparoscopic lavage is feasible and safe for the treatment of perforated diverticulitis with purulent peritonitis: the first results from the randomized controlled trial DILALA. Ann Surg 263(1):117–122
61. Swank HA, Vermeulen J, Lange JF, Mulder IM, van der Hoeven JA, Stassen LP, Crolla RM, Sosef MN, Nienhuijs SW, Bosker RJ, Boom MJ, Kruyt PM, Swank DJ, Steup WH, de Graaf EJ, Weidema WF, Pierik RE, Prins HA, Stockmann HB, Tollenaar RA, van Wagensveld BA, Coene PP, Slooter GD, Consten EC, van Duijn EB, Gerhards MF, Hoofwijk AG, Karsten TM, Neijenhuis PA, Blanken-Peeters CF, Cense HA, Mannaerts GH, Bruin SC, Eijsbouts QA, Wiezer MJ, Hazebroek EJ, van Geloven AA, Maring JK, D'Hoore AJ, Kartheuser A, Remue C, van Grevenstein HM, Konsten JL, van der Peet DL, Govaert MJ, Engel AF, Reitsma JB, Bemelman WA, Dutch Diverticular Disease (3D) Collaborative Study Group (2010) The ladies trial: laparoscopic peritoneal lavage or resection for purulent peritonitis and Hartmann's procedure or resection with primary anastomosis for purulent or faecal peritonitis in perforated diverticulitis (NTR2037). BMC Surg 10:29
62. Bemelman WA. Laparoscopic peritoneal lavage or resection for generalised peritonitis for perforated diverticulitis (ladies). Available from: http://clinicaltrials.gov/ct2/show/NCT01317485
63. Schultz JK, Yaqub S, Wallon C, Blecic L, Forsmo HM, Folkesson J, Buchwald P, Körner H, Dahl FA, Øresland T, SCANDIV Study Group (2015) Laparoscopic lavage vs primary resection for acute perforated diverticulitis: The SCANDIV Randomized Clinical Trial. JAMA 314:1364–1375
64. Winter DC. LapLAND laparoscopic lavage for acute non-faeculant diverticulitis. Available from: http://clinicaltrials.gov/ct2/show/NCT01019239
65. Feingold D, Steele SR, Lee S, Kaiser A, Boushey R, Buie WD, Rafferty JF (2014) Practice parameters for the treatment of sigmoid diverticulitis. Dis Colon Rectum 57:284–294

Laparoscopy in Small Bowel Obstruction 9

Mauro Zago, Diego Mariani, Hayato Kurihara, Gianluca Baiocchi, Nereo Vettoretto, Carlo Bergamini, Fabio Cesare Campanile, and Ferdinando Agresta

9.1 Introduction

Small bowel obstruction (SBO) due to adhesions is a common disease, accounting for about 75 % of small bowel obstruction. Incidence, natural history, treatment approach, and preventability of SBO have very little changed over the years. Little progresses have been made in prevention and treatment until around 15 years ago. More recently, the introduction of the laparoscopic approach, the availability

M. Zago, MD, FAAST (✉)
General Surgery Department, Minimally Invasive Surgery Unit, Policlinico San Pietro, Via Forlanini, 15, 24036 Ponte San Pietro, BG, Italy
e-mail: maurozago.md@gmail.com

D. Mariani, MD
General Surgery Department, Ospedale Civile, AO Legnano, Via Papa Giovanni Paolo II, 20025 Legnano, MI, Italy

H. Kurihara, MD
General Surgery Department, Emergency and Trauma Surgery Section, Istituto Clinico Humanitas, Via Manzoni, 56, 20089 Rozzano, MI, Italy

G. Baiocchi, MD
Department of Clinical and Experimental Sciences, University of Brescia, Italy

N. Vettoretto, MD
Montichiari Surgery Department, ASST Spedali Civili di Brescia, via G. Ciotti 154, 25018 Montichiari, BS, Italy

C. Bergamini, MD
General Surgery Unit, Ospedale di Montichiari, AO Spedali Civili, Brescia, Italy

F.C. Campanile, MD
General Surgery Department, Ospedale Andosilla, Civita Castellana, VT, Italy

F. Agresta, MD
Department of General Surgery, Azienda ULSS19 del Veneto, Adria (RO), Italy

F. Agresta et al. (eds.), *Emergency Laparoscopy*,
DOI 10.1007/978-3-319-29620-3_9

of more established criteria for conservative management, and improvement in imaging techniques have all contributed to advancements in this field. This chapter focuses on current evidences about laparoscopy for SBO, including its place in a comprehensive algorithm of management, and some technical tips and tricks to be respected when this surgical approach is adopted.

Topics such as pathophysiology, clinical presentation, and medical treatment of SBO are out of the objectives of this chapter.

9.2 General Issues: Epidemiology, Costs, Etiology, Classification

9.2.1 Epidemiology, Costs

In some papers of the first half of the last century, adhesions accounted for 7–27 % of intestinal obstructions, respectively, in the UK and USA [1–3]. Epidemiology of SBO has not significantly evolved over the years. Admissions for SBO range between 0.9 and 2 % of all hospital admissions [4, 5]. The incidence rate of SBO is not decreased [6–8], even if there is a growing evidence of a reduced rate of clinically relevant postoperative SBO due to adhesions after laparoscopic abdominal surgery. The burden of admissions for SBO entails an impressive impact on health budgets. Some studies revealed that the medical costs for SBO are so high to be comparable to those for some gastrointestinal malignancies [9]. Ray et al. reported about a yearly 948,000 hospital days of care required for the treatment of SBO [10]. They estimated that Medicare alone was paying $3.2 billion per year for treatment of SBO.

9.2.2 Etiology of SBO

Even though adhesions rarely lead to obstruction of the large bowel, they account for more than 70 % of all SBOs. Hernia, cancer, inflammatory bowel disease, intussusception, radiation, endometriosis, infection, and foreign body are other relatively common causes of SBO. In patients without previous operations, the most common cause of bowel obstruction is incarceration of small bowel in a hernia, but adhesions can occur even in patients without previous abdominal surgery.

9.2.3 Classification of SBO

Small bowel obstruction is generally classified as complete vs. partial, high grade vs. low grade, simple vs. closed loop, high vs. low, mechanical vs. ileus, and chronic vs. acute.

Even though the elements of definitions are not strict and they are often expressed in a subjective way (like "significant" or "less dramatic"), classification is useful for understanding the probability for surgery and the urgency for appropriate treatment.

Laparoscopic approach could be used in all types when surgery is indicated, but surgeons must consider the different risks of bowel injuries and or resection according to the preoperative classification.

Complete SBO is defined by significantly distended bowel, failure to pass stool or flatus, and lack of air in colon and rectum. It virtually always leads to surgical operation. *Partial SBO* is associated with less dramatic small bowel distention, evidence of flatus and/or stool passage, and evidence of gas throughout the entire bowel on plain film. Partial SBO can often be conservatively treated.

A *high-grade SBO* is essentially a complete SBO associated with abdominal pain and often an impressively distended abdomen. Successful conservative management is quite rare. A *low-grade SBO* has the features of a partial SBO and mild to no pain and discomfort. It frequently succeeds with watchful waiting.

A *simple SBO* is defined when the bowel is occluded at a single point along its length, whereas a *closed loop obstruction* occurs when both the afferent and efferent portions of a loop of bowel are occluded by a constrictive band, with higher risk of strangulation and bowel necrosis.

A *high SBO* is defined when obstruction occurs very proximally in the jejunum, whereas in a *low SBO* the occlusion is found in the distal ileum.

9.3 Pathophysiology of Adhesion Formation, SBO, and Laparoscopy

Attard and Maclean [7] have well depicted the main mechanisms by which adhesion formation can be avoided and prevented:

- Decreasing peritoneal damage
- Decreasing the early inflammatory response
- Prevention of fibrin formation
- Increasing fibrinolysis
- Preventing collagen deposition
- Providing barriers to adhesion formation

These issues pointed out that the growing use of laparoscopy in abdominal operations was expected to reduce the rate of postoperative adhesions and at the same time the incidence of SBO due to adhesions, due to lesser damage to the parietal and visceral peritoneum, lesser handling of tissues, and the well-known effect of laparoscopy in decreasing the inflammatory response.

9.3.1 Laparoscopic vs. Open Surgery and Adhesions

Laparoscopic surgery has potential theoretical advantages over open surgery in reducing the rate of adhesion formation, but very few comparative studies are available to prove this.

An animal experimental study performed by Tittel showed that laparoscopy decreased the incidence, extension, and strength of intraperitoneal adhesions compared with laparotomy [11]. A retrospective cohort of 716 consecutive patients undergoing either laparoscopic (211 pt) or open bowel resection (505 pt) suggested that postoperative SBO requiring hospitalization with conservative management was reduced in those patients who had laparoscopic surgery ($n = 4$) compared to the open surgery cases ($n = 31$; $p < 0.016$) [12] (LoE 3).

Gutt and coworkers [13] reviewed 15 papers published from 1987 to 2001, 3 clinical and 12 experimental. In the three clinical studies [14–16], adhesions following laparoscopy (mainly at the operative site) were less than after open surgery in comparable groups of patients. The problem of distant adhesions was poorly represented in the literature. Because of the important differences between studies with regard to the design, endpoints, and statistical calculations, a meta-analysis could not be achieved. The conclusions were based on the prevalence of evidence.

The authors anyway concluded that laparoscopic surgery was associated with a decrease in adhesion formation in all clinical and most of the experimental studies.

More recently, Schnüriger, in a collective literature review, found that the incidence of adhesion-related readmissions was 7.1 % in open vs. 0.2 % in laparoscopic cholecystectomy, 9.5 % vs. 4.3 % in respectively open and laparoscopic colectomy, 15.6 % vs. 0 % in hysterectomy, and 23.9 % vs. 0 % in adnexal surgery [17] (LoE 3). Angenete and coworkers published a population-based retrospective register study, including 108,141 patients. This large retrospective analysis showed a four times increased risk of SBO for open surgery compared with laparoscopy [18] (LoE 3).

We should desume that with the wider diffusion of laparoscopic surgery, the expected rate of this kind of SBO should decrease in the next years.

This seems not to be true for colorectal surgery. Two retrospective analysis of prospectively collected databases, including homogenous groups of patients submitted to open vs. laparoscopic colonic resections, showed a similar rate of SBO [19, 20] (LoE 3). In the latter study, with a long-term FU ranging between 36 and 46 months, the need for operative intervention was significantly lower (8 % vs. 2 %, $p = 0.006$) in the laparoscopic group.

9.4 Imaging of SBO, Decision Making, and Laparoscopy

Plain abdominal film remains the most employed imaging when an SBO is suspected (Fig. 9.1).

Even when the plain film confirms the diagnosis of SBO, the nature and the precise site of obstruction remain often only suspected and not confirmed. In case a laparoscopic approach is suggested, plain film is not enough for surgical planning in the vast majority of cases.

There are evidences that ultrasound (US) sensitivity in diagnosing SBO is comparable to plain film even when performed by non-radiologists [21–23] (LoE 3). Notwithstanding, US is unfortunately not widely used. The main US finding

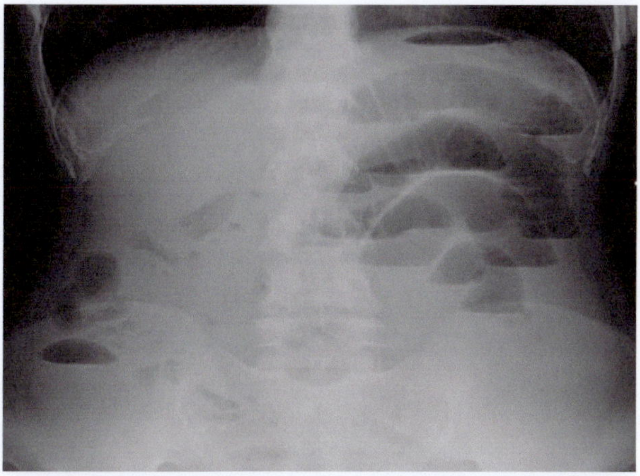

Fig. 9.1 Plain upright abdominal film, showing dilated small bowel loops with fluid levels. Neither the exact point of obstruction nor the etiology can be desumed

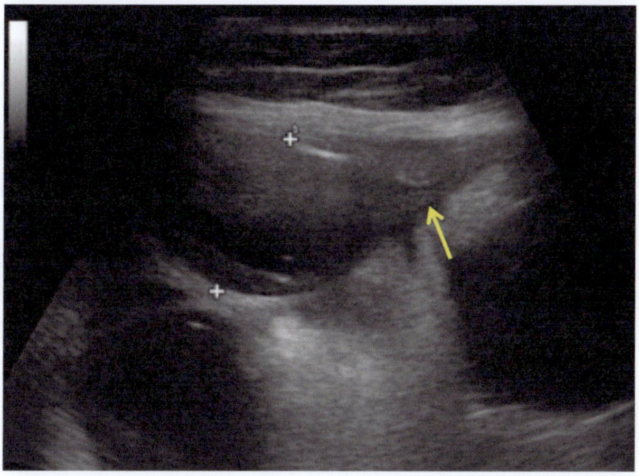

Fig. 9.2 Ultrasound view of a SBO. Detection of dilated (*white markers*), together with empty small bowel loops (*yellow arrow*), is a sensitive marker of SBO

confirming the presence of SBO is the visualization of both dilated and empty small bowel loops, which is highly sensitive for the diagnosis of SBO (Fig. 9.2). Additional findings are detection of free fluid, characters of fluid (by US-guided Diagnostic Peritoneal Aspiration, DPA), evaluation of peristalsis, mesurement of dilated loops, aspect of the bowel wall, aspect of plicae, and assessment of bowel viability with color flow mapping and power doppler. The main limit of US is to not be as sensitive as CT in detecting the site and the nature of the obstruction.

Contrast-enhanced CT (CECT) scan has become the imaging of choice for most patients with suspicion of SBO. A literature review performed by Mallo and coworkers analyzed that the accuracy of CT in identifying SBO associated with bowel ischemia or complete obstruction was very high [24]. Concerning bowel ischemia, CT aggregated positive predictive value (PPV) was 79 % (range 69–100 %), negative predictive value (NPV) 93 % (range 33–100 %), sensitivity (SN) 83 % (range 63–100 %), and specificity (SP) 92 % (range 61–100 %). The

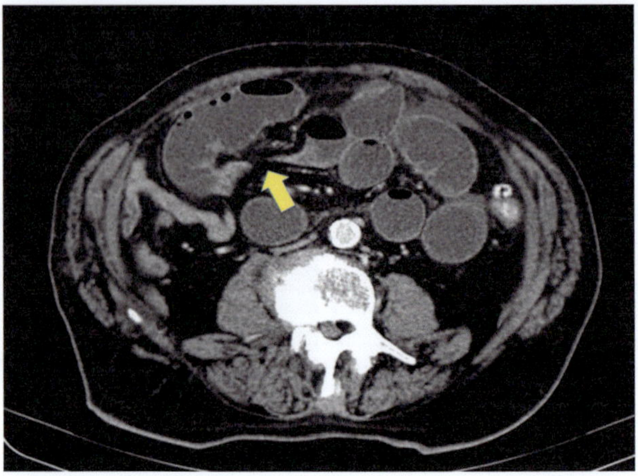

Fig. 9.3 CT has a high sensitivity for the identification of the transitional point due to a band adhesion (*arrow*). Empty small bowel loops are clearly evident on the left corner

aggregated PPV of CT for complete obstruction was 92 % (range 84–100 %), NPV 93 % (range 76–100 %), SN 92 % (range 81–100 %), and SP 94 % (range 68–100 %).

CECT scan (with or without oral contrast) shows proximal dilated small bowel, distal collapsed small bowel, and an empty colon. The presence of a transition point, usually due to an adhesion band (Fig. 9.3), does not predict neither the need for surgery nor the failure of nonoperative management [25]. CT scan can identify the vast majority of causes of the SBO (neoplasms, internal hernias, IBD, estrinsic stricture, etc.) and a careful identification of some CT signs can help in predicting the right and successful indication for the laparoscopic approach.

The main CT signs to be searched and interpreted are listed here:

- free fluid
- bowel loop caliper
- reduced bowel wall enhancement
- bowel loop thickness
- mesenteric swirl
- small bowel feces sign

Looking at CT findings, Schwenter showed that the need for bowel resection in SBO was significantly predicted in multivariate analysis by the presence of more than 500 mL of free fluid, reduction bowel wall enhancement, and mesenteric swirl. Adding clinical and biochemical criteria like WBC > 10,000/mmc, CRP > 75 mg/L, abdominal guarding, and pain lasting for more than 4 days, patients with four or more of these variables required resection. The presence of fever and the detection of a transition point on CT were not independent predictors of ischemic bowel [26].

Zielinski and coworkers confirmed that fever and transition point on CT were not independent predictors of operation. In a further prospective study, Zielinski highlighted that the lack of small bowel feces sign on CT scan was predictive for operation [27, 28]. The "small bowel feces sign" is the presence of particulate material in dilated small bowel loops on CT. Around 50 % of patients with SBO show it. The so-called whirl sign is defined as "swirl of mesenteric soft tissue and fat attenuation with adjacent loops of bowel surrounding rotated intestinal vessels" (Fig. 9.4).

In a retrospective study, Duda was able to identify the "whirl sign" in 20 % of CT of a large series of patients with SBO. When detected, the whirl sign should be carefully considered because it could be an ominous sign. Eighty percent of the Duda's series with the "whirl sign" required operation (PPV 80 %), whereas only 14 % without the sign underwent surgery (NPV 86 %) [29].

A comparative list of findings useful for both diagnosis and surgical planning is depicted in Table 9.1.

As discussed below in this chapter, safety and effectivenes of the laparoscopic approach are strictly related to careful patient selection. The use of laparoscopy as a

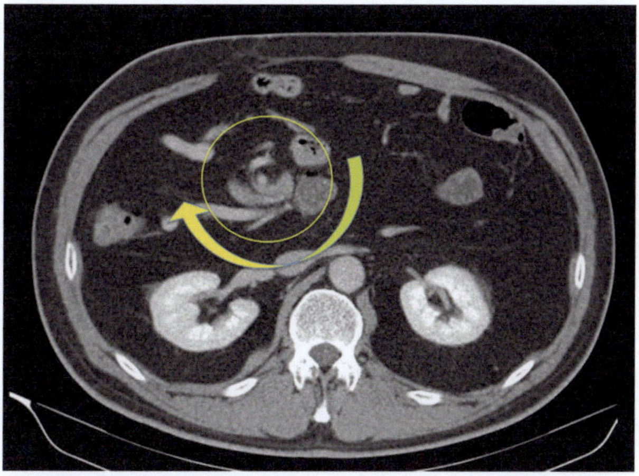

Fig. 9.4 The whirl sign (*circle*). This finding is better detected by an "up&down" scrolling of CT axial images on the screen

Table 9.1 Usefulness of imaging techniques for planning the laparoscopic approach for SBO

	Plain abdominal X ray	US	CECT
Diagnosis of SBO	+	+	++
Bowel peristalsis	–	+	–
Presence of free fluid	–	+	+
Characters of free fluid	–	++ [a]	±
Small bowel loops caliper	+	+	+
Bowel loops viability	–	+	++
Site of obstruction	–	±	++
Etiology	–	±	+
Preop. planning of trocars placement	–	+	++

US ultrasound, *CECT* contrast enhanced computed tomography
[a]By DPA

diagnostic tool without a full preoperative planning in this setting might be the door toward a disaster.

The need for a surgeon-performed interpretation of CT findings is evident. Items listed in Table 9.1, coupled with medical history, physiology, and clinical exam, are all needed for properly deciding the urgency of operation (presence and nature of free fluid, bowel viability), the probabilty of failure or intraoperative complications (loops caliper, etiology), and the proper trocar placement.

9.5 Evidences for the Laparoscopic Approach to SBO

The first reports of laparoscopic treatment date from the early 1990s, initially in the field of gynecologic surgery. In 1990, Clotteau first reported on laparoscopic adhesiolysis for SBO secondary to adhesions [30]. The main advantages of laparoscopy vs. open surgery for SBO concern the postoperative recovery, as well as the reduced rate of postoperative laparotomy-related adhesions and ventral hernia.

Neither RCTs nor prospective controlled studies are available in the scientific literature comparing open vs. laparoscopic approach for SBO [31]. A Finnish multicenter, prospective, randomized clinical trial was registered in 2013, comparing laparoscopic vs. open adhesiolysis for SBO, with the primary endpoint being the length of postoperative stay. Secondary endpoints include passage of stools, commencement of enteral nutrition, morbidity, and mortality. Results are expected in 2018 [32].

9.5.1 Guidelines

Some guidelines concerning laparoscopy and SBO are available in the literature and show a progressive trend toward a selected and more precise use of this appoach. The EAST Guidelines, published in 2008 [33], suggested that in a highly selected group of patients the laparoscopic treatment of SBO should be considered, leading to a shorter hospital length of stay. Notwithstanding, laparoscopy was not included in the proposed flowchart. The 2008 SAGES guidelines on diagnostic laparoscopy are very generic on this topic. They considered laparoscopy contraindicated in patients with a clear indication for surgical intervention such as massive bowel obstruction, perforated viscus (free air), and those with hemodynamic instability [34].

A group of experts published in 2013 an update of the Bologna Guidelines [35]. Laparoscopy is suggested as an option in highly selected patients. The open access technique is advised. The panel of an Italian consensus conference on laparoscopic adhesiolysis agreed to consider hemodynamic instability and/or cardiopulmonary impairment the only absolute contraindications to a minimally invasive approach [36].

Agresta and coworkers, on behalf of five Italian Scientific Societies and EAES, published in 2012 an update of the previous EAES guidelines on laparoscopy in abdominal emergencies [37, 38]. A mild advice supporting the selective use of laparoscopy in SBO was affirmed.

9.5.2 Conservative Management and Laparoscopy

The availability of the laparoscopic approach does not influence the current management of SBO suitable for conservative treatment. As specified above, the role and timing for nasogastric tube placement, Gastrografin® administration, antibiotic use, and time for oral intake resumption are not discussed here [35, 39, 40]. It is well known that surgery does not influence both the risk of recurrence and the need for a future operation [8] (LoE 3). Duron et al. found that the rates of primary or secondary recurrence (12 % and 18 %, respectively) were not different after open compared to laparoscopic surgery [41] (LoE 3).

In other words, laparoscopy is a minimally invasive surgical treatment with inherent morbidity and mortality, and according to present knowledge, it does not decrease the rate of recurrence of SBO after adhesiolysis.

9.5.3 Indications for Surgical Treatment and Selection for the Laparoscopic Approach

According to the above paragraph considerations, indications to surgical treatment do not change even if the patient is considered suitable for a laparoscopic approach.

An accurate and complete evaluation of the patient history, physiology, abdomen, and of the performed imaging must be performed. This is especially true for a patient with the classic tetrad frequently associated with bowel strangulation, namely, leukocytosis, tachycardia, fever, and severe unrelenting abdominal pain.

The management of patients with SBO is based on some critical issues: etiology, the degree of obstruction (partial or complete), and small bowel viability (ischemia or perforation). Therefore, CT plays a key role for a successful laparoscopic approach, as the majority of the morphological criteria associated with conversion to open surgery, intraoperative complications, and failure of laparoscopy are detectable on CT (axial, sagittal, and coronal views). Even in case of patients with bowel obstruction and a virgin abdomen, who virtually always undergo surgical exploration, a preoperative CT is advisable whenever the laparoscopic approach is evisageable.

Theoretically, all etiologies of SBO could be an indication to the laparoscopic approach, but the best and more successful situation is a SBO due to a single adhesion. It is an additional reason for a careful preoperative workup. A special situation is SBO occurring in patients with known intra-abdominal malignancy, for whom recurrent malignancy is possible. Although there is a comprehensible reluctancy to operate, 30 % of patients will have a simple adhesion amenable to simple lysis, 30 % have a resectable obstructing malignancy, and only 30 % have carcinomatosis not suitable for any surgical solution. It is probably the only setting of SBO for which laparoscopy, when feasible, should be considered as a diagnostic tool, in order to minimize the surgical trauma in very frail patients.

The only *absolute contraindication* to the laparoscopic approach is a physiologic status (hemodynamics, respiratory) which makes impossible the pneumoperitoneum [36]. Even the impossibility to get a sufficient peritoneal space (often related to bowel loops dilation) is a technical contraindication [42].

One of the main concern about the laparoscopic approach for SBO is the high *conversion rate*: complete laparoscopic treatment has been reported possible in the past in only 50–60 % of patients. Papers published in the last decade, in an era of a more standardized laparoscopic techniques and criteria, have shown a trend toward a reduction in conversion rate, in the laparoscopically treated patients, constantly lower than 50 % [42–50] (LoE 3).

A systematic review including all papers published up to 2007 (1236 patients) found a successful therapeutic laparoscopy rate in the range of 40–88 % and a conversion rate ranging from 0 to 52 %. Positive predictive factors for success are less than two previous laparotomies and the absence of peritonitis [51] (LoE 3). More recently, O'Connor et al. published a more comprehensive systematic review, reporting a conversion rate of 29 % [52] (LoE 3).

Conversion can be due to many reasons [52–65]:

- Inability to visualize and control the operative field (massive loops dilation)
- Neoplasms
- Dense adhesions
- Intestinal ischemia with bowel infarction
- Iatrogenic bowel injury
- Inability to find the point of obstruction
- Inability to achieve pneumoperitoneum

Overall morbidity after laparoscopic adhesiolysis ranges between 15 and 39 % [51, 53, 55, 56, 62, 63].

Inadvertent enterotomy rate is around 6.5 % and did not statiscally differ from open surgery [48, 53, 55, 56, 65]. It could be repaired laparoscopically in half of cases. The analysis of outcomes is discussed below. A bowel injury may be missed at the time of operation. Although a missed enterotomy can occur during laparotomy too, the incidence is reported to be higher with the laparoscopic approach. A careful surgical technique (see below) is the only method for preventing the risk.

Laparoscopy should not be used as a first step tool for the diagnosis of SBO without intention to treat.

Many studies have identified the factors that proved to be statistically significantly associated with failure of the laparoscopic approach.

These criteria should be kept in mind and accurately considered in order to optimize the selection of patient to be submitted to laparoscopy and are listed below:

- Small bowel loop diameter >4–5 cm
- More than two previous abdominal operations

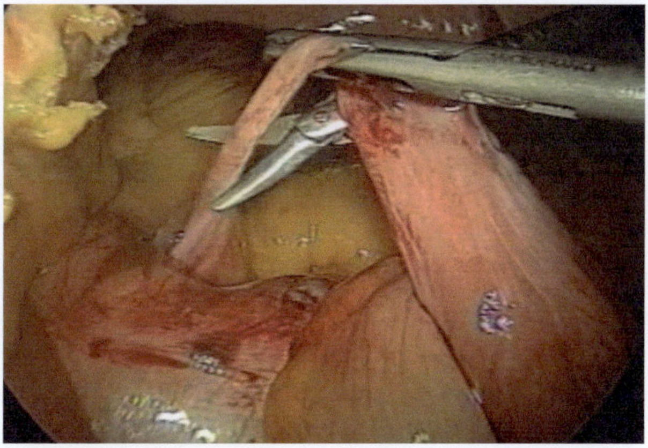

Fig. 9.5 Intraoperative view. Single band adhesion cut with cold scissors

- Operation after more than 24 h from diagnosis
- Duration of surgery
- Dense and extensive adhesions

Previous appendectomy was statistically associated with a higher rate of successful laparoscopic management, with the single band adhesion as the ideal condition for the laparoscopic approach [54–61, 66] (LoE 3) (Fig. 9.5).

The authors, in a retrospective study over 100 consecutive patients [59], reported a conversion rate of 34.2 % and found as statistically significant factor for conversion a small bowel caliper >4 cm. Notwithstanding, the analysis of the series revealed that 17.5 % of successful laparoscopic operations were performed in patients with bowel loops larger than 4 cm.

Reduced port and single-port laparoscopic adhesiolysis has been reported, but experiences are limited and only feasibility could be assessed. It is of interest to note that preoperative imaging identifying a single band adhesion is deemed a prerequisite for some authors [67] (LoE 4).

In pediatric patients, experience on the laparoscopic treatment of SBO is very limited. Recent literature shows a trend in considering laparoscopy the first option for adhesive small bowel obstruction in children [68, 69] (LoE 4).

9.5.4 Laparoscopy in the SBO Algorithm

In the last few years, many articles were published suggesting comprehensive algorithms for SBO management, including paths for nonoperative management, water-soluble contrast administration, timing for expectant management, and criteria for immediate or delayed surgery [35, 36, 62, 63, 70]. This chapter is specifically devoted to the role of laparoscopy in SBO, and a careful analysis and comparison among them is mandatorily skipped.

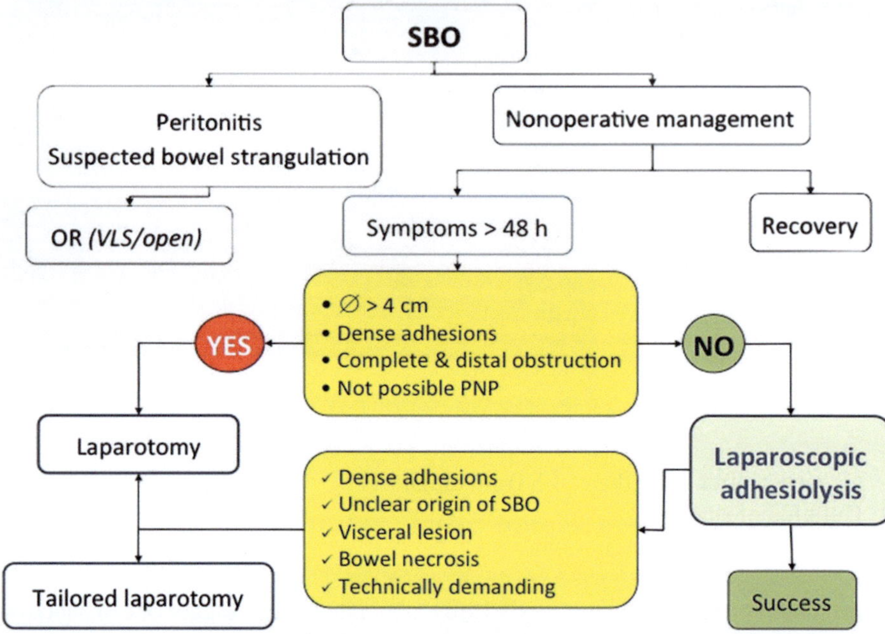

Fig. 9.6 Proposal of a simplified algorithm for the management of SBO, focused on the criteria for successful laparoscopic approach. Preoperative and intraoperative findings (midline boxes) guide the choice for laparoscopy or open approach

A simplified original algorithm focused on laparoscopic criteria for conversion to open surgery is proposed in Fig. 9.6 and could be used to integrate a more comprehensive protocol. Preoperative and intraoperative criteria obtained by the updated literature review and useful for the critical choice of the laparoscopic approach are highligted.

9.5.5 Laparoscopy and Clinical Outcomes

Laparoscopy adhesiolysis reveals advantages in most of the surgical outcomes.

A systematic review and meta-analysis, pooling the effects of outcomes of a total of 334 patients in four retrospective comparative studies using meta-analytic methods, showed that laparoscopic adhesiolysis was associated with a reduction in overall complication rate ($p<0.01$), prolonged ileus rate ($p<0.01$), and pulmonary complication rate ($p<0.04$), compared with open approach. No differences were observed for intraoperative bowel injuries, wound infection, and mortality [71] (LoE 2). Saleh and coworkers [64] analyzed data of the ACS NSQIP between 2005 and 2010, collecting 4616 patients submitted to surgery for SBO (3697 open, 919 laparoscopic). They excluded the sicker patients, the converted operations, and those with formal bowel resection in order to reduce potential biases.

Laparoscopy, in considering both unadjusted and adjusted odd ratios, revealed a statistically significant advantage over open surgery in terms of morbidity and 30-day postoperative morbidity ($p < 0.01$) and overall complications ($p < 0.01$). The mean postoperative length of stay (LOS) was 8.4 compared to 3.8 days in the open and laparoscopic groups, respectively ($p < 0.01$). The same group performed a retrospective review about the outcome of their own series of 269 patients, 83 of whom (30.9 %) were managed laparoscopically, with a conversion rate of 38.6 %. Laparoscopy allowed a quicker recovery (time of passage of flatus, $p < 0.005$), LOS (5 vs. 7 days, $p < 0.031$), and overall complication rate (27.7 vs. 43.6 %, $p < 0.014$). The same results were obtained following exclusion of bowel resections [65] (LoE 4). A significant reduction of 30-day mortality and of major complication rate with the laparoscopic approach was confirmed in a further analysis of the ACS NSQIP database done by Kelly and coworkers [72] (LoE 3).

The use of a tailored laparotomy (i.e., a reduced incision placed according to laparoscopic findings) would be a potential benefit of the laparoscopic approach, but this item has not been demonstrated yet. The use of a tailored mini-laparotomy (less than 10 cm) is reported ranging from 20 to 35 % of cases [59, 73].

Even though successful laparoscopic treatments of patients with negative predictive criteria are described without complication in some papers [59, 73], there is a current agreement among experts that a low threshold for open conversion remains recommended, especially facing with dense adhesions (LoE 5). Provided a full workup and a critical decision making have been done, conversion should not be considered a failure, but simply the further and wise step in the optimal management of a patient with SBO. From the other side, any surgeon with developed laparoscopic skills who has performed a standard midline incision to release a single adhesive band normally regrets that the laparoscopic approach was not chosen.

9.6 Technical Tips and Tricks

As stated by Azagury et al. [70], the ideal successful surgical management of SBO should be defined as "a laparoscopic lysis of adhesions without inadvertent enterotomy or laparoscopic with conversion to laparotomy before any intraoperative complication."

9.6.1 Equipment

No special laparoscopic instrumentation is needed for SBO adhesiolysis. Well-functioning atraumatic graspers (Johanne like) and cold scissors are the most important instruments. Recording any procedure is advisable, especially for reviewing the procedure in case of complications and when inadvertent enterotomy occurs, in order to improve the awareness and the skills of the entire surgical team. Advanced sealing instruments (radiofrequency dissector, ultrasonic scalpel) could be helpful but not indispensable and should be used in selected situations. The use of a 30° telescope is the rule.

9.6.2 Positioning of the Patient

Patient positioning strongly affects the feasibility of laparoscopic adhesiolysis. A bad placing of the patient on the table might be the main cause of conversion. You would need to tilt the table in every position during the operation for pulling away the dilated loops and sometimes even to change the side where you started to work.

Check that all the following issues were done:

- Both arms should be put along the patient's sides (assistant is almost always beside you).
- Always install shoulder keepers (and feet keepers if the patient is obese) to be prepared for steep positions if needed.
- Control the table remote control is working.

9.6.3 Trocar Placement and Access

Nasogastric tube and Foley catheter should already be in place.

First access to the peritoneal cavity should be placed far from the scars of previous surgery.

A preoperative individual planning, namely, a surgeon performed examination of preoperative CT, is essential for a safe trocar placement and effective surgery.

No evidences support the use of open laparoscopy vs. Veress needle vs. optic trocar for the induction of pneumoperitoneum. Some guidelines suggest the use of open laparoscopy as the preferred method [35, 36, 70]. A muscle splitting incision for the Hasson trocar insertion can be performed everywhere in the lateral abdominal quadrants, except in morbid obese patients.

Gentle blunt dissection with a 30° telescope directly against parietal adhesions is a smart trick for getting space enough for the positioning of the second trocar. The goal is to place at least three ports with a good triangulation. Additional ports should be inserted as needed.

A smart choice is to use a 5-mm angled scope that could be inserted in any port.

9.6.4 Surgical Technique

Adhesiolysis should start where adhesions are thinner, the bowel is easily identified, and loops are empty. Pulling away dilated loops by gravity and gaining the workspace is the first step, with the aim to focus on the transition point. For dissection, prefer cold scissors and blunt dissection whenever possible. Be aware about the high risk of immediate and/or delayed thermal injuries when using energy devices.

Nomally, identification of the last ileal loop allows to proceed back toward the occlusive point, gently handling empty loops. When the distal ileum is undetectable, work handling collapsed loops and moving in both directions, searching for the transition point.

The basic technique is an alternate mix of sharp and blunt dissection (cut the adhesion, push away the adjacent loop, etc.), with the help of the countertraction created by the tented abdominal wall.

Fear about handling dilated loops, as the risk of tearing and contamination is very high. If unavoidable, try to grasp the mesentery or pericolic fat rather than the bowel itself. Grasping of the bowel should be large, in order to widen the area of grasping and decreasing the pressure on the wall.

If serosal rents occur, they should be immediately fixed with absorbable sutures.

As the obstruction is satisfactorily identified and fixed, a complete adhesiolysis entails the risk of bowel injury and it is discouraged.

An inadvertent enterotomy can be laparoscopically repaired, provided it is small, contamination is controlled, and the repair is technically satifactory.

A low threshold for conversion, through a midline or a tailored mini-laparotomy, must be considered facing with inadvertent enterotomy, when the transition point is not clearly recognized and dense adhesions make laparoscopy unsafe and uncomfortable.

The key techical points summarized in Box 1 can help in maximizing the laparoscopic approach.

Box 1. Key Technical Points for Laparoscopic Adhesiolysis

- Patient positioning
  - Arms along the body
  - Shoulder keepers (steep tilting of the table would be needed)
- Trocars placement
  - Preoperative individual planning (CT)
  - Open laparoscopy or optic trocar preferred
  - First trocar far from scars
  - First trocar in the opposite side of the transitional point
- 30° scope
- Cold scissors for sharp dissection
- Minimal/no use of electrocautery
- Atraumatic forceps or suction cannula for blunt dissection
- Gentle handling of empty loops
- Avoid handling dilated loops

References

1. Wiseman DM (1998) Adhesion prevention: past the future. Perit Surg 39:1–38
2. Moss W, McFetridge EM (1934) Acute intestinal obstruction: a comparative study of 511 cases, with special reference to the lowered mortality achieved by modern methods of therapy. Ann Surg 100:158–166
3. Dayton MT et al (2012) New paradigms in the treatment of small bowel obstruction. Curr Prob Surg 49(11):642–717
4. Bevan PG (1984) Adhesive obstruction. Ann R Coll Surg Engl 66:164–169
5. Menzies D, Ellis H (1990) Intestinal obstruction from adhesions: how big is the problem? Ann R Coll Surg Engl 72:60–63
6. Scott FI, Oserman MT, Mahmoud NN, Lewis JD (2012) Secular trends in small bowel obstruction and adhesiolysis in the United States: 1988–2007. Am J Surg 204:315–320
7. Attard JP, MacLean AR (2007) Adhesive small bowel obstruction: epidemiology, biology and prevention. Can J Surg 50(4):291–300
8. Miller G, Boman J, Shrier J, Gordon PH (2000) Etiology of small bowel obstruction. Am J Surg 180:33–36
9. Kössi J, Salminen P, Rantala A et al (2003) Population-based study of the surgical workload and economic impact of bowel obstruction caused by postoperative adhesions. Br J Surg 90:1441–1444
10. Ray NF, Larsen JW, Stillman RJ et al (1993) Economic impact of hospitalizations for lower abdominal adhesiolysis in the United States in 1988. Surg Gynecol Obstet 176:271–276
11. Tittel A (2001) Comparison of adhesion reformation after laparoscopic and conventional adhesiolysis in an animal model. Langenbeck's Arch Surg 386:141–145
12. Duepree HJ, Senagore AJ, Delaney CP, Fazio VW (2003) Does means of access affect the incidence of small bowel obstruction and ventral hernia after bowel resection? Laparoscopy versus laparotomy. J Am Coll Surg 197:177–181
13. Gutt CN, Oniu T, Schemmer P, Mehrabi A, Büchler MW (2004) Fewer adhesions induced by laparoscopic surgery? Surg Endosc 18(6):898–906
14. Lundorff P, Hahlin M, Källfelt B et al (1991) Adhesion formation after laparoscopic surgery in tubal pregnancy: a randomized trial versus laparotomy. Fertil Steril 55:911–915
15. Milingos S, Kallipolitis G, Loutradis D et al (2000) Adhesions: laparoscopic surgery versus laparotomy. Ann NY Acad Sci 900:272–285
16. Polymeneas G, Theodosopoulos T, Stamatiadis A et al (2001) A comparative study of postoperative adhesion formation after laparoscopic vs open cholecystectomy. Surg Endosc 15:41–43
17. Schnüriger B, Barmparas G, Branco BC et al (2011) Prevention of postoperative peritoneal adhesions: a review of the literature. Am J Surg 201:111–121
18. Angenete E, Jacobsson A, Gellerstedt M, Haglind E (2012) Effect of laparoscopy on the risk of small-bowel obstruction. Arch Surg 147:359–365
19. Saklani AP, Naguib N, Shah PR, Makhail P, Winstanley S, Masoud AG (2012) Adhesive intestinal obstruction in laparoscopic vs open colorectal resection. Colorectal Dis 15:80–84
20. Reshef A, Hull TL, Kiran RP (2013) Risk of adhesive obstruction after colorectal surgery: the benefits of the minimally invasive approach may extend well beyond the perioperative period. Surg Endosc 27:1717–1720
21. Unlüer EE, Yavaşi O, Eroğlu O, Yilmaz C, Akarca FK (2010) Ultrasonography by emergency medicine and radiology residents for the diagnosis of small bowel obstruction. Eur J Emerg Med 17(5):260–264
22. Jang TB, Schindler D, Kaji AH (2011) Bedside ultrasonography for the detection of small bowel obstruction in the emergency department. Emerg Med J 28(8):676–678
23. Guttman J, Stone MB, Kimberly HH, Rempell JS (2015) Point-of-care ultrasonography for the diagnosis of small bowel obstruction in the emergency department. CJEM 17(2):206–209

24. Mallo RD, Salem L, Lalani T et al (2005) Computed tomography diagnosis of ischemia and complete obstruction in small bowel obstruction: a systematic review. J Gastrointest Surg 9(5):690–694
25. Colon MJ, Telem DA, Wong D et al (2010) The relevance of transition zones on computed tomography in the management of small bowel obstruction. Surgery 147:373–377
26. Schwenter F, Polleti PA, Platon A et al (2010) Clinicoradiological score for predicting the risk of strangulated small bowel obstruction. Br J Surg 97:1119–1125
27. Zielinski MD, Eiken PW, Bannon MP et al (2010) Small bowel obstruction—who needs an operation? A multivariate prediction model. World J Surg 34(5):910–919
28. Zielinski MD, Eiken PW, Lohse HSF et al (2011) Prospective, observational validation of a multivariate small-bowel obstruction model to predict the need for operative intervention. J Am Coll Surg 212(6):1068–1076
29. Duda JB, Bhatt S, Dogra VS (2008) Utility of CT whirl sign in guiding management of small-bowel obstruction. Am J Roentgenol 191(3):743–747
30. Clotteau JE, Premont M (1990) Occlusion by adhesions treated by celioscopic section [in French]. Presse Med 19(25):1196
31. Cirocchi R, Abraha I, Farinella E, Montedori A, Sciannameo F (2010) Laparoscopic versus open surgery in small bowel obstruction (Review). The Cochrane Collaboration. Cochrane Database Syst Rev 2, CD007511
32. Sallinen V, Wikstrom H, Victorzon M, Salaminen P, Koivukangas V, Haukijarvi E, Enholm B, Leppaniemi A, Mentula P (2014) Laparoscopic versus open adhesiolysis for small bowel obstruction – a multicentre, prospective, randomized, controlled trial. BMC Surg 14:77
33. Diaz JJ Jr, Bokhari F, Mowery NT, Acosta JA, Block EFJ, Bromberg WJ, Collier BR, Cullinane DC, Dwyer KM, Griffen MM, Mayberry JC, Jerome R (2008) Guidelines for management of small bowel obstruction. J Trauma 64:1651–1664
34. SAGES (2008) Diagnostic laparoscopy guidelines. Surg Endosc 22:1353–1383
35. Di Saverio S, Coccolini F, Galati M, Smerieri N, Biffl WL, Ansaloni L, Tugnoli G, Velmahos GC, Sartelli M, Bendinelli C, Fraga G, Kelly M, Moore FA, Mandalà V, Mandalà S, Masetti M, Jovine E, Pinna AD, Peitzman AB, Leppaniemi A, Sugarbaker PH, Van Goor H, Moore EE, Jeekel J, Catena F (2013) Bologna Guidelines for diagnosis and management of adhesive small bowel obstruction (ASBO): 2013 update of the evidence-based guidelines from the world society of emergency surgery ASBO working group. WJES 8:42
36. Vettoretto N, Carrara A, Corradi A, De Vivo G, Lazzaro L, Ricciardelli L, Agresta F, Amodio C, Bergamini C, Borzellino G, Catani M, Cavaliere D, Cirocchi R, Gemini S, Mirabella A, Palasciano N, Piazza D, Piccoli M, Rigamonti M, Scatizzi M, Tamborrino E, Zago M (2012) Laparoscopic adhesiolysis: consensus conference guidelines. Colorectal Dis 14:e208–e215
37. Sauerland S, Agresta F, Bergamaschi R, Borzellino G, Budzynsky A, Champault G, Fingerhut A, Isla A, Johansson M, Lundorff P, Navez B, Saad S, Neugebauer EA (2006) Laparoscopyfor abdominal emergencies: evidence based guidelines of the European Association for Endoscopic Surgery. Surg Endosc 20(1):14–29
38. Agresta F, Ansaloni L, Baiocchi L, Bergamini C, Campanile FC, Carlucci M, Cocorullo G, Corradi A, Franzato B, Lupo M, Mandalà V, Mirabella A, Pernazza G, Piccoli M, Staudacher C, Vettoretto N, Zago M, Fingerhut A, Uranues S (2012) Laparoscopic approach to acute abdomen. Consensus Dev Conf Surg Endosc 26:2134–2164
39. Branco BC, Barmparas G, Schnüriger B et al (2010) Systematic review and meta-analysis of the diagnostic and therapeutic role of water-soluble contrast agent in adhesive small bowel obstruction. Br J Surg 97:470–478
40. Abbas S, Bissett IP, Parry BR (2007) Oral water soluble contrast for the management of adhesive small bowel obstruction. Cochrane Database Syst Rev 3, CD004651
41. Duron JJ, Jourdan-Da Silva N, Tezenas du Montcel S, Berger A, Muscari F, Hennet H, Veyrieres M, Hay JM (2006) Adhesive postoperative small bowel obstruction: incidence and risk factors of recurrence after surgical treatment. A multicenter prospective study. Ann Surg 244:750–757

42. Zerey M, Sechrist CW, Kercher KW, Sing RF, Matthews BD, Heniford BT (2007) Laparoscopic management of adhesive small bowel obstruction. Am Surg 73:773–778
43. Iorgulescu R, Iordache M, Ilie R, Dragomirescu C (2005) Laparoscopic Surgery for small bowel obstruction. Chirurgia 101:313–318
44. Khaikin M, Schneidereit N, Cera S, Sands D, Efron J, Weiss G, Nogueras JJ, Vernava AM, Wexner SD (2007) Laparoscopic vs. open surgery for acute adhesive small-bowel obstruction: patient' outcome and cost-effectiveness. Surg Endosc 21:742–746
45. Cavaliere D, Schirru A, Caristo I, Bianchi M, Cosce U, Cavaliere P (2005) La laparoscopia nell'occlusione intestinale del tenue. Chir It 57:215–220
46. Johanet H, Marmuse JP (2005) Occlusion aigue du grele sur bride. Prevention et traitement des occlusions du grele su bride. Referentiel Association Française de Chirurgie (A.F.C.) n°4513 créé(e) le 28/04/05 par Pr Denis Collet
47. Cirocchi R, Giustozzi G, De Sol A et al (2007) Laparoscopic adhesiolysis in acute small bowel obstruction. Minerva Chir 62(6):477–488
48. Binenbaum SJ, Goldfarb A (2006) Inadvert enterotomy in minimally invasive abdominal surgery. JSLS 10:336–340
49. Qureschl I, Awad ZT (2010) Predictors of failure of the laparoscopic approach for the management of small bowel obstruction. Am Surg 76(9):947–950
50. Grafen FC, Neuhaus V, Schob O, Turina M (2010) Management of acute small bowel obstruction from intestinal adhesions: indications for laparoscopic surgery in a community teaching hospital. Langenbecks Arch Surg 395(1):57–63
51. Farinella E, Roberto Cirocchi R, La Mura F, Morelli U, Cattorini L, Delmonaco P, Migliaccio C, De Sol AA, Cozzaglio L, Sciannameo F (2009) Feasibility of laparoscopy for small bowel obstruction. World J Emerg Surg 4:3
52. O'Connor DB, Winter DC (2012) The role of laparoscopy in the management of acute small bowel obstruction: a review of over 2000 cases. Surg Endosc 26:12–17
53. Chopra R, McVay C, Phillips E et al (2003) Laparoscopic lysis of adhesions. Am Surg 69(11):966–968
54. Tierris I, Mavrantonis C, Stratoulias C et al (2011) Laparoscopy for acute small bowel obstruction: indication or contraindication? Surg Endosc 25:531–535
55. Ghosheh B, Salameh JR (2007) Laparoscopic approach to acute small bowel obstruction: review of 1061 cases. Surg Endosc 21:1945–1949
56. Franklin ME, Gonzalez JJ, Miter DB et al (2004) Laparoscopic diagnosis and treatment of intestinal obstruction. Surg Endosc 18:26–30
57. Levard H (2001) Laparoscopic treatment of acute small bowel obstruction: a multicentre retrospective study. ANZ J Surg 71:641–646
58. Suter M, Zermatten P, Halkic N, Martinet O, Bettschart V (2000) Laparoscopic management of mechanical small bowel obstruction. Are there predictors of success or failure? Surg Endosc 14:478–483
59. Zago M, Mariani D, Kurihara H, Turconi MG, Poldi D, Rosati R (2010) Selection criteria analysis for laparoscopic treatment of small bowel obstruction on a 100 patients series. Eur J Trauma Emerg Surg 36:120
60. Navez B, Arimont JM, Guit P (1998) Laparoscopic approach in acute small bowel obtructio. A review of 68 patients. Hepatogastroenterology 45:2146–2150
61. Léon EL, Metzger A, Tsiotos GG et al (1998) Laparoscopic management of small bowel obstruction: indication and outcomes. J Gastrointest Surg 2:132–140
62. Maung AA, Johnson DC, Piper GL, Barbosa RR, Rowell SE, Bokhari F, Collins JN, Gordon JR, Ra JH, Kerwin AJ et al (2012) Evaluation and management of small-bowel obstruction: an Eastern Association for the Surgery of Trauma practice management guideline. J Trauma Acute Care Surg 73:S362YS369
63. Loftus T, Moore F, VanZant E, Bala T, Brakenridge S, Croft C, Lottenberg L, Richards W, Mozingo D, Atteberry L et al (2015) A protocol for the management of adhesive small bowel obstruction. J Trauma Acute Care Surg 78(1):13–19

64. Saleh F, Ambrosini L, Jackson T, Okrainec A (2014) Laparoscopic versus open surgical management of small bowel obstruction: an analysis of short term outcomes. Surg Endosc 28:2381–2386
65. Byrne J, Saleh F, Ambrosini L, Quereshy F, Jackson TD, Okrainec A (2014) Laparoscopic versus sopen surgical management of adhesive small bowel obstruction: a comparison of outcomes. Surg Endosc. doi:10.1007/s00464-014-4015-7
66. Navez B, Navez J (2014) Laparoscopy in the acute abdomen. Best Pract Res Clin Gastroenterol 28:3–17
67. Hiro J, Inoue Y, Okugawa Y, Kawamoto A, Okita Y, Toiyama Y, Tanaka K, Uchida K, Mohri Y, Kusunoki M (2014) Single port laparoscopic management of adhesive small bowel obstruction. Surg Today 44:586–590
68. Apelt N, Featherstone N, Giuliani S (2013) Laparoscopic treatment for adhesive small bowel obstruction: is it the gold standard in children too? Surg Endosc 27:3927–3928
69. Aguayo P, Fraser JD, Ilyas S et al (2011) Laparoscopic management of small bowel obstruction in children. J Laparoendosc Adv Surg Tech A 21(1):85–88
70. Azagury D, Liu RC, Morgan A, Spain D (2015) Small bowel obstruction: a practical step-by-step evidence-based approach to evaluation, decision making, and management. J Trauma Acute Care Surg 79:661–668
71. Li MZ, Lian L, Xiao L, Wu W, He Y, Song X (2012) Laparoscopic versus open adhesiolysis in patients with adhesive small bowel obstruction: a systematic review and meta-analysis. Am J Surg 204:779–786
72. Kelly KN, Iannuzzi JC, Rickles AS, Garimella V, Monson JRT, Fleming FJ (2014) Laparotomy for small-bowel obstruction: first choice or last resort for adhesiolysis? A laparoscopic approach for small-bowel obstruction reduces 30-day complications. Surg Endosc 28:65–73
73. Lujan HL, Oren A, Plasencia G et al (2006) Laparoscopic management as the initial treatment of acute small bowel obstruction. JSLS 10:466–472

Incarcerated Hernias

10

Giovanni Alemanno, Riccardo Somigli, Paolo Prosperi, Mario Campli, Alberto Arezzo, Andrea Valeri, Carlo Bergamini, and Mauro Zago

10.1 Introduction

The lifetime risk of having a groin hernia repair has been estimated to be 27 % for men and 3 % for women. In the natural history of the inguinal or femoral hernia, 0.29–2.9 % of cases become incarcerated. Incarceration is the state of an external hernia which cannot be reduced into the abdomen. It implies an increased risk of small bowel obstruction, being the second most common cause of it [1]. Furthermore, among incarcerated hernias, 10–15 % become strangulated and gangrenous, which is a severe complication with a mortality rate of up to 5 % in the elderly. Incarceration has, therefore, great importance and should be considered a surgical emergency [2]. Actually, roughly 5 % of all patients having an operation for external hernia are explored as an emergency.

In 1993, Watson and colleagues demonstrated the feasibility of laparoscopic groin hernia repair (GHR). A modified pre-peritoneal femoral hernia repair with mesh and resection of incarcerated small bowel was been successfully completed by these authors under laparoscopic guidance in a 64-year-old patient with incarcerated femoral hernia [3].

G. Alemanno (✉) • R. Somigli • P. Prosperi • A. Valeri • C. Bergamini
Careggi University Hospital, Florence, Italy
e-mail: g.alemannomd@gmail.com

M. Campli
Division of Surgery, "Nuova Itor" Private Health Facility, Rome, Italy

A. Arezzo
Department of Surgical Science, University of Torino, Italy

M. Zago
General Surgery Department, Minimally Invasive Surgery Unit, Policlinico San Pietro, Via Forlanini 15, 24036 Ponte San Pietro, BG, Italy

F. Agresta et al. (eds.), *Emergency Laparoscopy*,
DOI 10.1007/978-3-319-29620-3_10

10.2 Literature Supporting the Role of Laparoscopy in Emergency GHR

In 2003, a Cochrane library study showed that the outcome of elective laparoscopic GHR is at least equivalent to that of the open approach. Indeed, the use of mesh during laparoscopic hernia repair seemed to be associated with a relative reduction in the risk of hernia recurrence of around 30–50 %. Furthermore, a less persisting pain and numbness following laparoscopic repair was suggested and the return to usual activities was faster. However, operation took a longer time and there appeared to have a higher risk of serious complication rate in respect of visceral (especially bladder) and vascular injuries [4].

This study was confirmed in 2010 by an extensive meta-analysis of randomized controlled studies (RCT) and comparative studies concerning patients treated for recurrent inguinal hernia with laparoscopic procedures versus open mesh repair. Significantly, fewer cases of hematoma/seroma formation were observed in the laparoscopic group in comparison with the Lichtenstein group, whereas the relative risk of overall recurrence of the laparoscopic versus the Lichtenstein group was comparable [5].

Concerning the incarcerated hernia, many non-comparative low-evidence level studies have been published so far. A review of cohort studies on laparoscopic repair of incarcerated groin hernias was published in 2010 by Deeba et al., updating the information given in the previous guidelines on laparoscopic emergency [6]. It reviews seven articles on this topic dating from 1989 to 2008, reporting on 328 cases treated with total extra-peritoneal (TEP) or trans-abdominal pre-peritoneal (TAPP) repair (Table 10.1). Of these seven articles, two are LE 3 prospective cohort studies and five are LE 4 small case series. The overall results of the Deeba et al.'s study were that average operative time was 61.3 min, average hospital stay was 3.8 days, mortality rate was 0.28 %, complication rate was 10.3 %, conversion rate was 1.8 %, intestinal laparoscopic or mini-laparotomy resection rate was 5.1 %, and reoperation rate was 0.9 %. The most serious complications consisted of two colonic lesions and one divided vas deferens. The others were infected mesh (0.6 %), wound infection (0.3 %), deep venous thrombosis (0.3 %), and other minor complications. The highest recurrence rate at 7 years was 5.8 %. The authors concluded that the laparoscopic approach, either TEP or TAPP, is possible for repairing incarcerated hernia taking into account the knowledge of anatomy and expertise needed to dissect and reduce the sac. Laparoscopy can also be used to resect bowel, if necessary, or to repair an occult contralateral hernia, present in 11.2–50 % of cases. The overall complication rate, recurrence rate, and length of hospital stay seem to be very similar to those documented for open repair of strangulated/incarcerated hernias.

The only comparative study so far available has been recently published by Yang et al. These authors have described the low middle-term outcome of open compared to laparoscopic strangulated groin hernia repair in adults [7]. In this series of 188 cases, retrospectively studied, Yang et al. reported that the laparoscopic group had a much lower wound infection rate compared to the open group. The mean

Table 10.1 Included studies with their respective data in the paper by Deeba et al.

Country	Author	Publication year patients	Approach	No. of patients	Conversion rate (%)	Operative time stay (min)	Length of stay	Complications	Intraoperative resection[a]
USA	Ferzli	2004	TEP	11	27.2	50	5.4	2	1
Germany	Leibl	2001	TAPP	194	0	55	NA	7	6
India	Saggar	2005	TEP	34	0	84.4	76,4 % of patients 24h	23 minor	NA
Japan	Ishihara	1996	TAPP	6	0	88	NA	1	NA
Italy	Legnani	2007	TAPP	9	0	72	2.7	0	1
Italy	Rebuffat	2006	TAPP	28	10.7	72	3.9	1	9
Germany	Mainik	2005	TEP	46	NA	NA	4.7	NA	NA
Total	7			328	6			34	17

Table 10.2 Operative details in the study by Yang et al.

	Laparoscopic group	Open group	*P* value
Operative time, mean ± SD (min)	79.82 ± 29.571	80.75 ± 35.161	0.863
TEP (*n*)	48	–	–
TAPP (*n*)	5	–	–
Laparoscopic plication with brad ligment (*n*)	3	–	–
Lichtenstein repair (*n*)	–	107	–
Tissue/suture repair (*n*)	–	10	–
Mesh plug repair (*n*)	–	14	–
Conversion (*n*)	1 open lichtenstein	19 laparotomies	0.009
Bowel resection (*n*)	1	10	0.117

Table 10.3 Post-operative results and follow-up in the study by Yang et al.

	Laparoscopic group	Open group	*P* value
Hospital stay, mean ± SD	4.39 ± 1.99	7.34 ± 2.354	0.307
Wound infection (*n*)	0	12	0.018
		4 laparotomy wounds	
		8 groin wound	
Hematoma (*n*)	2	5	0.918
Seroma (*n*)	8	7	0.074
Chronic pain (*n*)	0	0	–
Mesh infection (*n*)	0	0	–
Recurrence (*n*)	1	3	0.815
Follow-up, mean ± SD (months)	24 ± 15.24	25.095 ± 14.48	0.421
Loss at follow-up (*n*)	4 (7 %)	6 (4.58 %)	0.494

hospital stay was also shorter in this cohort, but this was not statistically significant (Tables 10.2 and 10.3).

With the important bias of a retrospective design and the presence of some difference between the two groups, such as the ASA grade and the mean age which were higher in the open group, the authors feel to conclude that laparoscopic repair for the treatment of strangulated groin hernias is feasible and appears to have lower morbidity compared to open repair. Interestingly, in their opinion, the necessity of bowel resection does not seem to significantly affect the laparoscopic outcome (EL4).

10.3 Laparoscopic Techniques

Concerning the different laparoscopic approaches to the emergency GHR, apart from the classical TAPP and TEP methods alone (se below), many variants have been described, which are known as "combined" or "hybrid" treatment where laparoscopy may have many possible roles, from the simple diagnostic evaluation

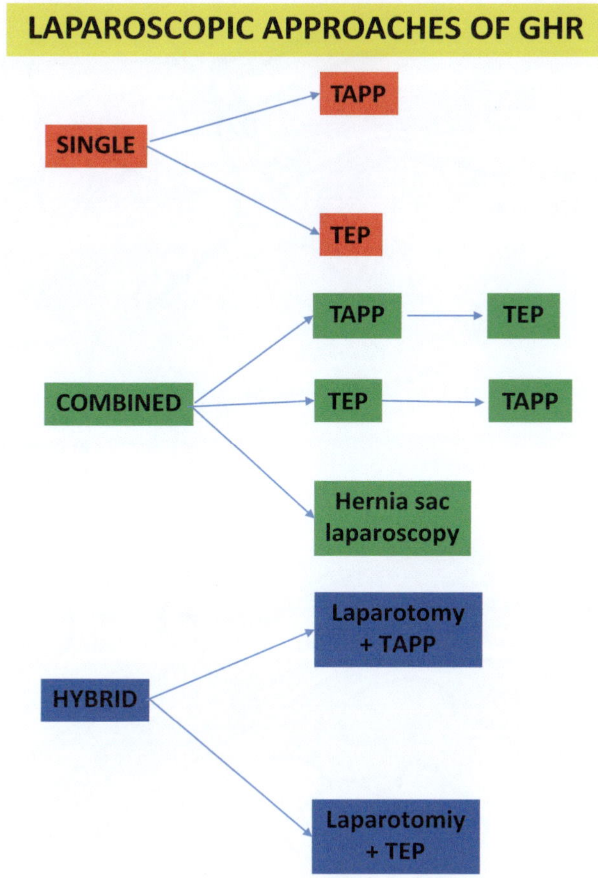

Fig. 10.1 Summary of laparoscopic approaches of GHR

of the bowel viability to a time of the surgical manipulation (Fig. 10.1). These composed techniques allow the surgeon to achieve an adequate peritoneal dissection of the cord in cases of long-standing nature of these hernias with the attendant anatomic distortion and an appropriate distension of the mesh.

1. *The Hybrid laparoscopic/laparotomic approach using the TAPP*. Some authors support the use of a TAPP, after an intra-abdominal reduction of the hernia sac through a scrotal incision, since in these cases the extra-peritoneal space is always limited even when the incarcerated hernia has been reduced, as the sac is often very large and requires extensive dissection from the cord structures. Another argument in favor of TAPP for such authors is the fact that, unlike TEP or open technique where the surgeons have a few minutes to make a decision on bowel resection, trans-abdominal approach allows the reassessment of the

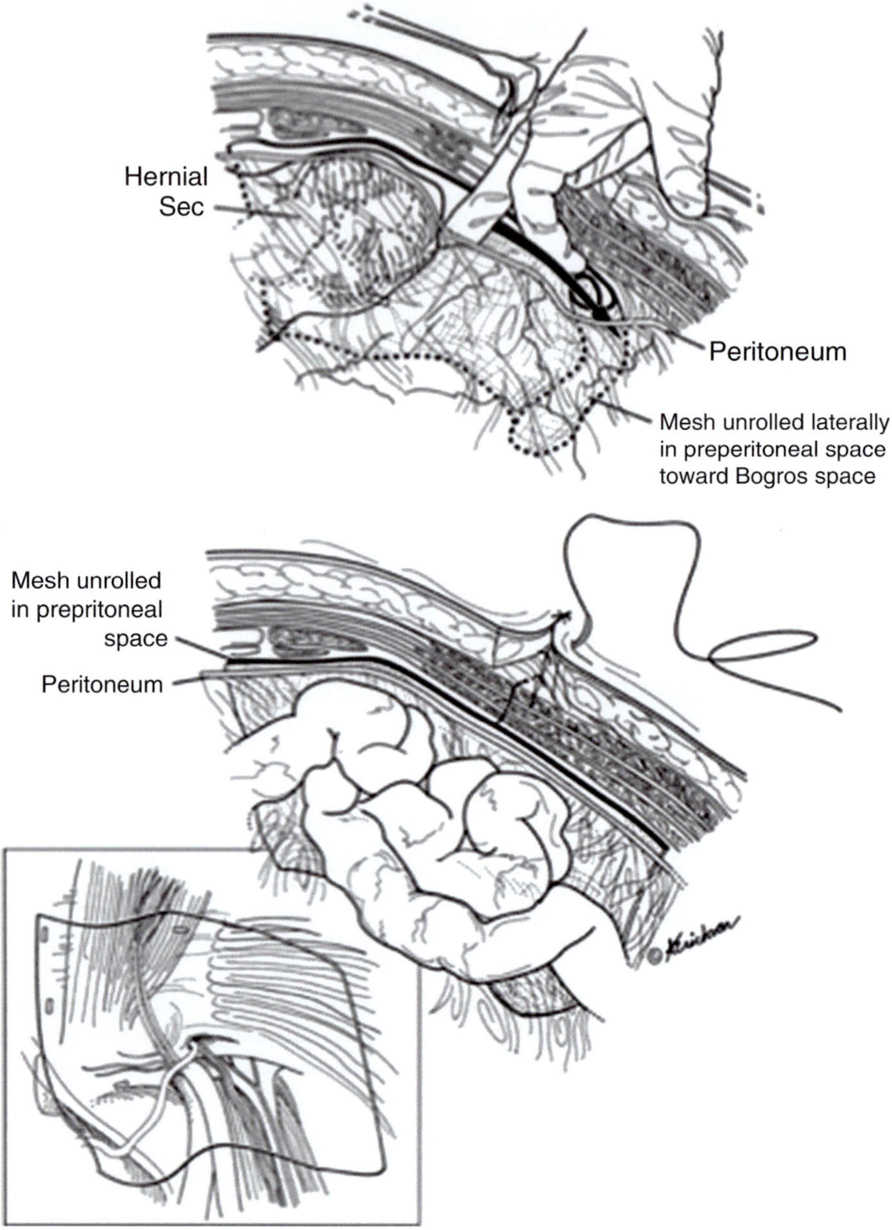

Fig. 10.2 Completing placement of the mesh

viability of bowels at the end of the procedure, thereby avoiding unnecessary bowel resection [8] (Fig. 10.2).

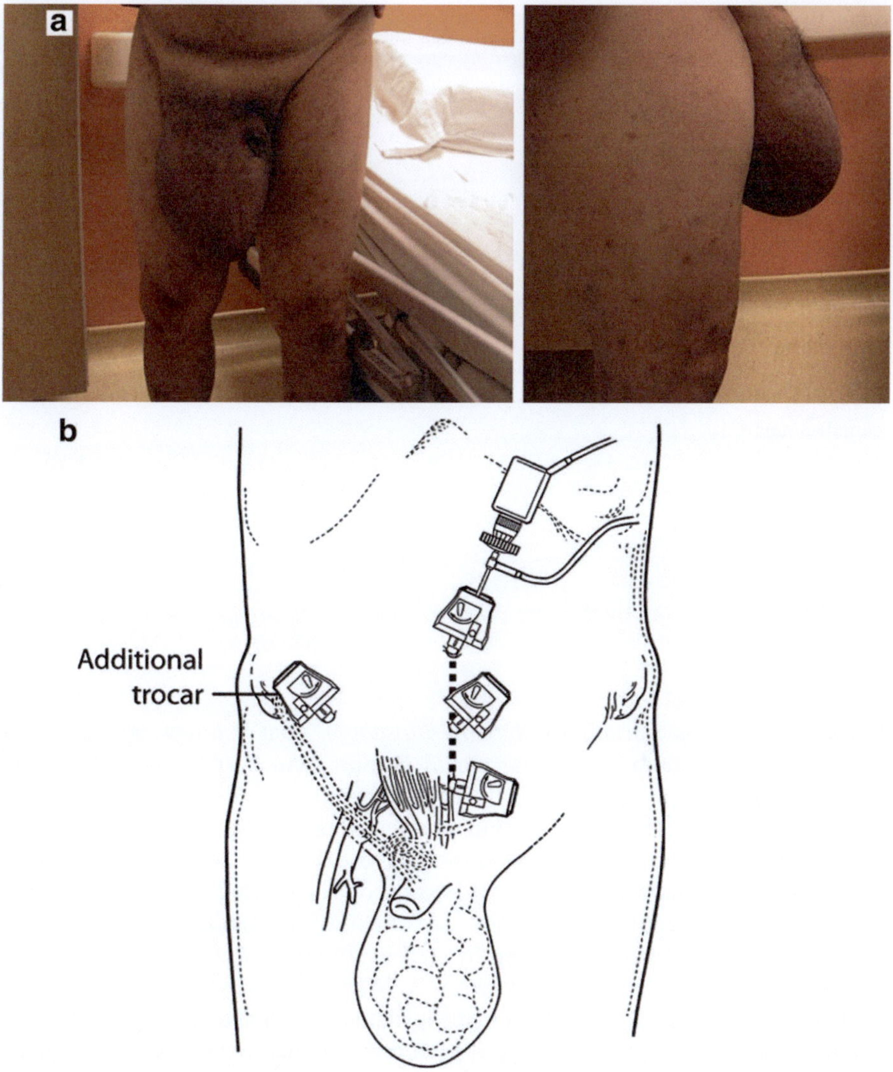

Fig. 10.3 (**a**) Giant inguino-scrotal hernia. (**b**) Placement of ports

2. *Hybrid laparoscopic/laparotomic using the TEP*. Other authors prefer the TEP because they feel that laparoscopic extra-peritoneal preparation of the pre-peritoneal floor avoids the usual struggle of an open pre-peritoneal repair and results in a larger and better positioned mesh than in an open anterior approach. In addition, dissection of the cord structures does not rely on invagination of the sac which makes the dissection more difficult when dealing with the scrotal hernia [9] (Fig. 10.3a, b)

Table 10.4 Outcome and follow-up in the study by Sgourakis et al.

	Laparoscopic group	Open group	*P* value
Operstive time (min)	67.78 ± 12.39	82.84 ± 21.08	<0.05
Presence of hemorrhagic fluid	8	7	0.885
Extension of the operation (no. of patients)	2 (2 resections)	4 (4 standard laparotomies, 2 resections)	0.413
Median hospital stay (h)	28	34	0.044
Hospital stay over 36 h	3	9	0.108
Major complications	0	4 (20 %)	<0.05
Minor complications	3 (14 %)	3 (15 %)	0.955
Deaths	0	2	0.157
Return to ordinary and professional activities (days)	17.28 ± 5.34	24.23 ± 9.14	0.017
Recurrent hernia	0	0	-

3. *The new "hernia sac laparoscopy (hernioscopy)"* that is a new mixed laparoscopic/open technique for incarcerated hernias, which spontaneously reduce during the surgical manipulations. This technique consists of inserting a 10-mm trocar through the internal inguinal ring and place a tight purse-string suture on the hernia sac. Patient is placed in the Trendelenburg position and pneumoperitoneum is established. A 10-mm laparoscope is inserted for the inspection of the incarcerated content and for the assessment of its viability (color, swelling, peristalsis, and ischemia). A step-by-step exploration of the whole abdominal cavity is to be subsequently performed. When detecting gangrenous hernia content an additional 10-mm port in the ipsilateral lower abdomen quadrant helps retrieve the hernia content through the internal inguinal ring by using a clamp for fixing the specimen. By pushing the hernia content through the internal inguinal ring the laparoscope is simultaneously withdrawn. Alternatively, an open mini-laparotomy may be performed at the site of the second trocar for retrieval and resection. A randomized controlled study suggested that this was effective in avoiding unnecessary laparotomy (Table 10.4) [10].
4. *Combined "one stage" sequential TAPP/TEP*. In this technique an intra-peritoneal laparoscopic exploration and hernia reduction (followed by mini-laparotomic bowel resection if necessary) is followed by a subsequent TEP repair (Fig. 10.4). The results of the preliminary report suggest that this approach is safe, feasible, and effective, offering an easy reduction of the hernia content with a superb view for assessing its viability, followed by a standard TEP repair,

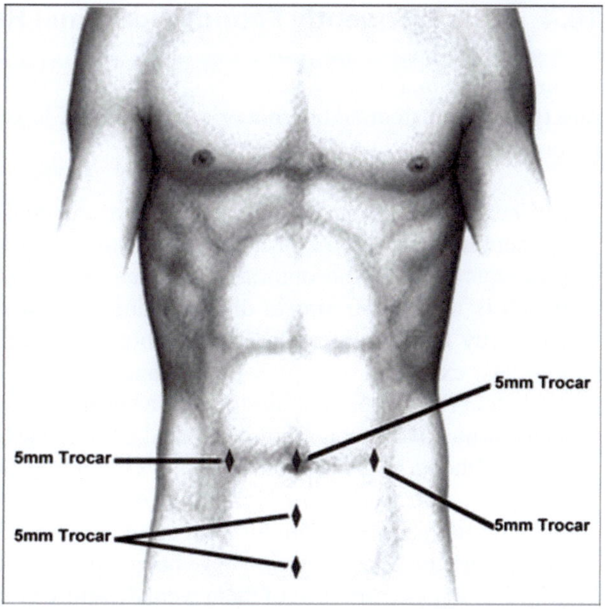

Fig. 10.4 Placement of trocars. After completion of intraperitoneal laparoscopic reduction, the umbilical 5-mm trocar is removed, a Hasson trocar is introduced into the pre-peritoneal space, and a standard total extra-peritoneal (TEP) repair is performed

with minimal risk of major complications such as wound and mesh infection. It also offers the opportunity to repair a concurrent bilateral hernia if found. The authors answer to the predictable opposition that abdominal exploration should naturally be followed by TAPP procedure and that this approach may allow to perform a safer technique in urgent cases for such surgeons who are used to perform TEP in their practice in elective cases. Furthermore, in their series, despite incarceration of bowel in the inguinal canal, not a single case of postoperative mesh infection was recorded. They attribute this positive result to the particularities of TEP technique in which the post-reduction empty hernia sac usually can be easily reduced unopened,and theoretically may serve as a barrier between the intra-peritoneal portion of the sac containing the incarcerated bowel and the pre-peritoneal space, in which the mesh is placed [9].

5. *Combined "two-stage" laparoscopic hernioplasty*. In this kind of approach, which has been introduced for the first time by Ginestà and Sasaki [11, 12], the second TEP procedure might be recommended within a week after first operation and possible resection of the strangulated viscous, if inflammatory response of the first surgery is settled and patient's condition is fit for general anesthesia. In such a way the inflammatory response of the first surgery is settled and patient's condition is fit for a second general anesthesia. Therefore, this treatment is particularly suggested for elderly patients, in poor general health, and in case of with femoral or obturator hernias requiring intestinal resection. Sometimes, when the patients are particularly high aged and have relatively hyponutrition, duration between first and second surgery may be longer.

10.4 Less Frequently Found Abdominal Hernias

A number of small case-series or single-case reports have been reported on other rare types of incarcerated hernia or other types of laparoscopic techniques that are reported below.

1. Most case reports concern emergency *obturator hernioplasties* [13]. The obturator hernia is a rare type of abdominal wall hernia in which abdominal content protrudes through the obturator foramen (Fig. 10.5). The obturator foramen, which is usually 10 mm in diameter and oval in shape, is almost completely closed by the obturator membrane, obturator internus, and obturator externus muscles, except at the upper part. Emaciation has been known to be the most important risk factor of obturator hernia because massive weight loss leads to loss of the protective effect of pre-peritoneal fat over the obturator canal and increases the likelihood of herniation. Thus, it commonly occurs in debilitated elderly people in their seventh or eighth decades and is sometimes called the "skinny old lady hernia." Up to 50–60 % of cases present with partial bowel obstruction in Richter's type incarceration have been reported. Bowel resection is required in 25–75 % of cases, as most of them were diagnosed too late. The mortality rate has

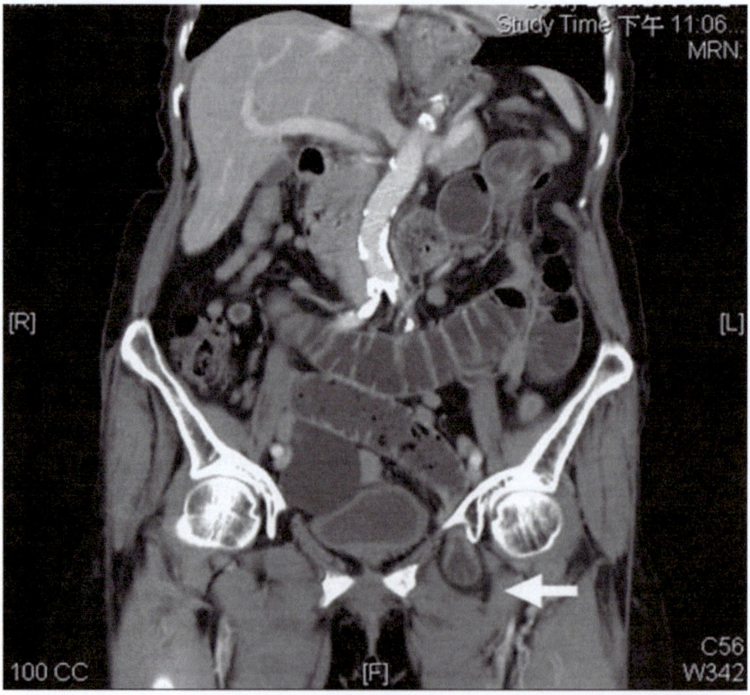

Fig. 10.5 Incarcerated left obturator hernia on CT coronal reconstruction. The *arrow* indicates the location of the left obturator hernia

been reported to be between 12 and 70 %. Unfavorable outcomes are commonly associated with delay in diagnosis and surgical intervention. The laparoscopic approach may be advantageous for both early diagnosis and treatment with good results in terms of resolution of symptoms and hospital stay. It enables clear bilateral visualization of all of the potential hernia orifices of the region. It has a lower rate of postoperative ileus due to gentler manipulation of the intestine, decreased pulmonary complications, less postsurgical pain resulting in shorter postoperative hospital stays, and better esthetic results. These advantages are especially important in these old-aged, fragile, and malnourished patients.

2. The *spigelian hernia*, which is a rare condition that requires a low degree of suspicion to diagnose because of the overlying intact external oblique and vague presenting symptoms [14] (Fig. 10.6). It accounts for 2 % of all the emergency surgeries with a high incarceration and strangulation rate (17–33 % according to the literature). The laparoscopic approach may accurately and quickly localize the obstruction site, which sometimes is a challenge in an open repair of this type of hernia, especially in an obese individual. Laparoscopic repair has lower recurrence rates, is associated with a quicker recovery, and has a shorter hospital stay compared with open techniques also according to the literature (5.2 vs. 1.4 days). This is true even in the elderly patients undergoing laparoscopic repair of spigelian hernias. TEP has been the method of choice in elective cases, whereas a combined laparotomy after a laparoscopic diagnosis or an IPOM-like totally laparoscopic treatment has been the preferred method in emergency settings, mainly because of small bowel incarceration and distension in emergency presentation.
3. The *De Garangeot hernia*, consisting of a concomitant inflamed appendix incarcerated within the hernia sac [15]. Acute appendicitis within a femoral hernia

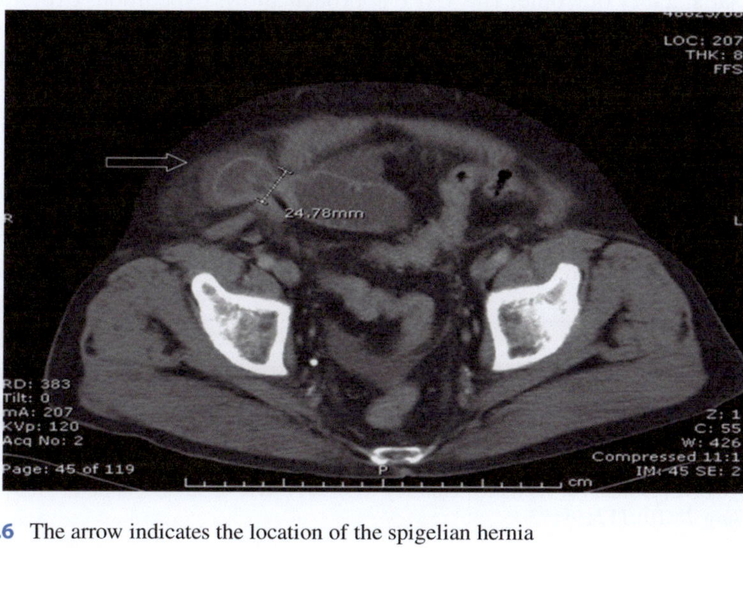

Fig. 10.6 The arrow indicates the location of the spigelian hernia

accounts for 0.13 % of all cases of acute appendicitis. Usually, inflammation of the appendix is attributed to intraluminal obstruction or obstruction at the opening with the cecum. However, it is thought that external compression of the appendix at the neck of the hernia explains the cause of acute appendicitis in femoral hernia. The anatomy of the femoral canal usually prevents intraperitoneal spread of infection, and hence, the patient will not present with symptoms of peritonitis but rather local signs such as erythema and groin tenderness. The use of imaging in these cases is controversial. CT scanning has been shown to be of benefit in some studies; however, it is quite unlikely and difficult to diagnose appendicitis within the groin mass itself. The laparoscopy is therefore the best modality of investigation when the clinical suspect is present and, at the same time, it allows the contemporary resection of the appendix and repair of the hernia defect. It is not recommended to place synthetic mesh plugs within the defect because of the infective and inflammatory processes involved in appendicitis.

4. The *"reduction en masse" incarcerated hernia*, a rare complication of an incarcerated inguinal hernia, occurring in approximately 1 of 13,000 hernias [16]. It arises when the incarcerated sac is reduced into the pro-peritoneal space with forcible manipulation or during the operation. The intestinal loop remains trapped in the sac, however, and obstruction persists. If left unrecognized and untreated, strangulation may develop and result in significant morbidity and mortality. Reduction en masse occurs because repeated difficult reductions cause trauma to the neck of the sac. Subsequent scarring makes it unyielding to the incarcerated bowel. A relatively lax hernial ring allowing the passage of the sac through it conjointly facilitates the development of reduction en masse. A delay in diagnosis is not infrequent because of the ambiguous presentation. If suspected, computed tomography of the abdomen helps to confirm the diagnosis. A TAPP hernioplasty can be used for managing incarcerated inguinal hernias with satisfactory outcome. The TAPP approach allows expeditious exploration of the abdominal cavity for concomitant defects. The incarceration can be promptly relieved and the viability of the bowel observed while performing hernioplasty. Unnecessary bowel resections can therefore be avoided. In cases of irreversible ischemia of the bowel, a resection can be performed after the conclusion of the hernioplasty.

Diaphragmatic and internal incarcerated hernias are beyond the scope of this chapter.

References

1. Kulah B, Kulacoglu IH, Oruc MT, Duzgun AP, Moran M, Ozmen MM, Coskun F (2001) Presentation and outcome of incarcerated external hernias in adults. Am J Surg 181(2):101–104
2. Gallegos NC, Dawson J, Jarvis M, Hobsley M (1991) Risk of strangulation in groin hernias. Br J Surg 78(10):1171–1173

3. Watson SD, Saye W, Hollier PA (1993) Combined laparoscopic incarcerated herniorrhaphy and small bowel resection. Surg Laparosc Endosc 3(2):106–108
4. McCormack K, Scott NW, Go PM, Ross S, Grant AM, EU Hernia Trialists Collaboration (2003) Laparoscopic techniques versus open techniques for inguinal hernia repair. Cochrane Database Syst Rev 1, CD001785
5. Dedemadi G, Sgourakis G, Radtke A, Dounavis A, Gockel I, Fouzas I, Karaliotas C, Anagnostou E (2010) Laparoscopic versus open mesh repair for recurrent inguinal hernia: a meta-analysis of outcomes. Am J Surg 200(2):291–297
6. Deeba S, Purkayastha S, Paraskevas P, Athanasiou T, Darzi A, Zacharakis E (2009) Laparoscopic approach to incarcerated and strangulated inguinal hernias. JSLS 13(3):327–331
7. Yang GP, Chan CT, Lai EC, Chan OC, Tang CN, Li MK (2012) Laparoscopic versus open repair for strangulated groin hernias: 188 cases over 4 years. Asian J Endosc Surg 5(3):131–137
8. Siow SL, Mahendran HA, Hardin M, Chea CH, Nik Azim NA (2013) Laparoscopic transabdominal approach and its modified technique for incarcerated scrotal hernias. Asian J Surg 36(2):64–68
9. Hoffman A, Leshem E, Zmora O, Nachtomi O, Shabtai M, Ayalon A, Rosin D (2010) The combined laparoscopic approach for the treatment of incarcerated inguinal hernia. Surg Endosc 24(8):1815–1818
10. Sgourakis G, Radtke A, Sotiropoulos GC, Dedemadi G, Karaliotas C, Fouzas I, Karaliotas C (2009) Assessment of strangulated content of the spontaneously reduced inguinal hernia via hernia sac laparoscopy: preliminary results of a prospective randomized study. Surg Laparosc Endosc Percutan Tech 19(2):133–137
11. Ginestà C, Saavedra-Perez D, Valentini M, Vidal O, Benarroch G, García-Valdecasas JC (2013) Total extraperitoneal (TEP) hernioplasty with intestinal resection assisted by laparoscopy for a strangulated Richter femoral hernia. Surg Laparosc Endosc Percutan Tech 23(3):334–336
12. Sasaki A, Takeuchi Y, Izumi K, Morimoto A, Inomata M, Kitano S (2014) Two-stage laparoscopic treatment for strangulated inguinal, femoral and obturator hernias: totally extraperitoneal repair followed by intestinal resection assisted by intraperitoneal laparoscopic exploration. Hernia, Jun 8:1–6
13. Maricevich M, Farley D (2011) A pseudo-TEP repair of an incarcerated obturator hernia. Int J Surg Case Rep 2(8):290–292
14. Subramanya MS, Chakraborty J, Memon B, Memon MA (2010) Emergency intraperitoneal onlay mesh repair of incarcerated spigelian hernia. JSLS 14(2):275–278
15. Shah A, Sira Janardhan H (2013) De garengeot hernia: a case report and review of literature. Indian J Surg 75(Suppl 1):439–441
16. Wu CC, Kang JC, Huang YM (2012) Laparoscopic transabdominal preperitoneal hernioplasty for reduction en masse of an incarcerated inguinal hernia: a case report. J Gastrointest Surg 16(7):1433–1435

Incarcerated Incisional and Ventral Hernias 11

Micaela Piccoli, Grazia Maria Attina', Vincenzo Trapani, Domenico Marchi, Barbara Mullineris, and Bruno Scotto

11.1 Introduction

Laparoscopic repair of ventral and incisional hernia has gained wider acceptance among surgeons than the open technique, due to the favorable results in terms of incidence of recurrences, complications, and patient satisfaction. After postoperative peritoneal adhesions, these diseases are the second most common cause of occlusion of the small intestine and therefore deserve some considerations aside [1]. Complications such as incarcerations or strangulation may occur in 5 % of cases [2, 3]. Urgent surgical procedures may be required in 5–13 % of incarcerated abdominal wall hernia cases and intestinal resections may be required in 10–15 % [4].

The emergency laparoscopic treatment of incarcerated incisional and ventral hernias seems to be one of the most interesting and debated topics [2]. Apart from case reports and few case series, the role of the laparoscopic treatment of ventral/incisional hernias in emergent situations for strangulation and/or incarceration has not been established to date, due to the reluctance to use this approach in such situations [2–5].

In these instances, a traditional open approach is preferred without placing a mesh in most of the cases, aiming at the resolution of the life-threatening condition and delaying the definitive repair. On the other hand, there are available evidences that demonstrate the superiority of laparoscopic approach in various abdominal emergencies [5].

M. Piccoli (✉) • G.M. Attina' • V. Trapani • D. Marchi • B. Mullineris • B. Scotto
Dipartimento di Chirurgia. UOC di Chirurgia Generale, d'Urgenza e Nuove Tecnologie, Nuovo Ospedale Civile Sant'Agostino Estense (NOCSAE), 41126 Modena, Italy
e-mail: m.piccoli@ausl.mo.it; graziamaria.attina@gmail.com; v.trapani@ausl.mo.it; d.marchi@ausl.mo.it; b.mullineris@ausl.mo.it; dr.brunoscotto@gmail.com

F. Agresta et al. (eds.), *Emergency Laparoscopy*,
DOI 10.1007/978-3-319-29620-3_11

11.2 Incarcerated Ventral and Incisional Hernia

In 2005 [6], the previous International Consensus Conference of the European Association of Endoscopic Surgery (EAES) stated that the open approach remains the standard treatment for incarcerated hernia, although laparoscopic surgery may be considered in selected patients and restricted to surgeons with maximum expertise in this field.

In 2010 [7], an Italian Consensus Conference of the main national scientific societies (SIC, ACOI, SICE, and the Italian Chapter of Hernia Society) on laparoscopic treatment of ventral and incisional hernia underlined that the incidence of intra- and postoperative complications and recurrences in emergency cases was the same as in elective cases. Good experience in emergency surgery and in laparoscopic repair of the abdominal wall in elective patients is always strictly required.

In 2012 [8], the Consensus Development Conference on Laparoscopic approach to acute abdomen (SICE, ACOI, SIC, SICUT, SICOP, EAES) confirmed that the laparoscopic approach to incarcerated ventral and incisional hernias may be performed in selected patients.

In these three Consensus, the grade of recommendation was GoR C.

The objective of this study is to evaluate recent and relevant news about laparoscopic approach to incarcerated ventral and incisional hernia repair with respect to previous Consensus Development Conference on *"Laparoscopic approach to acute abdomen"* of 2012.

The main points were:

- Selection criteria for patients undergoing laparoscopic repair in emergency
- Surgical details
- Use of biological prosthesis in contaminated field

11.2.1 Selection Criteria for Patients Undergoing Laparoscopic Repair in Emergency

Incarcerated or strangulated ventral/incisional hernias are due to small bowel obstruction (SBO). In these cases, safety and feasibility of the laparoscopic approach has been reported in several studies with various outcomes. According to the previous recommendations (EAES 2005, Italian Consensus Conference of laparoscopy in acute abdomen 2012, SICE 2013), laparoscopic treatment of incarcerated or strangulated ventral/incisional hernia can be successfully accomplished in selected patients [6–8] .

Either randomized control trials or prospective controlled studies are available in the literature [9], and laparoscopy remains contraindicated in these cases [9] :

- High operative risk
- Hemodynamic instability
- Massive abdominal distension
- Perforation and/or bowel necrosis
- Limited laparoscopic experience

Best cases for laparoscopy are patients with incarcerated ventral incisional hernia in these situations [9–11]:

- Absence of *marked abdominal distension* with reduced working space that precludes entry into the peritoneal cavity. Moderate abdominal distension and bowel distension with a diameter <5 cm are favorable situations with low risk of conversion (Fig. 11.1). Laparoscopic management of acute SBO caused by an incarcerated incisional hernia is challenging because of the reduced working space due to ileus, the fragility of dilated intestinal loops, and the difficulty to identify the cause of obstruction in some cases. Manipulation of bowel should be done very carefully as intestinal injuries can have disastrous consequences (conversion rates ranging from 0 % to 52 % according to surgeon's skill and patient selection) [9–14].

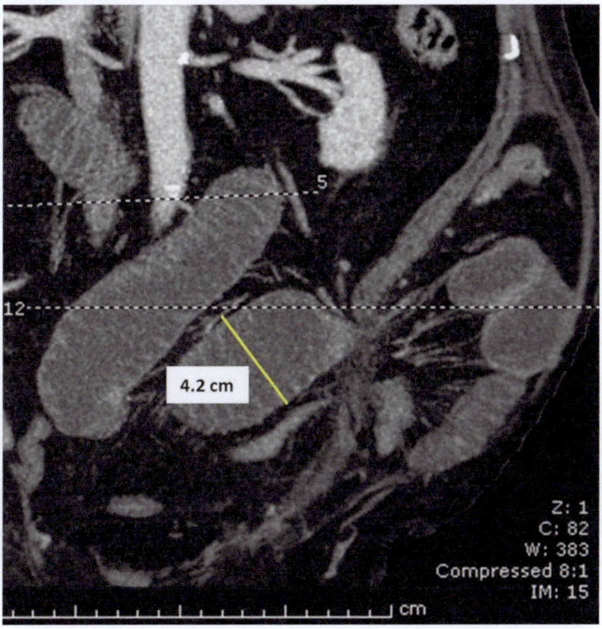

Fig. 11.1 Abdomen CT: incarcerated ventral hernia with moderate abdominal distension and bowel distension with a diameter of 4.2 cm

- Some authors introduce the *number (>4) of previous laparotomies* as a predictive factor of conversion [5]. However, not only the number but also the type of previous procedure and the location of the surgical scars are very important. As far as adhesiolysis is concerned, one surgical xipho-pubic scar following an abdominal trauma or massive peritonitis will often give rise to more difficulties than three scars (for example, in the right subcostal area, in the hypogastrium, and in the right iliac region) resulting from elective and uncomplicated surgery [15];
- Absence of peritonitis with the need for bowel resection and bowel handling in a highly inflamed environment and absence of clinical signs of intestinal ischemia [2, 3, 5];
- Absence of high septic-risk situations, for example, concomitant execution of contaminated abdominal procedures and the presence of contaminated skin lesions or enterocutaneous fistulas [2, 3, 5] ;
- Absence of major defects with loss of domain or hernias that do not allow the laparoscopic approach with adequate overlap of the mesh [2];
- Morbid obesity, old age, and debilitation are not considered contraindications to laparoscopy [16, 17].

11.2.2 Details of Surgical Technique

The search showed no studies directly comparing different methods of adhesiolysis and their risks, although the 2012 Italian Consensus Conference recommended cold and sharp adhesiolysis. In an animal model, ultrasonic coagulating shears, electrothermal bipolar vessel sealer, titanium laparoscopic clips, and plastic laparoscopic clips show safe hemostasis. In order to reduce the thermal damage on the intestine, we reiterate the concept that it is safer to use cold and sharp adhesiolysis or ultrasonic dissection [18, 19].

When an incisional hernia is found to be the cause of obstruction, all incarcerated or strangulated intestinal contents are reduced back into the abdominal cavity and inspected for viability [14]. The hernial contents are reduced by a combination of manual external pressure, internal traction, and adhesiolysis.

As in open surgery, adequate traction and countertraction are the key elements for a successful procedure, facilitating the identification of the avascular plane of dissection [3, 13, 14, 20–22].

The best way to release the bowel is the enlargement of the hernia's port using careful incision of the fascia at the edge of the hernia's ring. It is essential to use atraumatic grasper and cold scissors close to bowels (Fig. 11.2A–D). The next step is similar to the elective treatment: positioning of intraperitoneal mesh fixed with tacks.

The dangerous part of the laparoscopic approach consists in the adhesiolysis because it may lead to bowel perforation [2]. Most series reveal no differences

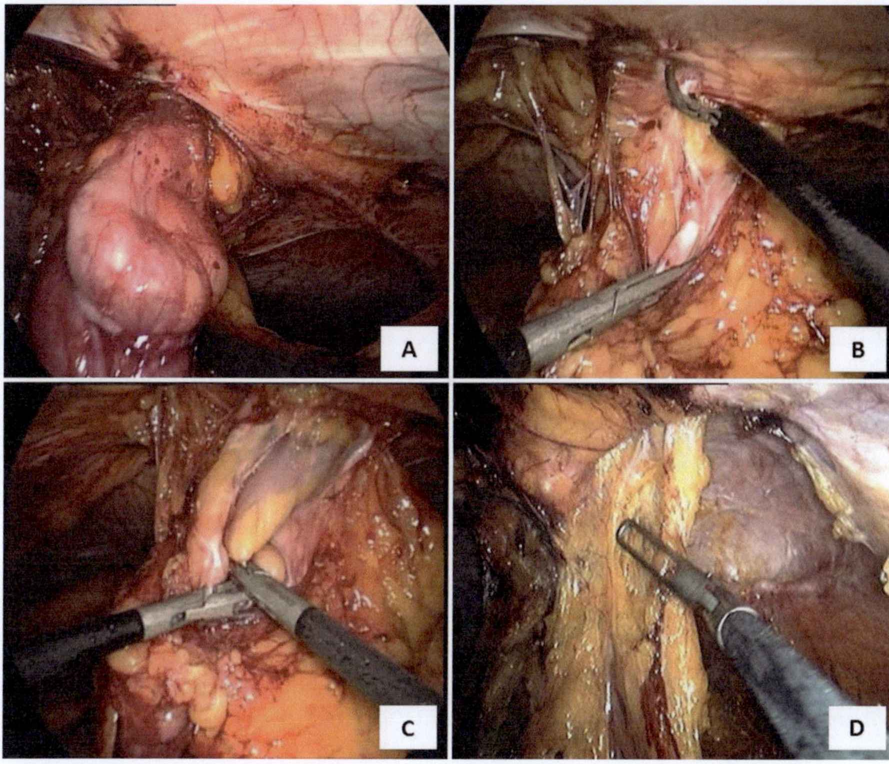

Fig. 11.2 (**a–d**) Laparoscopic view of the incarcerated incisional hernia of the middle line: reduction of the intestinal contents with enlargement of the hernia's port using careful incision of the fascia at the edge of the hernia's ring

between open and laparoscopic groups with respect to iatrogenic injuries to bowel. In general, iatrogenic injuries were more likely in the presence of dense and extensive adhesions [13]. Two bowel injury mechanisms have been described: direct trauma by scissor with no intraoperative recognition and an indirect lesion due to energy source with subsequent necrosis causing the perforation [15].

The need to perform proper adhesiolysis, in order to adequately identify the hernia defect allowing the placing of the mesh, represents a crucial point [2]; this is particularly important in the emergency setting due to the bowel distension of the incarcerated bowel loops, associated with the vascular compromise with possible development of necrosis and contaminated effusion and the impossibility to perform an adequate preoperative bowel cleaning [22].

The incidence of recognized enterotomies varies from 6 to 14.3 %; the management of this condition is somewhat controversial: in many centers the hernia procedure is terminated and the injury is repaired both laparoscopically and by conversion to open technique and the hernia repair deferred [23]. Most recently, some authors have reported the feasibility to repair the enterotomy laparoscopically and to complete the procedure with the application of mesh in cases where the injury is not associated with a large amount of spillage of intestinal content [12, 20, 24]. We suggest to repair the lesions laparoscopically if the iatrogenic lesion involves the small bowel, without fecal contamination of the abdomen, and to proceed in positioning the mesh. If the lesion involves the colon or if there is a fecal contamination, we prefer to suture the perforation, clean the abdomen, and place the mesh during a second operation [3, 14, 22].

Moreover, surgeons must be very careful and check the bowel at the end of the procedure to avoid any undiscovered lesion that, in the postoperative period, can cause peritonitis. The peritonitis is the major complication that occurs in up to 6 % of patient and can lead to fatal consequences involving a 0.3 % of mortality [25]. This implies a strict early postoperative follow-up to identify suspicious symptoms and signs like fever, leukocytosis, increasing abdominal pain to establish a correct diagnosis, and an early reoperation. Some authors identified three categories of patients with high risk of visceral injury [5]:

1. *Hernias with multiple bowel loops*
2. *Previous recent repair with intraperitoneal polypropylene mesh*
3. *Previous episodes of severe peritonitis*

In the presence of incarceration under these circumstances, laparoscopy still can be attempted. However, if release of the incarcerated bowel or release of the bowel adherent to the peritoneum around the hernia's defect cannot be performed safely, conversion to open repair must be considered [13, 20].

Reasons for conversion are: 1. Reduced working space because of intestinal distension; 2. Dense adhesions; 3. Iatrogenic perforation; 4. Bowel necrosis [3, 12, 14, 20, 26].

Iatrogenic perforation and bowel necrosis are relative reasons because they could be managed laparoscopically [14].

The conversion is not a failure, but simply the necessary sequence of events in the optimal management of these patients [13].

11.2.3 Surgical Experience

In several studies on laparoscopic repair in emergent situations, the authors talk about "learning curves" and "experienced surgeon" without defining them evenly. Studies, concerning elective surgery, suggest that the incidence of major complications such as a missed enterotomy and mortality tends to decrease as surgeon's experience increases after at least 50 cases [22, 25, 27]. Institutional and individual learning curves had no significant influence on clinical outcomes, although improved experience was reflected in improved operation time, conversion rate, and hospital stay [28].

However, this type of surgery requires experience in both laparotomic and laparoscopic emergency surgery, as well as a comprehensive experience in elective laparoscopic repair techniques. It is not possible to define the clinical competence because of too many variables: experience in previous different operations, high/low volume surgeon, and center.

11.2.4 Risk of Infection of the Mesh and Use of Biological Meshes

The Consensus Development Conference on laparoscopic treatment of ventral hernias (SICE 2013) reported the following data [2, 3, 5]:

- the presence of nonviable bowel (ischemic bowel or intestinal necrosis) has not to be considered as a contraindication for prosthetic repair and the immediate mesh repair is preferably deferred only in cases of abundant peritoneal contamination [11].
- The biological meshes provide a new prospective in the contaminated surgical field, in laparoscopic emergency hernia repair too, with good results in terms of recurrence and wound infection [12]. Nowadays, even if their laparoscopic implant is feasible, the use of biological prosthesis should be restricted to contaminated field in open surgery. Their laparoscopic use is recommended in controlled trials [29, 30].

The introduction of such materials in clinical practice has provided a new prospective for abdominal wall defect repair in contaminated surgical field [31]. Few authors suggest the use of biomaterial in the laparoscopic emergency hernia repair with good results in terms of recurrence rate and wound infection [26, 29]. There are no comparative trials evaluating each of the commercially available biological mesh products and their application in laparoscopic repair of potentially contaminated ventral hernias. Further studies are still required to establish the efficacy of biological mesh in laparoscopic repair in potentially contaminated fields.

References

1. Ghezzi TL, Moschetti L, Corleta OC, Abreu GP, Abreu LP (2010) Analysis of the videolaparoscopy potentiality in the surgical treatment of the bowel obstruction. Arq Gastroenterol 47(2):148–151
2. Olmi S, Cesana G, Eba L, Croce E (2009) Emergency laparoscopic treatment of acute incarcerated incisional hernia. Hernia 3:605–608
3. Shah RH, Sharma A, Khullar R, Soni V, Baijal M, Chowbey PK (2008) Laparoscopic repair of incarcerated ventral abdominal wall hernia. Hernia 12:457–463
4. Derici H, Unalp HR, Bozdag AD et al (2007) Factors affecting morbidity and mortality in incarcerated abdominal wall hernias. Hernia 11:341–346
5. Landau O, Kyzer S (2004) Emergent laparoscopic repair of incarcerated incisional and ventral hernia. Surg Endosc 18:1374–1376
6. Sauerland S et al (2006) Emergent laparoscopic repair of incarcerated incisional and ventral hernia. Surg Endosc 20(1):14–29

7. Agresta F et al (2012) Laparoscopic approach to acute abdomen from the Consensus Development Conference of the Società Italiana di Chirurgia Endoscopica e nuove tecnologie (SICE), Associazione Chirurghi Ospedalieri Italiani (ACOI), Società Italiana di Chirurgia (SIC), Società Italiana di Chirurgia d'Urgenza e del Trauma (SICUT), Società Italiana di Chirurgia nell'Ospedalità Privata (SICOP), and the European Association for Endoscopic Surgery (EAES). Surg Endosc 26(8):2134–2164
8. Cuccurullo D, Piccoli M, Agresta F, Magnone S, Corcione F, Stancanelli V, Melotti G (2013) Laparoscopic ventral incisional hernia repair: evidence-based guidelines of the first Italian Consensus Conference. Hernia 17(5):557–566
9. Navez B, Navez J (2014) Laparoscopy in the acute abdomen. Best Pract Res Clin Gastroenterol 28(1):3–17
10. Consensus Development Conference on laparoscopic treatment of ventral hernias (SICE 2013)
11. Bessa SS, Abdel-Razek AH (2013) Results of prosthetic mesh repair in the emergency management of the acutely incarcerated and/or strangulated ventral hernias: a seven years study. Hernia 17(1):59–65
12. Grafen FC, Neuhaus V, Schob O, Turina M (2010) Management of acute small bowel obstruction from intestinal adhesions: indications for laparoscopic surgery in a community teaching hospital. Langenbecks Arch Surg 395(1):57–63
13. Lujan HJ, Oren A, Plasencia G, Canelon G, Gomez E, Hernandez-Cano A, Jacobs M (2006) Laparoscopic management as the initial treatment of acute small bowel obstruction. JSLS 10:466–472
14. Franklin ME, Gonzalez JJ, Miter DB, Glass JL, Paulson D (2004) Laparoscopic diagnosis and treatment of intestinal obstruction. Surg Endosc 18:26–30
15. Piccoli M, Marchi D, Abati G, Melotti G (2008) Laparoscopic Approach in intestinal obstructions: indications, techniques, advantages and constraints. In: Sartelli M, Catena F (eds) Emergency surgery manual. Alpes, Rome, pp 227–238
16. Raftopoulos I, Courcoulas AP (2007) Outcome of laparoscopic ventral hernia repair in morbidly obese patients with a body mass index exceeding 35 kg/m2. Surg Endosc 21(12):2293–2297
17. Carlson MA, Frantzides CT, Shostrom VK, Laguna LE (2008) Minimally invasive ventral herniorrhaphy: an analysis of 6,266 published cases. Hernia 12:9–22
18. Bittner R, Bingener-Casey J, Dietz U et al (2014) Guidelines for laparoscopic treatment of ventral and incisional abdominal wall hernias (International Endohernia Society (IEHS)) – Part 1.2.3. Surg Endosc 28:2–29
19. Pawlak M, Bury K, Śmietański M (2015) The management of abdominal wall hernias – in search of consensus. Videosurgery Miniinv 10(1):49–56
20. Kirshtein B, Roy-Shapira A, Lantsberg L, Avinoach E, Mizrahi S (2005) Laparoscopic management of acute small bowel obstruction. Surg Endosc 19:464–467
21. Szomstein S, Lo Menzo E, Simpfendorfer C, Zundel N, Rosenthal R (2006) Laparoscopic lysis of adhesions. World J Surg 30:535–540
22. Sharma A, Mehrotra M, Khullar R, Soni V, Baijal M, Chowbey PK (2008) Limited-conversion technique: a safe and viable alternative to conversion in laparoscopic ventral/incisional hernia repair. Hernia 12:367–371
23. Assalia A, Gagner M, Shein M, Monson JR (eds) (2006) Controversies in laparoscopic surgery. Springer, New York, NY. ISBN: 3-540
24. Il trattamento laparoscopico del laparocele. Prima Consensus Conference Italiana. Allegato al n. 22 del 8-14 Giugno 2010. il Sole 24 ore. Sanità 5-41
25. Piccoli M, Ferronato M, Morici R, Gentile I, Mecheri F, Melotti G (2008) Emergency laparoscopic repair of complicated ventral and incisional hernias. Surgery 2:227–235
26. Parra MW, Rodas EB, Niravel AA (2010) Laparoscopic repair of potentially contaminated abdominal ventral hernias using a xenograft: a case series. Hernia 11:687
27. Salameh JR, Sweeney JF, Graviss EA, Essien FA, Williams MD, Awad S, Itani KM, Fisher WE (2006) Laparoscopic ventral hernia repair during the learning curve. Hernia 6(4):182–187

28. Neo EL, Zingg U, Devitt PG, Jamieson GG, Watson DI (2010) Learning curve for laparoscopic repair of very large hiatal hernia. Surg Endosc 7:1461–1468
29. Franklin ME Jr, Trevino JM, Portollo G, Vela I, Glass JL, Gonzalez JJ (2008) The use of porcine small intestinal submucosa as a prosthetic material for laparoscopic hernia repair in infected and potentially contaminated fields: long-term follow up. Surg Endosc 22:1941–1946 (EL 4)
30. Catena F, Coccolini F, Ansaloni L, Di Saverio S, Pinna AD (2011) Closure of the LAPSIS trial (Br J Surg 2010; 97: 1598). Br J Surg 98(2):319
31. Campanelli G, Catena F, Ansaloni L (2008) Prosthetic abdominal wall hernia repair in emergency surgery: from polypropylene to biological meshes. World J Emerg Surg 3:33

Emergency Laparoscopy for Abdominal Trauma

12

Salomone Di Saverio, Arianna Birindelli, Andrea Biscardi, Matteo Mandrioli, Luca Di Donato, Antonio Tarasconi, Roberto Cirocchi, Carlo Coniglio, Giovanni Gordini, and Gregorio Tugnoli

12.1 Introduction

Although the first experiences of trauma laparoscopy were reported in the early 1920s [1], the technique did not become immediately popular due to concerns on the effects of pneumoperitoneum on such delicate patients and because of the relative inexperience in this procedure and limited laparoscopic skills among the surgeons.

Starting from the second part of the twentieth century, laparoscopy has been increasingly used in elective surgery, and, from the beginning of the twenty-first century, it has been introduced also in emergency surgery [2] and finally in trauma surgery.

Trauma patients are particularly frail since most of them have multiple organ injuries. Several advantages of the minimally invasive approach such as decreased postoperative pain and less adhesion formation, faster recovery and shorter length of

---

Author's Contribution: AB and SDS wrote the chapter; AB searched and revised the literature; SDS has described the surgical techniques and performed all laparoscopic procedures; SDS provided patients materials and pictures; all authors critically revised the chapter and gave the final approval of manuscript.

S. Di Saverio, MD, FACS, FRCS (✉) • A. Birindelli, MD • A. Biscardi, MD • M. Mandrioli, MD • L. Di Donato, MD • A. Tarasconi, MD • G. Tugnoli, MD, PhD
Maggiore Hospital Regional Emergency Surgery and Trauma Center – Bologna Local Health District, AUSL Bologna, Bologna, Italy
e-mail: salo75@inwind.it; salomone.disaverio@gmail.com

R. Cirocchi, MD
Department of Surgery, Hospital of Terni, University of Perugia, Perugia, Italy

C. Coniglio, MD • G. Gordini, MD, PhD, MPH
Trauma ICU, Trauma Center – Department of Emergency, Maggiore Hospital – Bologna Local Health District, Bologna, Italy

F. Agresta et al. (eds.), *Emergency Laparoscopy*,
DOI 10.1007/978-3-319-29620-3_12

hospital stay, earlier return to work and daily physical activities, fewer postoperative wound infections, incisional hernias, and better cosmetic results are already well known and are easily reproducible also in the setting of trauma patients. Moreover, in the injured patients the use of minimally invasive surgery is particularly valuable since it is able to decrease the systemic inflammatory response with lower risk of secondary organ injury (especially lungs and kidneys) [3, 4]. Diagnostic laparoscopy seems to significantly reduce the rate of negative laparotomies [5–14], having high sensitivity, specificity, and accuracy [6, 7, 9, 13, 15, 16], especially in penetrating abdominal trauma, with better cost-effectiveness when compared to open surgery [12, 13, 17].

Despite these potential benefits, laparoscopy has not yet gained widespread acceptance within the trauma community and its role in this area is still under strong debate. The most relevant criticisms have been raised are about the longer time needed in laparoscopy to set up the equipment, enter the abdomen, and control the injury but also the risk of missed injuries that are particularly high if the surgeon has minimal experience in minimally invasive surgery.

Provided a careful selection of patients and advanced laparoscopic surgical training, this technique can be then extremely useful in trauma patients both as a diagnostic and, eventually, a therapeutic tool.

12.2 Diagnostic Laparoscopy

Laparoscopy may be an accurate diagnostic tool for abdominal trauma, having nowadays replaced Diagnostic Peritoneal Lavage (DPL) being much more accurate and representing as well a minimally invasive alternative to exploratory laparotomy.

Laparoscopy revealed to be particularly useful in the diagnosis of intra-abdominal organ injuries for hemodynamically stable trauma patients with doubtful clinical or imaging findings and it has been already demonstrated to be able to greatly decrease the rate of nontherapeutic laparotomies, with obvious benefits for both the patient's health and cosmesis and the economy, in terms of morbidity, length of stay, and return to work [6, 9, 11, 12, 14, 17–23]. Despite the clear advantages of the procedure, it is very important to perform it only in correctly selected patients and by experienced and laparoscopically skilled surgeons [7, 9, 10, 18, 19, 24, 25].

12.2.1 Patient Selection

The first step in order to safely perform a diagnostic laparoscopy in trauma patients is the correct selection of candidates.

First of all, the absolute need of hemodynamic stability is widely accepted, in terms of selecting as candidates for trauma laparoscopy those patients having hypovolemic shock no higher than ATLS class I (see Table 12.1) or patients fully responders to initial small-volume fluid bolus administration. Class

Table 12.1 ATLS classification of hemorrhagic shock

	Class I	Class II	Class III	Class IV
Blood loss (ml)	<750	750–1500	1500–2000	>2000
Pulse rate (per min)	<100	>100	>120	>140
Blood pressure	Normal	Normal	Decreased	Decreased
Pulse pressure (mmHg)	Normal	Decreased	Decreased	Decreased
Respiratory rate (per min)	14–20	20–30	30–40	>40
Urine output (ml/h)	>30	20–30	5–15	Negligible
Central venous system (mental status)	Slightly anxious	Mildly anxious	Anxious confused	Lethargic

II–III–IV hypovolemic shock patients, transient or nonresponders to fluid resuscitation, septic shock patients, or those with cardiorespiratory contraindications to pneumoperitoneum are not suitable for laparoscopy. Another absolute contraindication to laparoscopy is a severe traumatic brain injury, since it has been reported that pneumoperitoneum may increase the intracerebral pressure [26].

FAST US followed by a total body CT scan is recommended in every stable patient with blunt abdominal trauma, or with penetrating abdominal trauma after gunshot wound or after stab wound on the lower quadrants or on the back, in order to assess the site and extent of injuries. However, it has been demonstrated that both US and CT scan have low sensitivity and specificity in diagnosing diaphragmatic, mesentery, and hollow viscus injuries [27, 28], with significant negative impact on patient outcome. On the other hand, laparoscopy has been reported to be highly sensitive and specific as well as accurate, in the presence of appropriate surgical skills [7, 9, 13, 19].

Diagnostic laparoscopy is indicated either in blunt or penetrating abdominal trauma, in case of CT scan equivocal findings or discrepancy between the clinical examination and the imaging, the so-called unclear abdomen, but also in case of unclear source of potentially active bleeding.

Another common indication to diagnostic laparoscopy in blunt trauma is the finding of unexplained free abdominal fluid with the suspicion of a hollow viscus injury or a mesenteric laceration on a CT scan.

In case of penetrating trauma, laparoscopy can be used to investigate the presence of abdominal free fluid in the absence of parenchymal injuries and to rule out the suspicion of peritoneal penetration (Fig. 12.1), hollow viscus injury, or diaphragmatic injury (Fig. 12.2). A further indication for diagnostic laparoscopy in penetrating abdominal trauma is the suspicion of an occult diaphragmatic injury, even in the presence of a spleen or liver injury successfully managed with observation +/− angioembolization.

In case of a stable patient with isolated penetrating abdominal trauma after stab wound of the anterior and upper quadrants and a suspected diaphragmatic injury, the CT scan can even be avoided and a straight diagnostic laparoscopy may be performed.

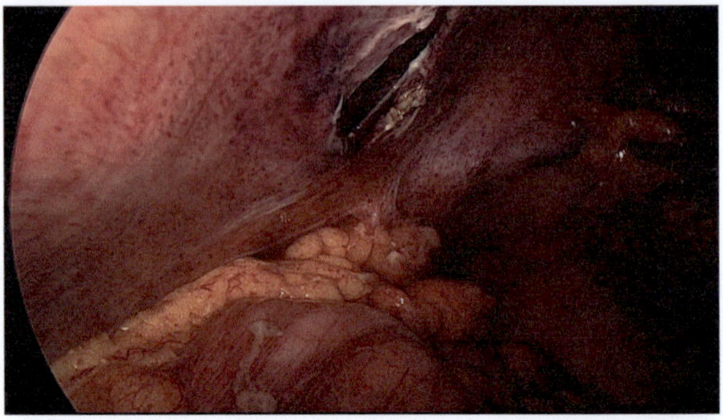

Fig. 12.1 Laparoscopic diagnosis of peritoneal violation after a penetrating left flank trauma (intraoperative picture courtesy from Dr. S. Di Saverio surgical procedures logbook)

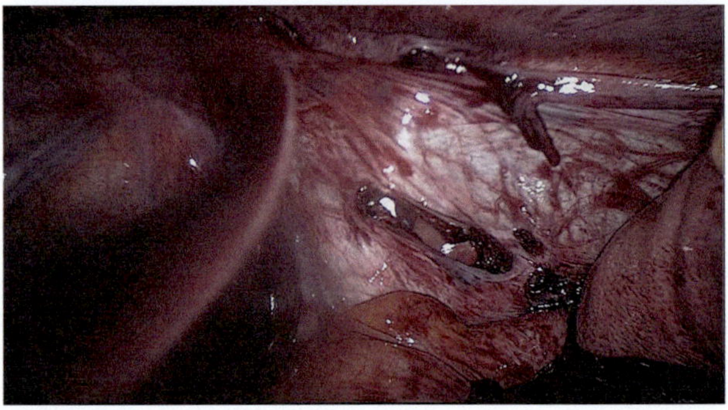

Fig. 12.2 Laparoscopic diagnosis of a left diaphragmatic tear after an abdominal penetrating trauma, note the thoracic drain (intraoperative picture courtesy from Dr. S. Di Saverio surgical procedures logbook)

In a later stage, laparoscopy can be useful to diagnose a post-traumatic acute pancreatitis development.

In pediatric trauma, where the physical examination is often unreliable and the radiation exposure should be avoided or minimized, diagnostic laparoscopy can be particularly useful and safe. Similar indications can be seen in pregnant patients and in geriatric or mentally impaired.

Large vessel, retroperitoneal, and renal injuries should not be diagnosed laparoscopically as their diagnosis is easier and more reliable with three-phase contrast-enhanced CT scan, including urogram.

12.2.2 Surgical Technique

Many studies have already stated the high efficacy of diagnostic laparoscopy in precisely recognizing the abdominal injuries, as well as significantly reducing the rate of nontherapeutic laparotomies for trauma up to 73 % [15]. However, in order to perform a correct and safe diagnosis and avoid missed injuries, it is extremely important that the surgeon is properly trained and confident in laparoscopy [7, 9, 10, 18, 19, 24, 25]. Both the presence of appropriate support and collaboration of the operating room staff and the availability of proper theater equipment play an important role in performing such procedures.

Apart from occasional experiences of local anesthesia with intravenous sedation ("awake laparoscopy") in emergency department [29], diagnostic laparoscopy for trauma is usually performed under general anesthesia.

The patient should be in a supine position, the same as for a trauma open approach in order to be prepared for immediate conversion to laparotomy or/and thoracotomy, in case of abdominal injuries that cannot be treated laparoscopically or sudden onset of hemodynamic instability or suspicion of thoracic injuries. In addition, as for every laparoscopic procedure, the patient should be fully secured and tight with belts on every side, in order to be able to safely achieve a moderate tilt in all directions and shift of the abdominal organs during the exploration to guarantee an adequate laparoscopic intraoperative view and exposure. A further reason for using supine position with legs straight and extended is because trauma patients often have concomitant orthopedic fractures involving the pelvis and/or the long bones of the extremities.

The first access is best achieved at the navel with an open technique (we do not recommend using Verres needle in trauma patients who may have a distended bowel) using a 10/12 mm trocar. Pneumoperitoneum should be slowly and progressively established, avoiding hyperpressure (reaching no more than 12–14 mmHg), and insufflation should be suddenly interrupted in case of abrupt rise in respiratory pressure, blood hypotension, or tachycardia. If the patient's stability rapidly restores, laparoscopy can be carefully and slowly resumed. Either 30° or 0° laparoscope can be used in diagnostic procedures, whereas 30° scope is better performing in case of operative laparoscopy, in our experience. Once preliminary exploration of the abdominal cavity has shown no urgent need to convert to laparotomy, we suggest to insert two further trocars (5 or 12 mm), preferably bladeless, under direct vision in left-upper and lower quadrants, in order to start a systematic exploration of the abdomen and run the entire bowel. Two more trocars in the right quadrants can be added in order to explore the left quadrants, if needed. In penetrating injuries, peritoneal violation (Fig. 12.1) and diaphragmatic injuries (Fig. 12.2) can be reliably determined with laparoscopy. A diaphragmatic injury can occur also after a blunt thoracoabdominal trauma (Fig. 12.3). Similarly to what is usually done in the open approach, the peritoneal cavity is examined systematically,

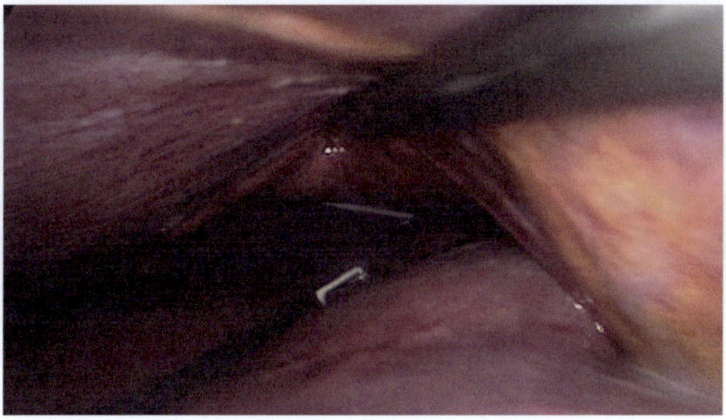

Fig. 12.3 Laparoscopic diagnosis of a right diaphragmatic large tear after an abdominal blunt trauma; the thoracic drain can be seen in the chest (intraoperative picture courtesy from Dr. S. Di Saverio surgical procedures logbook)

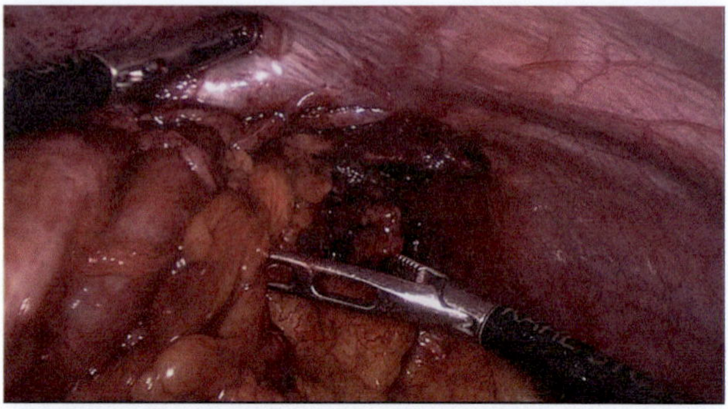

Fig. 12.4 Laparoscopic diagnosis and reduction of a diaphragmatic posttraumatic hernia (intraoperative picture courtesy from Dr. S. Di Saverio surgical procedures logbook)

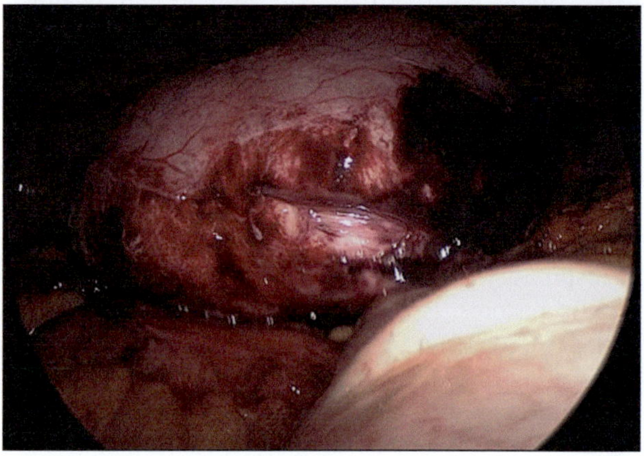

Fig. 12.5 Laparoscopic diagnosis of a colic serosal tear after a blunt abdominal trauma (intraoperative picture courtesy from Dr. S. Di Saverio surgical procedures logbook)

beginning with the right-upper quadrant and proceeding clockwise. To explore the supramesocolic region the patient is tilted in reverse Trendelenburg position and liver, gallbladder, spleen, diaphragm (Fig. 12.4), and stomach and duodenum should be carefully inspected. Especially the deepest areas of the diaphragm can be better seen laparoscopically than with a laparotomy. Afterward, the transverse and descending colon and the mesocolon are carefully inspected; then, moving the patient to a Trendelenburg position, the exploration moves to the rectum and Douglas pouch along with the pelvic organs, the cecum, and right colon (Fig. 12.5). After cranially moving the omentum, the small bowel is entirely run with two atraumatic grasping forceps, in a retrograde fashion from the ileocecal region to the duodenal–jejunal flexure, always exploring both sides of the bowel wall and both mesenteric and antimesenteric borders. During laparoscopy, we should also be looking for either mesenteric lacerations and hematomas or bowel injuries such as blast full thickness laceration (Fig. 12.6) or tears as well as through-and-through lesions (Fig. 12.7) or superficial serosal injuries. It is always advisable to run the bowel by grabbing the mesenteric fat and to avoid grasping the bowel wall loops as much as possible. The lesser sac should always be opened and explored in every penetrating abdominal trauma, or even in blunt trauma whenever an injury to the

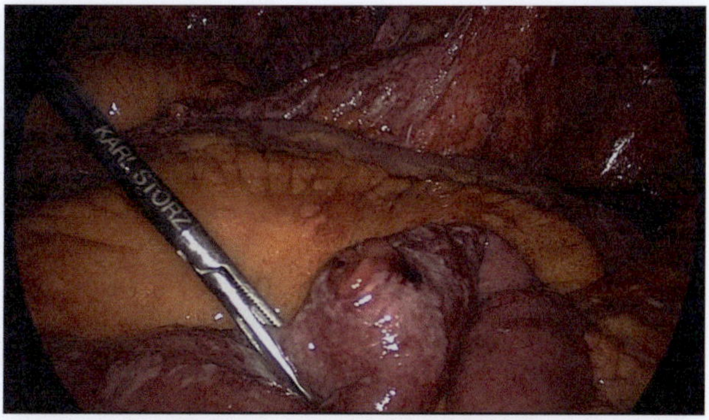

Fig. 12.6 Laparoscopic diagnosis of a small bowel blast perforation after a blunt abdominal trauma; note the diffuse peritonitis (intraoperative picture courtesy from Dr. S. Di Saverio surgical procedures logbook)

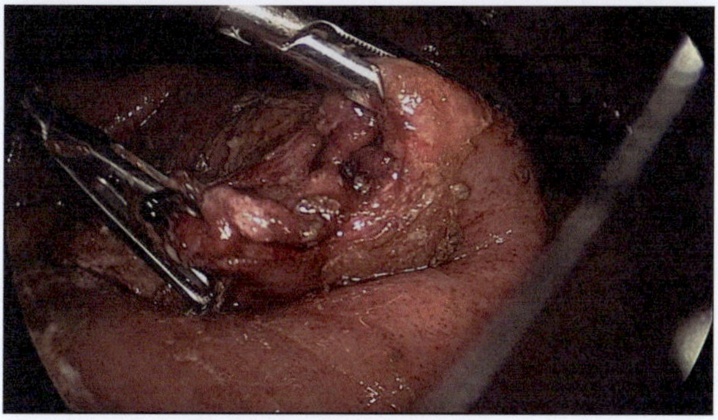

Fig. 12.7 Laparoscopic diagnosis of small bowel through-and-thorugh laceration after penetrating abdominal trauma (intraoperative picture courtesy from Dr. S. Di Saverio surgical procedures logbook)

posterior gastric wall, duodenum, or pancreas is suspected, when unclear findings or hematomas of these organs are seen on CT images or if a proper i.v. contrast CT scan was not obtained preoperatively.

Thorough suction and/or peritoneal irrigation may be needed for optimal visualization; methylene blue can be administered transanally, through the NGT, or intravenously to help identifying colorectal, gastroduodenal, or urinary tract injuries, respectively. A low threshold for open conversion should be maintained if the surgeon is not confident and missing injuries are suspected.

We do not recommend laparoscopic exploration and opening of the retroperitoneum in trauma patients setting. Hemodynamically stable patients with expanding or pulsating retroperitoneal or pelvic hematomas should be immediately converted to open surgery. Non-expanding retroperitoneal or pelvic hematomas in stable patients should never be explored or the retroperitoneum opened neither laparoscopically nor in open surgery.

12.2.3 Pitfalls

It is very important to maintain correct indications for diagnostic laparoscopy by carefully selecting suitable patients (e.g., exclude hemodynamically unstable patients) but also performing this procedure only in the presence of a properly trained and experienced operator and having carefully considered the accuracy of diagnostic alternatives such as CT scan and angiography.

Diagnostic laparoscopy-related complications are reported up to 2.8 % of patients [7]. The most common complication of laparoscopy is tension pneumothorax due to pneumoperitoneum in patients with unexpected diaphragmatic injuries. This condition can be easily treated with the suture of the injury and placement of a thoracostomy tube. Other complications might be iatrogenic perforation of a hollow viscus, laceration of a solid organ, and vascular injuries during trocar insertion or abdominal exploration and bowel manipulation. Another possible, although rare, complication is gas embolism in patients with intra-abdominal venous injuries, especially in liver lacerations; the transperitoneal absorption of carbon dioxide (which may cause metabolic and hemodynamic changes such as acidosis, cardiac suppression, atelectasis, subcutaneous emphysema, and increased intracranial pressure) may lead to life-threatening consequences.

Missing injuries are the most feared complication of diagnostic laparoscopy and range between 0 % [8] and 77 % [10]: its rate is directly proportional to the surgeon's laparoscopic expertise and it can be significantly reduced if the operator adheres to a standardized laparoscopic exploration technique and does not hesitate to convert to open surgery if he/she does not feel confident in the diagnostic procedure performed.

12.3 Therapeutic Laparoscopy

Once the diagnosis is achieved, either by CT scan or by diagnostic laparoscopy, the possibility of performing a laparoscopic treatment depends on the type and extent of the injuries, on the patient's hemodynamic stability, and, last but not least, on the surgeon's technical laparoscopic skills. The laparoscopic treatment of traumatic injuries provides all the advantages of the minimally invasive approach. These benefits are particularly remarkable in trauma patients. In these patients in fact, inflicting less trauma by using laparoscopy may represent a significant potential for decreasing the further release of proinflammatory elements with secondary injury to lungs and kidneys, in addition to what is already caused by their primary traumatic injury [3, 4].

12.3.1 Patient Selection

As already stated in the section on diagnostic laparoscopy, also in therapeutic laparoscopy the first condition required is the absolute patient's hemodynamic stability, the absence of severe cardiorespiratory contraindications to laparoscopy, and the absence of severe brain traumatic injury. Further conditions for using therapeutic laparoscopy in approaching abdominal trauma are the experience of the surgeon with advanced laparoscopic skills and being confident in his/her ability to adequately inspect the abdominal cavity and assess potential injuries, the adequate support by the staff and the equipment availability. If all these conditions are present, several abdominal traumatic injuries can be safely treated laparoscopically. We recommend to carefully assess large vessel, retroperitoneal, and renal injuries with the CT scan, explore and treat them only in highly selected cases, and never approach them laparoscopically.

12.3.2 Surgical Techniques

Therapeutic laparoscopy should be performed under general anesthesia and by a highly experienced laparoscopic surgeon. According to the expertise and confidence of the surgeon, many abdominal injuries can be treated laparoscopically. If the injury was detected preoperatively on CT scan, then it is possible to adjust and tailor the position of both the patient and the trocars according to the location and type of injury (Fig. 12.8). The therapeutic procedures most commonly laparoscopically performed are diaphragmatic suturing or prosthetic repair, gastrointestinal suturing, stapling or resection, hemostasis or resection of bleeding liver lacerations,

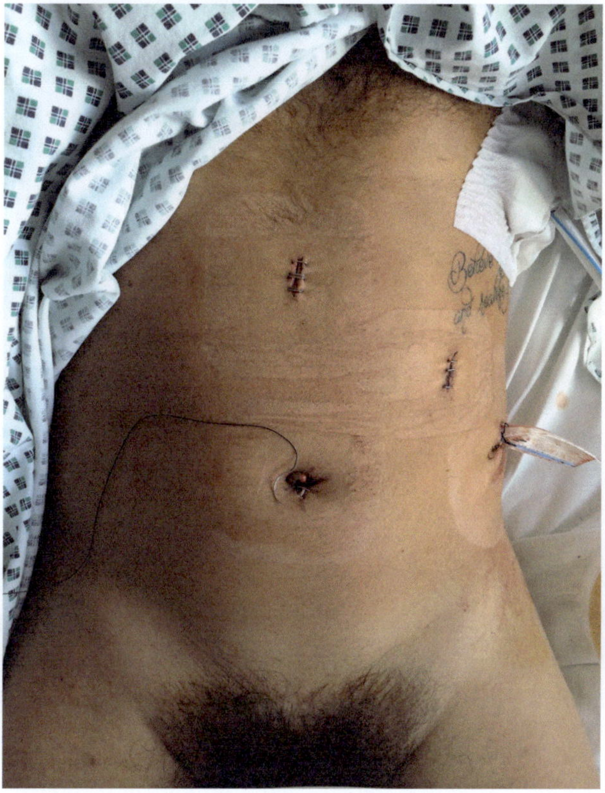

Fig. 12.8 Position of trocars and cosmetic outcome after laparoscopic splenectomy after a blunt abdominal trauma (picture courtesy of Dr. S. Di Saverio from his patients follow-up)

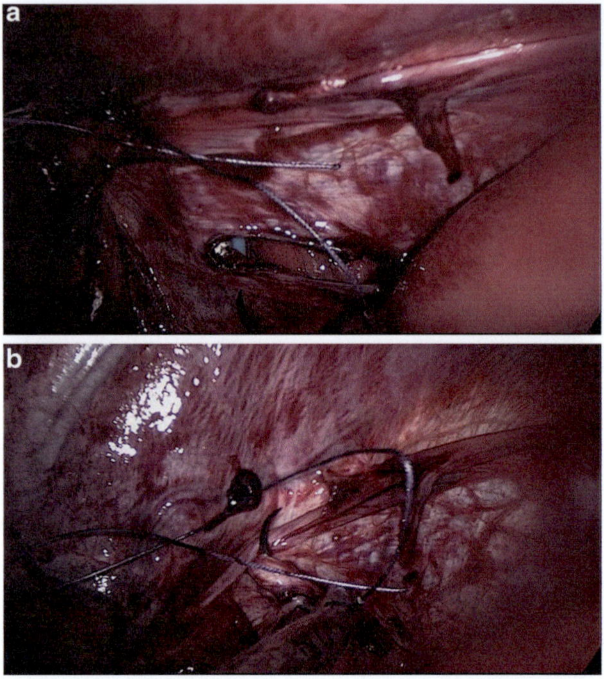

Fig. 12.9 (a,b) Laparoscopic simple repair of a diaphragmatic laceration after a penetrating abdominal trauma (intraoperative picture courtesy from Dr. S. Di Saverio surgical procedures logbook)

hemostasis and drainage of distal pancreatic injuries, spleen-preserving surgery with laparoscopic hemostasis or repair, or splenectomy.

Diaphragmatic injuries are typical of penetrating upper quadrant trauma and can be repaired either with single stitches or running suture, preferring nonabsorbable thread (Fig. 12.9a,b); however, in case of diaphragmatic disruption, prosthetic nonabsorbable mesh is used to reconstruct the diaphragm. In the majority of cases chest tube drainage is required.

Gastric injuries occur more often in case of penetrating abdominal trauma. These injuries can be treated laparoscopically with a simple repair with or without omental patch, followed by intraoperative testing for leaks using methylene blue injection through NGT for verifying the effective closure.

Laparoscopy does not play an important role in the treatment of duodenal injuries. In fact, low-grade duodenal injuries do not usually need any surgical treatment, while in high-grade duodenal injuries laparotomy is the treatment of choice because of the involvement of the pancreatic head and since the diagnosis is frequently late, and the patient is in septic shock.

The treatment of small bowel injuries depends on the extent of the damage: little perforations with vital margins can be repaired with double layer suturing (Fig. 12.10); destructive injuries or large defects in the mesenteric side should be resected and anastomosed (intra- or extracorporeally).

Colon serosal tears usually require just a simple laparoscopic repair (Fig. 12.11), but if destructive, larger, and full thickness injuries are found, resection and

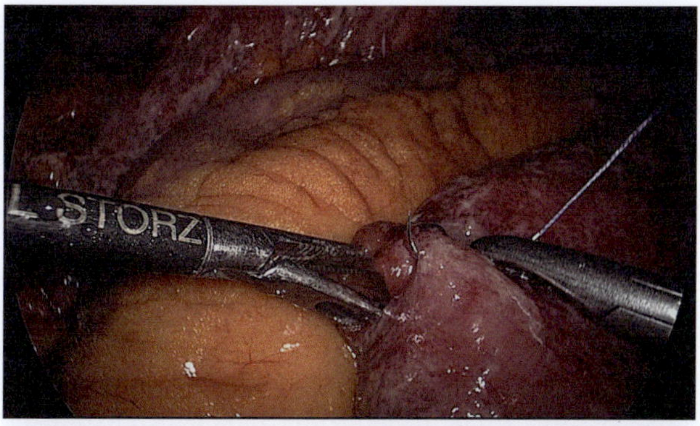

Fig. 12.10 Laparoscopic simple repair of small bowel blast injury after blunt abdominal trauma (intraoperative picture courtesy from Dr. S. Di Saverio surgical procedures logbook)

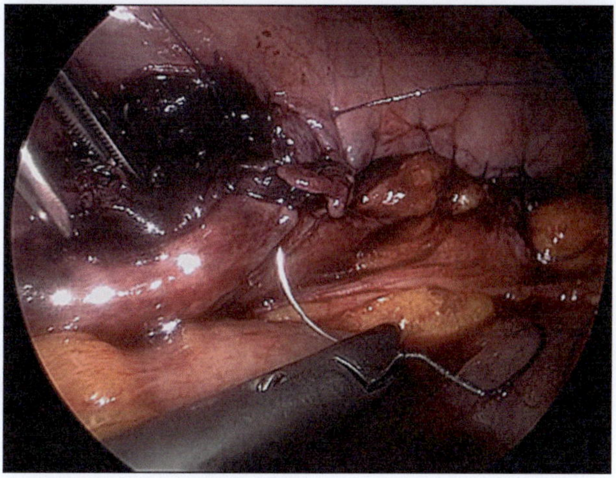

Fig. 12.11 Laparoscopic simple repair (running suture) of a colic serosal tear after a blunt abdominal trauma (intraoperative picture courtesy from Dr. S. Di Saverio surgical procedures logbook)

anastomosis (intra- or extracorporeal) or stoma diversion must be performed, according to patient's general conditions and the location of the perforation.

Small liver lacerations with active bleeding, found during diagnostic or therapeutic laparoscopy for other indications, can be controlled laparoscopically with hemostatic agents or figure-of-eight stitches, but arterial hepatic bleeding is usually primarily eligible for NOM +/− angiography and embolization, if available. Hepatic resection may be indicated if large hepatic necrosis develops after trauma or as a complication of angioembolization but requires a significant hepatobiliary and minimally invasive expertise to be safely performed laparoscopically.

Gallbladder lacerations can be diagnosed intraoperatively and treated with laparoscopic cholecystectomy.

AAST grade I–II pancreatic injury can be nonoperatively managed, but if found during diagnostic laparoscopy, hemostasis and drain placement can be performed with a minimally invasive procedure. The treatment of grade III pancreatic injuries depends on the location of the ductal tear along the organ, traumas of the pancreatic head are preferably just drained, while those of the tail can be treated with a laparoscopic distal pancreatectomy ("suck the head and eat the tail"). Grade IV and V pancreatic injuries are usually hemodynamically unstable and cannot be treated laparoscopically. However, laparoscopy can be useful in controlling eventual postoperative low output fistulas.

Laparoscopic splenectomy can be performed in case of stable high-grade injuries, unavailable or contraindicated embolization, failed NOM, or need for other urgent surgeries in a multiple trauma patient expecting a prolonged orthopedic surgery or a spinal surgery in prone position. Spinal surgery is known to be long and blunt, so, in this case, even if the patient is hemodynamically stable and a splenic angioembolization has been performed, we do not feel comfortable in leaving inside the abdomen a high-grade ruptured spleen and prefer to perform a laparoscopic splenectomy. After cleaning the hemoperitoneum we recommend to isolate the spleen and mobilize it, bluntly suspend it, and then resect the splenic hilum with a flexible endo-stapler (Fig. 12.12a,b). As it is commonly done in elective laparoscopic splenectomy, the specimen can be then completely morcellated and extracted through the umbilical access.

Bladder blast lacerations, most frequently found in blunt abdominal traumas, can be safely repaired by laparoscopic simple suturing.

Mesenteric lacerations may not require any procedure, but if active bleeding is found, hemostasis or suturing should be accomplished; if signs of bowel ischemia are found, bowel resection and anastomosis (intra- or extracorporeal) should be performed.

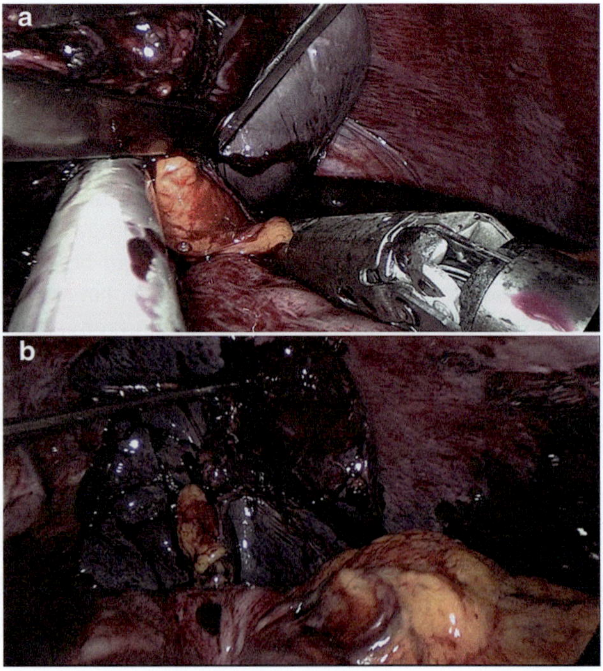

Fig. 12.12 (a,b) Laparoscopic splenectomy in abdominal blunt trauma (intraoperative picture courtesy from Dr. S. Di Saverio surgical procedures logbook)

Minor vascular injuries can be laparoscopically treated with coagulation, hemostatics, hemoclips, or suturing.

12.3.3 Pitfalls

Before attempting a laparoscopic treatment of arterial bleeding, we suggest to always keep in mind the chance of better treating this type of injuries with angioembolization, if available, and eventually consider a laparoscopic approach only if this first option fails and if the patient remains perfectly hemodynamically stable. Large vessel injuries are usually associated with hemodynamic instability and there is no role at all for laparoscopy in such patients.

Once again, we recommend avoiding to explore laparoscopically the retroperitoneal traumatic injuries.

The operator should be particularly careful avoiding iatrogenic vascular or intestinal injuries, especially when handling small bowel loops or using coagulating devices which can cause intestinal thermal injuries. We recommend to convert to open surgery as soon as the operator feels he/she loses the control of the injuries or is not sure of the complete and safe assessment of the whole abdomen. The rate of treatment success without iatrogenic injuries is directly related to the surgeon's experience.

12.4 Literature Review

In recent years, trauma laparoscopy has increasingly gained interest and a large number of studies have been published in the literature. However, due to the acute and complex type of patients, most of the series are retrospective and the data quality is limited and inhomogeneous.

Only two RCTs on trauma patients were ever performed: the first one compared laparoscopy with peritoneal lavage and found higher diagnostic specificity in the laparoscopic group [30], while the second one found a significant reduction of nontherapeutic laparotomy rate ($p = .016$) and hospital length of stay ($p = .049$) in patients with abdominal penetrating trauma managed with diagnostic laparoscopy if compared to laparotomy [5].

The most widely accepted and reported indication to diagnostic laparoscopy is the assessment of occult diaphragmatic injury in penetrating left-upper quadrant traumas, since radiological findings are usually not reliable in predicting diaphragmatic injury, which occur in up to 30 % of such patients [31]. This type of injury can usually be successfully repaired laparoscopically [32].

In the retrospective study by Chestovich et al., with a total of 518 patients with penetrating trauma, in the laparoscopic group the length of stay has been found to be shorter ($p < .001$) and there were no missed injuries; on the other hand, wound infections ($p = .002$) and ileus and small bowel obstruction ($p = .018$) were more common with the open procedure [8].

Similar results were reported on a large Russian population who underwent laparoscopic surgery for penetrating trauma, with quicker recovery time, less pain, shorter hospital stay, and lower complication rate ($p < .0001$) compared to open surgery, with no missed injuries [12].

According to the European Association for Endoscopic Surgery, laparoscopy may be useful in hemodynamically stable patients with abdominal trauma (with a B and C grade of recommendation for penetrating and blunt trauma, respectively) [33].

Diagnostic laparoscopy has been included in the Eastern Association for the Surgery of Trauma Guidelines in penetrating abdominal trauma, when there is a suspicion of intraperitoneal penetration or diaphragmatic injury (Class 2 recommendation) [34].

On the other hand, conflicting results are from a multicenter, institutional review board-approved prospective study, which enrolled 160 stable patients with anterior abdominal stab wounds. In this study, only nine laparoscopic explorations were performed and it did not appear that the minimally invasive approach had a role in management of this kind of patients and was not cost-effective [35]. Also in the Leppaniemi prospective randomized study of 43 patients with abdominal stab wounds, no statistically significant difference in the total hospital costs of the two strategies was found [5], but a retrospective cost analysis comparing the total hospital costs of exploratory laparotomy versus diagnostic laparotomy in 37 patients with penetrating abdominal trauma showed that laparoscopy was 1136 € cheaper than exploratory laparotomy [17].

One large series (131 patients) of both penetrating and blunt abdominal traumas from a Level 1 Trauma Center confirmed the diagnostic efficacy and safety of laparoscopy, with a rate of nontherapeutic laparotomy for patients sustaining penetrating vs. blunt injury of 1.8 % and nil, respectively [20].

The largest study ever published analyzed the United States National Trauma Data Bank between 2007 and 2010 and identified 4755 patients, with either penetrating or blunt trauma, who underwent a diagnostic laparoscopy at 467 trauma centers. A therapeutic laparoscopic intervention was performed in 916 (19.3 %) patients and the conversion to open surgery rate was 20.2 % (961 patients), of which 581 laparotomies were therapeutic. The most common laparoscopic procedure performed was repair of the diaphragm, followed by gastrostomies, large bowel repairs, small bowel repairs, liver laceration repairs, splenectomies, and small and large bowel resections. Mortality was not statistically different between the open and the laparoscopic groups, but patients undergoing laparoscopic surgery had a significantly shorter length of stay (5 vs. 6 days; $p < .001$) [23].

A recent systematic review on laparoscopy in penetrating abdominal trauma showed a range of sensitivity from 66.7 % to 100 %, specificity from 33.3 % to 100 %, and accuracy from 50 % to 100 % and confirmed its role in avoiding negative laparotomy, decreasing morbidity, shortening hospital stay, and increasing cost-effectiveness [16].

In a previous systematic review by O'Malley et al. including 51 studies (13 prospective) with 2569 patients who underwent diagnostic laparoscopy for penetrating abdominal trauma, 44 % were positive for intra-abdominal injuries, 13.8 % had a therapeutic laparoscopy, and 58.3 % were spared a nontherapeutic laparotomy. Overall, 72 patients (2.8 %) suffered complications, there were three mortalities (0.1 %), and 83 missed injuries (3.2 %). Sensitivity ranged from 66.7 to 100 %, specificity from 33.3 to 100 %, and accuracy from 50 to 100 %. Twenty-three of the 51 studies reported sensitivity, specificity, and accuracy of 100 %. The authors concluded that laparoscopy may have an important role in selected patients with penetrating abdominal trauma, especially with diaphragmatic injuries, and that the surgeon expertise plays an important role [7]. According to Lin et al., the surgeon's ability and experience is described as at least 20 laparoscopic procedures per month in acute care patients [6].

The systematic review on the use of laparoscopy in blunt abdominal trauma by Nicolau included 66 articles for a total of 343 patients and demonstrated a 0 % missed injury rate [36].

The use of laparoscopy for trauma in specific conditions like pregnancy and pediatric patients has been also reported in the last years [37–40], but deserves further investigation.

In conclusion, the current evidence shows that laparoscopy in selected hemodynamically stable trauma patients can significantly decrease nontherapeutic laparotomy rates, length of stay, and hospital costs and is highly sensitive and specific with very low missed injury rates, but adherence to a standardized laparoscopic examination technique and operator experience with routine use of laparoscopy in elective or acute care practice strongly influence positive results of minimally invasive surgery in trauma. Provided adequate surgical advanced skills, laparoscopy has been reported with impressive results in the treatment of a breadth of abdominal injuries [23].

To optimize results, the laparoscopy for trauma patients should be added to diagnostic and treatment algorithms at institutions where appropriate levels of laparoscopic expertise are available.

References

1. Short AR (1925) The uses of celioscopy. BMJ 2:254–255
2. Di Saverio S (2014) Emergency laparoscopy: a new emerging discipline for treating abdominal emergencies attempting to minimize costs and invasiveness and maximize outcomes and patients' comfort. J Trauma Acute Care Surg 77(2):338–350
3. Balogh ZJ, Reumann MK, Gruen RL, Mayer-Kuckuk P, Schuetz MA, Harris IA, Gabbe BJ, Bhandari M (2012) Advances and future directions for management of trauma patients with musculoskeletal injuries. Lancet 380(9847):1109Y1119
4. Manfredi AA, Rovere-Querini P (2010) The mitochondrion–a Trojan horse that kicks off inflammation? N Engl J Med 362(22):2132–2134
5. Leppaniemi A, Haapiainen R (2003) Diagnostic laparoscopy in abdominal stab wounds: a prospective, randomized study. J Trauma 55(4):636–645
6. Lin HF, Wu JM, Tu CC et al (2010) Value of diagnostic and therapeutic laparoscopy for abdominal stab wounds. World J Surg 34(7):1653–1662

7. O'Malley E, Boyle E, O'Callaghan A, Coffey JC, Walsh SR (2013) Role of laparoscopy in penetrating abdominal trauma: a systematic review. World J Surg 37(1):113–122
8. Chestovich PJ, Browder TD, Morrissey SL, Fraser DR, Ingalls NK, Fildes JJ (2015) Minimally invasive is maximally effective: diagnostic and therapeutic laparoscopy for penetrating abdominal injuries. J Trauma Acute Care Surg 78(6):1076–1085
9. Stefanidis D, Richardson WS, Chang L, Earle DB, Fanelli RD (2009) The role of diagnostic laparoscopy for acute abdominal conditions: an evidence based review. Surg Endosc 23:16–23
10. Villavicencio RT, Aucar JA (1999) Analysis of laparoscopy in trauma. J Am Coll Surg 189:11–20
11. Sosa JL, Baker M, Puente I, Sims D, Sleeman D, Ginzburg E, Martin L (1995) Negative laparotomy in abdominal gunshot wounds: potential impact of laparoscopy. J Trauma 38(2):194–197
12. Khubutiya MS, Yartsev PA, Guliaev AA, Levitsky VD, Tlibekova MA (2013) Laparoscopy in blunt and penetrating abdominal trauma. Surg Laparosc Endosc Percutan Tech 23(6):507–512
13. Choi YB, Lim KS (2003) Therapeutic laparoscopy for abdominal trauma. Surg Endosc 17:421–427
14. Lee PC, Lo C, Wu JM, Lin KL, Lin HF, Ko WJ (2014) Laparoscopy decreases the laparotomy rate in hemodynamically stable patients with blunt abdominal trauma. Surg Innov 21(2):155–165
15. Kawahara NT, Alster C, Fujimura I et al (2009) Standard examination system for laparoscopy in penetrating abdominal trauma. J Trauma 67:589–595
16. Uranues S, Popa DE, Diaconescu B, Schrittwieser R (2015) Laparoscopy in penetrating abdominal trauma. World J Surg 39:1381–1388
17. Marks JM, Youngelman DF, Berk T (1997) Cost analysis of diagnostic laparoscopy vs laparotomy in the evaluation of penetrating abdominal trauma. Surg Endosc 11(3):272–276
18. Lim KH, Chung BS, Kim JY, Kim SS (2015) Laparoscopic surgery in abdominal trauma: a single center review of a 7-year experience. World J Emerg Surg 10:16
19. Lin HF, Chen YD, Lin KL, Wu MC, Wu CY, Chen SC (2015) Laparoscopy decreases the laparotomy rate for hemodynamically stable patients with blunt hollow viscus and mesenteric injuries. Am J Surg 210(2):326–333. doi:10.1016/j.amjsurg.2014.11.009
20. Johnson JJ, Garwe T, Raines AR, Thurman JB, Carter S, Bender JS, Albrecht RM (2013) The use of laparoscopy in the diagnosis and treatment of blunt and penetrating abdominal injuries: 10-year experience at a level 1 trauma center. Am J Surg 205(3):317–320. doi:10.1016/j.amjsurg.2012.10.021, discussion 321
21. Smith RS, Fry WR, Morabito DJ, Koehler RH, Organ CH Jr (1995) Therapeutic laparoscopy in trauma. Am J Surg 170:632–637
22. Fabian TC, Croce MA, Stewart RM, Pritchard FE, Minard G, Kudsk KA (1993) A prospective analysis of diagnostic laparoscopy in trauma. Ann Surg 217:557–565
23. Zafar SN, Onwugbufor MT, Hughes K, Greene WR, Cornwell EE III, Fullum TM, Tran DD (2015) Laparoscopic surgery for trauma: the realm of therapeutic management. Am J Surg 209(4):627–632
24. Grushka J, Ginzburg E (2014) Through the 10-mm looking glass: advances in minimally invasive surgery in trauma. Scand J Surg 103(2):143–148
25. Zantut LF, Ivatury RR, Smith RS, Kawahara NT, Porter JM, Fry WR, Poggetti R, Birolini D, Organ CH Jr (1997) Diagnostic and therapeutic laparoscopy for penetrating abdominal trauma: a multicenter experience. J Trauma 42:825–831
26. Josephs LG, Este-McDonald JR, Birkett DH, Hirsch EF (1994) Diagnostic laparoscopy increases intracranial pressure. J Trauma 36:815–818, discussion 818–819
27. Bhagvan S, Turai M, Holden A, Ng A, Civil I (2013) Predicting hollow viscus injury in blunt abdominal trauma with computed tomography. World J Surg 37(1):123–126
28. Matsushima K, Mangel PS, Schaefer EW, Frankel HL (2013) Blunt hollow viscus and mesenteric injury: still underrecognized. World J Surg 37(4):759–765
29. Weinberg JA, Magnotti LJ, Edwards NM, Claridge JA, Minard G, Fabian TC, Croce MA (2007) "Awake" laparoscopy for the evaluation of equivocal penetrating abdominal wounds. Injury 38(1):60–64

30. Cuschieri A, Hennessy TP, Stephens RB, Berci G (1988) Diagnosis of significant abdominal trauma after road traffic accidents: preliminary results of a multicentre clinical trial comparing minilaparoscopy with peritoneal lavage. Ann R Coll Surg Engl 70(3):153–155
31. Berg RJ, Inaba K, Okoye O, Pasley J, Teixeira PG, Esparza M, Demetriades D (2014) The contemporary management of penetrating splenic injury. Injury 45(9):1394–1400
32. Mjoli M, Oosthuizen G, Clarke D, Madiba T (2015) Laparoscopy in the diagnosis and repair of diaphragmatic injuries in left-sided penetrating thoracoabdominal trauma: laparoscopy in trauma. Surg Endosc 29(3):747–752
33. Agresta F, Ansaloni L, Baiocchi GL, Bergamini C, Campanile FC, Carlucci M, Cocorullo G, Corradi A, Franzato B, Lupo M, Mandalà V, Mirabella A, Pernazza G, Piccoli M, Staudacher C, Vettoretto N, Zago M, Lettieri E, Levati A, Pietrini D, Scaglione M, De Masi S, De Placido G, Francucci M, Rasi M, Fingerhut A, Uranüs S, Garattini S (2012) Laparoscopic approach to acute abdomen from the Consensus Development Conference of the Società Italiana di Chirurgia Endoscopica e nuove tecnologie (SICE), Associazione Chirurghi Ospedalieri Italiani (ACOI), Società Italiana di Chirurgia (SIC), Società Italiana di Chirurgia d'Urgenza e del Trauma (SICUT), Società Italiana di Chirurgia nell'Ospedalità Privata (SICOP), and the European Association for Endoscopic Surgery (EAES). Surg Endosc 26(8):2134–2164. doi:10.1007/s00464-012-2331-3
34. Como JJ, Bokhari F, Chiu WC et al (2010) Practice management guidelines for selective nonoperative management of penetrating abdominal trauma. J Trauma 68(3):721–733
35. Biffl WL, Kaups KL, Pham TN, Rowell SE, Jurkovich GJ, Burlew CC, Elterman J, Moore EE (2011) Validating the Western Trauma Association algorithm for managing patients with anterior abdominal stab wounds: a Western Trauma Association multicenter trial. J Trauma 71(6):1494–1502
36. Nicolau AE (2011) Is laparoscopy still needed in blunt abdominal trauma? Chirurgia (Bucur) 106(1):59–66
37. Rolton DJ, Lovegrove RE, Dehn TC (2009) Laparoscopic splenectomy and diaphragmatic rupture repair in a 27-week pregnant trauma patient. Surg Laparosc Endosc Percutan Tech 19(4):e159–e160
38. Talutis SD, Muensterer OJ, Pandya S, McBride W, Stringel G (2015) Laparoscopic-assisted management of traumatic abdominal wall hernias in children: case series and a review of the literature. J Pediatr Surg 50(3):456–461
39. Rutkoski JD, Segura BJ, Kane TD (2011) Experience with totally laparoscopic distal pancreatectomy with splenic preservation for pediatric trauma–2 techniques. J Pediatr Surg 46(3):588–593
40. Sharp NE, Holcomb GW III (2013) The role of minimally invasive surgery in pediatric trauma: a collective review. Pediatr Surg Int 29(10):1013–1018

Update in Laparoscopic Approach to Acute Mesenteric Ischemia

13

Gianfranco Cocorullo, Nicola Falco, Tommaso Fontana, Roberta Tutino, Giuseppe Salamone, and Gaspare Gulotta

13.1 Introduction

The laparoscopic approach to Acute Mesenteric Ischemia is today unclear and less debated (AMI).

There are in fact no clinical evidences on this particular focus and only few articles can be found in several databases (pubmed, cochrane library, etc.), and the problem concerns both diagnostic and therapeutic utilization of the procedure.

These considerations were already taken into account in 2012 EAES guidelines where the Grade of Recommendation (GoR) of laparoscopy in AMI was low in both diagnostic and therapeutic aspects.

According to the new Oxford Classification [1], the use of laparoscopy in patients with suspicious or diagnosed AMI presents a weak GoR.

13.2 Epidemiology

AMI is an uncommon but serious disease often associated with a bad prognosis, accounting <1 in every 1000 hospital admissions. Women are more affected than men with 3:1 ratio. Epidemiological study attributes this difference to higher longevity of females vs. males. Clinical risk factors may provide some clues for AMI diagnosis. Patients with a history of atrial fibrillation, recent myocardial infarction, congestive heart failure, or peripheral arterial embolism have an higher risk for Superior Mesenteric Artery (SMA) embolism. History of postprandial abdominal pain, weight loss, and food intolerance in patients with acute abdominal

G. Cocorullo (✉) • N. Falco • T. Fontana • R. Tutino • G. Salamone • G. Gulotta
Department of Surgical Oncological and Stomatological Sciences, Unit of General and Emergency Surgery, University of Palermo, Palermo, Italy
e-mail: gianfranco.cocorullo@unipa.it

F. Agresta et al. (eds.), *Emergency Laparoscopy*,
DOI 10.1007/978-3-319-29620-3_13

pain could indicate an acute thrombotic occlusion of SMA. AMI in fact is associated with occlusion of SMA for arterial embolism or thrombosis in 67.2 % of cases, while mesenteric venous thrombosis occurs in 15.7 %. Only in remaining patients it is possible to find the third form of AMI without vessel obstruction, the so-called nonocclusive mesenteric ischemia (NOMI) [2].

13.3 Diagnosis

The diagnosis of AMI represent a very difficult diagnostic enigma; clinical markers are often aspecific but according to the literature severe and diffuse abdominal pain, bowel emptying, risk factor of embolism, arterial or venous thrombosis, and history of prior undiagnosed attacks of abdominal angina associated with specific laboratory tests (persistent $pH < 7.34$; plasmatic lactate level: 2.1 mmol/L, WBC: 12,000/mmc) could be highly suggestive of AMI [3].

According to the EAES guidelines and the latest articles of International literature, the gold standard for diagnosis of AMI is multidetector CT Angiography (CTA) with a sensibility of 93.3 % and a specificity of 95.9 % (Fig. 13.1) [4, 5].

In a recent review of more than 6000 patients, Acosta [5] underlines the secondary role of explorative laparotomy/laparoscopy to confirm cases of AMI without signs of SMA occlusion at CTA. Through the abdominal exploration, in fact, the surgeon could notice bowel aspect, its dilatation and peristaltism, the presence of evident pulsations in the mesenteric arcade arteries, and the bleeding from cut surfaces; the surgeon, moreover, could observe bowel wall necrosis and/or peritonitis in late form of AMI (Fig. 13.2).

Only few additional reports have been found on the diagnostic role of explorative laparoscopy. The laparoscopic diagnosis of AMI is clearly influenced by the stage of bowel damage, the etiology of the ischemia, and the experience of the surgeon. In fact, the ability to recognize signs of bowel ischemia depends on the

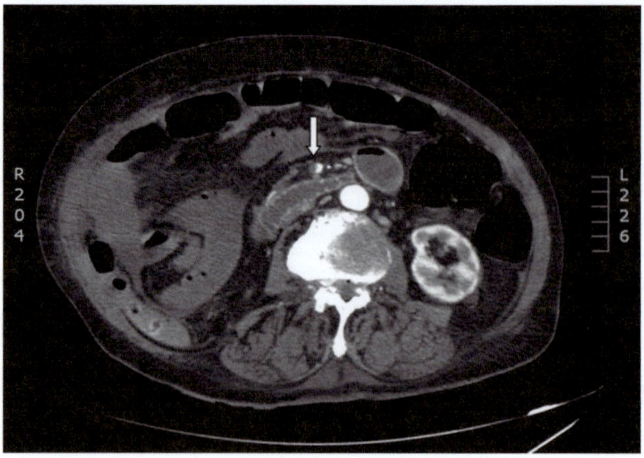

Fig. 13.1 CT angiography

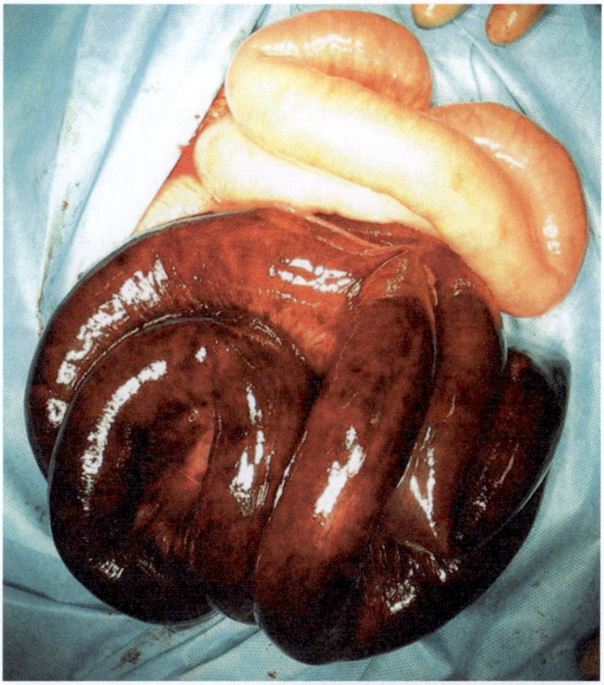

Fig. 13.2 Ischemic bowel

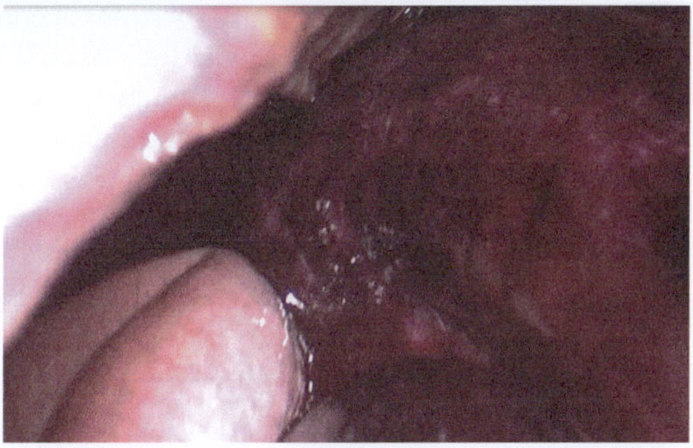

Fig. 13.3 Laparoscopic abdominal exploration

single operator's specific medical records and on the level of his learning curve, considering also that a low pressure of CO_2 pneumoperitoneum is advised if there is a suspicious AMI (Fig. 13.3).

In this way, since the first application of fluorescein proposed in 1993 by Kam and Scheeres to increase the sensibility of laparoscopy, several studies on canine or porcine models were proposed [6]. However, only few evidences are collected from these studies and in particular Paral Jiri et al. (2007) confirmed on porcine model the feasibility of this procedure using the specific optical system in the follow-up of AMI patients. Moreover, there are no trials or perspective studies on humans. The article of Paral represents the last important experience in the use of fluorescein, but the related level of evidence (LE) in the EAES guidelines, which was 2b in 2012, has been changed to LE 3 according to 2011 Oxford classification [7]. Unfortunately, in the last 2 years no studies have been produced on the primary diagnostic role of the laparoscopy and so the procedure maintains a weak GoR.

Most studies, instead, underline the possible role of laparoscopy with or without fluorescein in second-look exploration as "damage control surgery" [3, 5]. Nevertheless, in 2012, was published a study [3] that underlines the feasibility of a diagnostic laparoscopy in AMI in patients with Aortic Dissection (AoD). According to Tshomba Y et al that in patients with suspicious clinical signs of AMI without peritonitis if there are no conditions for rapid execution of CTA or a previous CTA had been not conclusive, an early diagnosis might be better than a clearer but late diagnosis. In this way, laparoscopy can reduce the number of unnecessary laparotomies overall in elderly critically ill patients. The study of Tshomba et al. [3] confirms that the best of laparoscopy in AMI diagnosis is the second look with the possibility of bedside use (directly in ICU). The author observed 202 consecutive AoD treated in the same center (71 acute type A AoD; 131 acute and chronic type B AoD) and only in 17 patients AMI was suspected. Diagnostic laparoscopy (DL) was performed in nine cases, in three cases during the medical treatment and in six patients after surgical or endovascular revascularization. In Tshomba's experience eight of nine DL were negative, but in one case AMI was diagnostic and the patient underwent revascularization in emergency. This experience is important, but it is based on few patients and so more studies need to confirm the feasibility and safeness of DL in AMI secondary to AoD; according to Tshomba the diagnostic power of DL increases in the second look overall in patients with aortic dissection type B (chronic type). In these cases, in fact, usually little time has been spent between starting of symptoms related to ischemic event and the evidence of bowel wall ischemia; therefore, it is known that sensitivity of diagnostic laparoscopy increases 24 hours after ischemic event. Moreover, according to the same article laparoscopy may be a feasible alternative to CTA in patients with kidney failure or other contraindications to injection of iodate CT contrast medium [3].

13.4 Treatment

Wyers in 2010 underlines that the first treatment of AMI is bowel revascularization. The second step is the reassessment of bowel viability. If possible the time of 20 or 30 min after revascularization should be spent before decision making about viability to evaluate signs of adequate perfusion as mesenteric vessel pulsation, normal color and appearance of the bowel serosa, peristalsis, and bleeding from cut surfaces [2]. Moreover, if an explorative diagnostic laparotomy (or laparoscopy) is performed as the first diagnostic step, an on-table SMA angiography should be performed at the same time. If no vascular surgeon is available, resection of obvious necrotic bowel should be performed and after the abdomen closure the patient should be transported to a vascular surgical center [5]. Main techniques to resolve the SMA occlusion are open SMA embolectomy for SMA embolism; other therapeutic options are hybrid or endovascular stenting in acute thrombotic occlusions, medical therapy with vasodilators and high dose of EBPM for thrombotic case, NOMI, and venous infarction [2].

In a limited number of cases when primary laparoscopy access is feasible and revascularization has been performed with endovascular access, it is possible to evaluate bowel perfusion laparoscopically and to perform at the same time a laparoscopical bowel resection of residual ischemic segments. The possibility of performing a "one-step anastomosis" will be evaluated each time by the surgeon, depending on the bowel presentation and the performance status (ASA score) of the patient. In nonpermissive patients, the surgeon should choose a two-step operation differing in performing anastomosis [8]. However, as suggested by the experience of Meriggi F et al. in their recent (2011) case report, laparoscopic primary access overall in AoD is an important tool for leading therapeutic decision and timing [9] (LE 4). It is clear that unfortunately there are no strong evidences about the therapeutic role of laparoscopy in AMI because only few experiences are published referring to a single center or more frequently to a single case report. More resources and efforts are needed in the evaluation of laparoscopic usefulness in AMI.

13.5 Follow-Up and Damage Control Surgery

Following the rule of damage control surgery a CTA is indicated for patients who underwent a stent positioning and it should be performed after the revascularization. The monitoring of restored bowel viability (second look) should be repeated two times in the postoperative time. Moreover, the second look is frequently performed also after surgical resection of necrotic bowel because an extension of ischemia is not rare in these patients and it requires further bowel resection. According to the literature in both cases a laparoscopic close exploration should represent a valid and more feasible technique than to perform an unsutured abdomen closure (Bogotà Bag, VA system, etc.) [5].

13.6 Conclusions

The gold standard for the primary diagnosis is CTA and laparoscopy has a limited rule. Fluorescein does not increase significantly the sensibility and specificity of the laparoscopy. The necessity to perform a low-pressure laparoscopy limits the diagnostic power of the procedure and reduces the feasibility and the diffusion of its execution. Nevertheless, the literature underlines the feasibility of a diagnostic laparoscopy in AMI after AoD when in the presence of suggestive clinical signs of AMI without peritonitis there are no conditions for the rapid execution of CTA or when a previous CTA had been nonconclusive. Laparoscopy may result in a feasible alternative to CTA also in patients with IRC that contraindicates injection of iodate CT contrast medium. Furthermore, laparoscopic primary access overall in AoD is an important tool for leading therapeutic decision and timing. The main rule of laparoscopy in AMI is the second look, in fact it should represent an alternative to multiple laparotomic explorations with less operation time and maintaining the closure of the abdomen. Another possible application of laparoscopy in the management of patient with AMI is the so-called bedside laparoscopy that for patients in ICU consents the repeatability of the procedure to follow the clinical course of patients. Referring to the therapeutic aspect, the usefulness of laparoscopy in AMI appears today limited only to few cases.

References

1. OCEBM Levels of Evidence Working Group. The Oxford levels of evidence 2. Oxford Centre for Evidence-Based Medicine, Oxford
2. Wyers MC (2010) Acute mesenteric ischemia: diagnostic approach and surgical treatment. Semin Vasc Surg 23(1):9–20
3. Tshomba Y, Coppi G, Marone EM, Bertoglio L, Kahlberg A, Carlucci M, Chiesa R (2012) Diagnostic laparoscopy for early detection of acute mesenteric ischaemia in patients with aortic dissection. Eur J Vasc Endovasc Surg 43(6):690–697
4. Agresta F, Ansaloni L, Baiocchi GL, Bergamini C, Campanile FC, Carlucci M, Cocorullo G, Corradi A, Franzato B, Lupo M, Mandalà V, Mirabella A, Pernazza G, Piccoli M, Staudacher C, Vettoretto N, Zago M, Lettieri E, Levati A, Pietrini D, Scaglione M, De Masi S, De Placido G, Francucci M, Rasi M, Fingerhut A, Uranüs S, Garattini S (2012) Laparoscopic approach to acute abdomen from the Consensus Development Conference of the Società Italiana di Chirurgia Endoscopica e nuove tecnologie (SICE), Associazione Chirurghi Ospedalieri Italiani (ACOI), Società Italiana di Chirurgia (SIC), Società Italiana di Chirurgia d'Urgenza e del Trauma (SICUT), Società Italiana di Chirurgia nell'Ospedalità Privata (SICOP), and the European Association for Endoscopic Surgery (EAES). Surg Endosc 26(8):2134–2164
5. Acosta S (2014) Surgical management of peritonitis secondary to acute superior mesenteric artery occlusion. World J Gastroenterol 20(29):9936–9941
6. Kam DM, Scheeres DE (1993) Fluorescein-assisted laparoscopy in the identification of arterial mesenteric ischemia. Surg Endosc 7(2):75–78
7. Paral J, Ferko A, Plodr M, Raupach J, Hadzi-Nikolov D, Dolezal D, Chovanec V (2007) Laparoscopic diagnostics of acute bowel ischemia using ultraviolet light and fluorescein dye: an experimental study. Surg Laparosc Endosc Percutan Tech 17(4):291–295
8. Palanivelu CI, Rangarajan M, Maheshkumaar GS, Rajan PS (2008) Relaparoscopy in the management of acute abdomen due to localized ischemic bowel: a novel technique–case report. Int J Surg 6(6):e89–e91
9. Meriggi F, Alloni A, Gramigna P, Tramelli P, Vigano M (2011) Acute aortic dissection with intestinal ischemia: what to do first. Ann Thorac Cardiovasc Surg 17(6):631–633

Anaesthesia and Emergency Laparoscopy 14

Riccardo Ragazzi, Marco Tartaglione, Savino Spadaro, Antonio Gioia, and Carlo Alberto Volta

14.1 The Pathophysiology of Pneumoperitoneum

Pneumoperitoneum [1] is the main cause of all the systemic pathophysiological changes that take place during laparoscopic surgery. Understanding normal variations allows us to understand some conditions in which it is advisable to avoid or interrupt a laparoscopic procedure and, secondly, to understand which anaesthesiological strategies are useful in managing critical patients.

To induce pneumoperitoneum, carbon dioxide is usually preferred over other gases [2] (azote, nitric oxide, helium, argon, or oxygen) due to its high level of solubility in the circulatory system, together with its inability to feed combustion, its low peritoneal absorption, and the availability of a chemical buffer in our bodies—bicarbonate—that neutralises it and allows it to be eliminated through the respiratory system.

When inducing pneumoperitoneum, carbon dioxide is insufflated into the peritoneal cavity at a speed of 4–6 l/min and a pressure of 10–20 mmHg. It is later maintained by a constant flow of 200–400 ml/min.

'Carboperitoneum' can be defined as a physiological condition, which is mainly responsible for mechanical changes, like the increase of intra-abdominal pressure (IAP), and chemical changes linked to insufflated CO_2 [3]. Recognising the physiological effects of carboperitoneum, which are negligible in generally healthy patients, can help reduce complications and make laparoscopy a safer technique, even for patients with serious respiratory and/or circulatory comorbidities.

R. Ragazzi • M. Tartaglione • S. Spadaro • A. Gioia • C.A. Volta (✉)
Anaesthesia and Intensive Care Unit, University of Ferrara, Ferrara, Italy
e-mail: carloalberto.volta@unife.it

F. Agresta et al. (eds.), *Emergency Laparoscopy*,
DOI 10.1007/978-3-319-29620-3_14

14.1.1 Cardiovascular Effects

Increased intra-abdominal pressure alters venous return, systemic vascular resistance (SVR), and cardiac function. With IAP values of less than 10 mmHg venous return increases: splanchnic circulation is compressed, with a consequent increase in the circulating haematic volume and therefore in cardiac output. With an IAP of 10–20 mmHg vena cava compression reduces the venous return and consequently diminishes cardiac output. Systemic vascular resistance is increased both due to the mechanical effect of increased IAP and increase in circulating catecholamines (adrenaline and noradrenaline). Arterial pressure is unaltered, or there may be slight hypertension, as this is determined by the product of systemic vascular resistance greatly increased by slightly diminished cardiac output, in the case of normal circulating volume.

Under normal working pressure during laparoscopy (10–15 mmHg of IAP), related to a slight reduction in venous return, there is always an increase in systemic vascular resistance which, in an euvolemic patient, tends to result in increased arterial pressure compared to the subject's normal values.

With levels of IAP greater than 15–20 mmHg, there is a drastic reduction in venous return caused by the compression of the inferior vena cava and the surrounding collateral vessels, which leads to marked hypotension and diminished cardiac output.

As well as IAP, haemodynamic alterations can also be affected by hypercapnia, caused by the insufflation of carbon dioxide, if followed by acidosis. A fall in myocardial contractility and a direct vasodilatory effect [4] can be seen in the case of moderate or severe hypercapnia ($PaCO_2$ greater than 60 mmHg), while the effects are modest at lower values.

Tachyarrhythmia can arise due to the increase of the haematic concentration of CO_2 and of catecholamine.

Finally, haemodynamic stability is influenced by the effect of the patient's position: falls in arterial pressure in the reverse Trendelemburg position and increases when the patient is in the Trendelemburg position are much more marked, the more the patient is hypovolemic and has a low cardio-circulatory reserve.

14.1.2 Effects on the Respiratory System

The main changes caused by pneumoperitoneum are in pulmonary volumes, pulmonary compliance, the resistance of the airways, and the alteration of the ventilation/perfusion ratio.

The diaphragm is pushed upwards and there is a reduction in its range, with a reduction in pulmonary volumes. Pulmonary compliance diminishes by 35–40 % [5], while the resistance of the airways increases. There is a reduction in functional residual capacity (FRC), with the possible closure of the small airways and pulmonary atelectasis. Raising the diaphragm promotes ventilation at the apex of the lungs, instead of the base, causing a possible alteration of the ventilation/perfusion ratio (V/Q). These conditions can aggravate the intrapulmonary shunt until it creates a condition of hypoxemia. The carbon dioxide absorbed in circulation through peritoneum causes hypercapnia; the absence of adjustment in pulmonary ventilation causes vasoconstriction of the pulmonary circulation and a condition of acidosis of varying severity. During an operation, performed with controlled mechanical ventilation, hypercapnia is contrasted by increasing alveolar ventilation by 10–25 % [6].

In patients with cardiopulmonary diseases who normally have an altered V/Q ratio, arterial CO_2 can be further increased, with a consequent increase in the gradient (normally between 2 and 9 mmHg) between $PaCO_2$ and CO_2 expired ($EtCO_2$) [7]. It is advisable for these patients to have invasive monitoring of $PaCO_2$ arterial cannulation for blood samples during the operation, to avoid a state of hypercapnia that is not detected using only $EtCO_2$.

14.1.3 The Effects of Pneumoperitoneum on Flow Limitation and the Use of PEEP

In a healthy patient, the pulmonary volume at the end of expiration corresponds to the point of equilibrium of the respiratory system, i.e. to the functional residual capacity (FRC). Inducing anaesthesia involves a reduction in FRC, which is further reduced by the presence of pneumoperitoneum. The consequence is a gradual reduction of expiratory flows to the point in which they become the same as the maximum, therefore creating an expiratory flow limitation (EFL). If EFL occurs, there will also be instability in the small airways, which represents a powerful proinflammatory mechanism.

The management of ventilation during laparoscopic procedures is a fundamental element in performing an operation without respiratory complications.

For example, it is useful to apply ‘extrinsic’ PEEP (PEEPe), generally of a value equal to or above 5 cm H_2O, able to produce a ‘volume effect’, increasing FRC and a ‘pressure effect’ to contrast flow limitation [8].

The benefits of PEEPe include the prevention of the closure of the small airways, to avoid alveolar collapse at the end of expiration and, as a result, atelectasis: the action of recruitment on non-ventilated but perfused alveoli and the reduction of perfusion in non-ventilated areas improve the ventilation/perfusion ratio and reduce pulmonary shunt [9].

14.1.4 Neurological Effects

Hypercapnia, increased systemic vascular resistance, increased intra-abdominal pressure, and phases of the operation that involve the use of the Trendelenburg position are all cofactors that can cause an increase in intracranial pressure (ICP) and therefore a decrease in cerebral perfusion pressure [10] (CPP). The latter also depends upon an eventual reduction in cardiac output. Therefore, an increase in ICP should be taken into account during laparoscopic surgery.

14.1.5 Effects on the Renal Apparatus

Increased intra-abdominal pressure increases renal vascular resistances and reduces the glomerular filtration rate, reducing renal function and diminishing diuresis, often creating oliguria. The effect is aggravated by a reduction in cardiac output.

14.1.6 Intraoperative Positions

The different positions of a patient and variations in the inclinations of the operating table can cause further physiopathological changes during laparoscopy or increase the effects already mentioned. The most widely used positions in laparoscopy are the Trendelenburg position (head down) and the reverse Trendelenburg position (head up).

In the first position there is a cephalic movement of the internal organs, with increased pressure exerted on the diaphragm. The effects on respiration include reduced FRC, a reduced ventilation/perfusion ratio (due to the increase in perfusion of spaces that are no longer opportunely ventilated), and an increased risk of atelectasis, i.e. an accentuation of the effects already foreseen for pneumoperitoneum alone [11]. These effects are more marked in obese patients and in subjects with a limited cardiorespiratory reserve, as well as in elderly and high-risk patients. The cardiovascular effects include an increase in venous return from the limbs, with a consequent increase in cardiac output. In patients who are not affected by cardiovascular diseases, the compensatory vasodilatation that results cancels out the consequences of this effect, altering arterial pressure only minimally. Attention should also be paid to possible movement upward of the carina of trachea, which may cause dislocation of the tracheal tube, whose end may locate itself in a main bronchus [12].

In the 'head up' position, the caudal movement of the internal organs reduces pressure on the diaphragm, increasing the current volume to equal the flow and improving respiratory function. It, therefore, produces the opposite cardiovascular effects. There is a reduction in venous return, cardiac output, and arterial pressure and also an increase in peripheral and pulmonary vascular resistance [13–15]. The lower limbs may be subject to venous stasis during long surgery. Greater attention must be paid to hypovolemic patients or cardiovascular compromised patients.

14.2 Contraindications

An absolute contraindication for laparoscopy is haemodynamic instability.

The Consensus Statement of the Italian Society of Endoscopic Surgery (SICE) 2012 on a laparoscopic approach to the acute abdomen, in accordance with the 2006 Guidelines of the European Association for Endoscopic Surgery (EAES), stresses that a necessary condition for a patient to undergo laparoscopic procedures is 'stable haemodynamic and respiratory parameters'. Patients admitted to hospital with 'major trauma' or 'serious' comorbidity become eligible for laparoscopic surgery if there is lasting stability of these parameters after reanimation and/or intensive medical care [16].

A patient defined as 'haemodynamically unstable' does not respond or responds only temporarily to an initial infusion of liquids if in a condition of shock.

Shock is defined as a condition of hypoperfusion in body tissue that leads to a state of hypoxia in cells and tissues due to the reduced amount of oxygen and/or increased consumption of oxygen or its inadequate use, necessary for maintaining the aerobic metabolism [17].

In order to reach a diagnosis of clinical shock, the following haemodynamic and biochemical parameters must be considered [18]:

1) The presence of systemic arterial hypotension (systolic arterial pressure of less than 90 mmHg or mean arterial pressure of less than 70 mmHg) with associated tachycardia (cardiac frequency of over 90 beats/min).
2) Clinical signs of hypoperfusion in body tissue, which can be seen at a cutaneous level (cold, sweaty, or cyanotic skin), at a renal level (diuresis of less than 0.5/kg/h or anuria), and at a neurological level (an altered mental state, obtundation of the senses, disorientation, and mental confusion).
3) An increase in serum lactates (over 1.5 mmol/L), indicating an alteration in the cellular metabolism of O_2

In patients in a state of shock a vital factor is the speed with which a source of blood loss or contamination is localised and controlled, and the presence of an expert surgeon and a trained team. When the time needed to prepare for laparoscopy may put the patient's life at risk, a laparotomic technique is preferable, to reduce delaying the operation as much as possible [19].

In more detail, according to other bibliographical sources, laparoscopy has contraindications in

- Patients with polytrauma, who may have multiple intrabdominal wounds, who would need complex laparoscopic procedures, with a consequent increase in the duration of these laparoscopies [19].
- Patients admitted for abdominal trauma, who have peritonitis with haemodynamic instability, haemorrhagic shock, or evisceration, who must undergo a laparotomy immediately [20].

The following conditions should be regarded as absolute (or if opportunely treated and evaluated relative) contraindications:

- Patients with non-correctable hypercapnia over 50 mmHg must be carefully evaluated [20].
- Patients with traumatic brain injury or neurological conditions in which intracranial pressure (ICP) must be carefully evaluated, as the induction of pneumoperitoneum causes an increase in intracranial pressure [21]. As well as the factors responsible for an increase in ICP already discussed, an extreme Trendelenburg position may cause a further increase in cerebral blood flow and intracranial pressure [22].

In these patients, IAP must be kept as low as possible, sudden increases in IAP must be avoided, and ICP monitoring should be evaluated [23].

- Patients with severe myopia or a detached retina. The increase in intraocular pressure (IOP) in the extreme Trendelenburg position, combined with the physiopathological effects caused by pneumoperitoneum and the effects of drugs used in general anaesthesia [24], may cause a drop in retinal perfusion and, in some cases, an increased risk of ischemic retinopathy. It has been demonstrated that an induction of general anaesthesia with propofol and maintenance through administering propofol under Totally Intravenous Anaesthesia, or TIVA, can control the increase of IOP during laparoscopic surgery [25].

The following may be regarded as relative contraindications:

- In glaucoma, the effects on ocular pressure do not seem to be clinically significant, but further confirmation is needed [26].
- An increase has been observed in sickling crises in a series of patients affected by Sickle-Cell disease who underwent laparoscopic cholecystectomy. In fact, insufflated CO_2 causes respiratory acidosis which, combined with the increase in IAP and consequent hypoventilation, may cause a sickling crisis due to acidosis and hypoxemia [27]. Both these effects, typical of pneumoperitoneum, can increase the risk of developing acute thoracic syndrome (ACS) in these patients [28]. It is, therefore, advisable that great attention is paid during the operation: using a medium-low working pressure (8–11 mmHg), extending the hospital stay beyond 3 days to identify possible ACS on the second or third day, mobilising the patient early, carrying out effective pain checks, and monitoring the patient's respiratory function to prevent pulmonary complications [29].
- Cardiac pathology in patients who undergo laparoscopic surgery is not an absolute contraindication if an adequate surgical and anaesthesiological strategy is adopted [30].
- Traumatic haemoperitoneum is a relative contraindication in terms of the patient's haemodynamics. Traumatic haemoperitoneum is not in itself a possible cause of haemorrhagic shock. The SICE Consensus Statement also underlines

that the induction of pneumoperitoneum must be slow, progressive, and carried out carefully. In the event of a sudden drop in blood pressure and an increase in respiratory pressure, insufflation of CO_2 must be stopped or pressure values reduced [31]. It should be underlined that the surgeon should not hesitate to convert the procedure into an exploratory laparotomy if he or she is not certain that there are no occult lesions [32]. It should also be underlined that in traumatised patients a minimally invasive approach may be useful and safe, as it has less potential risk than a negative laparotomy [33], but if shock occurs the possibility of converting the laparoscopy should be considered.

14.3 Considerations and Management of High-Risk Patients

14.3.1 Assessment of a 'High-Risk' Patient

Due to an increase in the average age in Europe (with the population over 65 increased by 16–18 %, and a forecast of 28.7 % by 2080) [34] and life expectancy in Italy (79.4 years for men and 84.5 for women 2013), there has been an increase in cases of comorbidity, prior abdominal surgery, and patients undergoing pharmaceutical combination therapy.

Those patients who have one or more of these characteristics are classified as 'high risk':

- Age > 80
- BMI > 30 kg/m^2
- Previous major pelvic or abdominal surgery
- ASA > 2

In the guidelines cited above some suggestions were made to manage the physiological effects of pneumoperitoneum in patients at greater risk during an operation [23].

The most pronounced cardiovascular effects can be seen when pneumoperitoneum is induced, with haemodynamic effects that are virtually irrelevant in ASA I–II patients with 12–14 mmHg of carboperitoneum, while they are relevant in ASA III–IV patients, who need at least invasive measurement of arterial pressure. They also require adequate preoperative volemic filling and beta-blockers [23]. If it is a long operation, intermittent pneumatic compression of the lower limbs should also be considered. Low-pressure insufflation should be maintained in the case of cardiac dysfunction. In the case of cardiopulmonary diseases, intra- and postoperative monitoring of haematic gases is recommended [23].

In ASA I–II patients a high IAP has no significant effects on renal, splanchnic, or hepatic perfusion, while in patients with hepatic or renal perfusion that is already compromised, medium-low pressure should be used and adequate volemic filling is recommended before and during the operation.

14.3.2 Patients with Serious Heart Disease

'*Heart disease is not an absolute contraindication for laparoscopic surgery*' according to the guidelines of the SICE 2012 Consensus Statement [16].

Laparoscopy is a safe technique that can be performed without absolute contraindications even in patients with terminal heart disease: the literature contains a recent description of a laparoscopic cholecystectomy in a patient with a left ventricular assist device (LVAD) awaiting a heart transplant [35].

14.3.3 Serious COPD

The main consequence of pre-existing pulmonary diseases before a laparoscopic operation is an increased risk of developing pulmonary complications.

These complications partly depend on the development of atelectasis under general anaesthetic, to which postoperative hypoventilation, a reduction in current volume, and residual functional capacity and altered pulmonary expansion contribute. There is a 4–10 % rate of COPD in Europe and therefore approximately one patient in ten is affected.

In urgent operations for these patients, an arterial blood gas (ABG) checking for haemoglobin before and after the operation and monitoring $PaCO_2$ and PaO_2 is essential. In elective surgery, a preoperative spirometric assessment is also fundamental. This investigation studies the patient's functional respiratory reserve.

14.3.4 Ventilatory Pulmonary Protection Strategies

All that is needed to contrast the increase of $PaCO_2$ and acidosis is moderate mechanical hyperventilation [36].

During assisted ventilation of the patient, a volume of air (or pressure) that is excessive for the lung during positive pressure ventilation may result in ventilator-induced lung injury (VILI), with possible rare but serious complications such as the rupture of the alveolar septum, pneumomediastinium, subcutaneous emphysema, pneumothorax, and/or air embolisms. This is often related to long surgery. The rupture of the alveolar septum can also occur with normal volumes and pressures in lungs with bullous disease.

Protective ventilation is born of a need to correct hypercapnia, increasing minute volume, but at the same time avoiding excessively high insufflation volumes and pressures that may cause lung damage. This is why mechanical ventilation that is correctly set and personalised is an important fact that the surgeon–anaesthetist team must be involved in and assess in order to decide whether or to interrupt or continue a surgical procedure when problems of ventilation arise.

14.3.5 Obese Patients

Obese patients are usually classified as ‘critical’ patients. As is known, obese patients have an increased risk of postoperative complications like infection at the site of surgery, dehiscence, pulmonary embolism, and renal insufficiency [37].

Respiratory function is seriously altered in pathologically obese patients (BMI ≥ 40 kg/m^2) who undergo laparoscopy. The main causes are the supine position, muscular paralysis due to the use of muscle relaxants, and pneumoperitoneum [38]. Reduced functional residual capacity and increased closing volume of the airways with consequent atelectasis increase the risk of postoperative respiratory complications and prolong hospital stays [39].

Perioperative risk can be increased by various associated comorbidities, like cardiocirculatory diseases and diabetes.

Elective laparoscopic bariatric surgery is widely practised and the knowledge acquired through this elective surgery for obese patients should be explored and evaluated also when the patient is operated on for other urgent reasons.

Physiologically, these patients have an IAP 2–3 times higher than healthy patients. During laparoscopy, they can absorb more CO_2 at a systemic level and therefore need more time to eliminate it [40].

Increased IAP also increases venous stasis more than in a normal patient; it reduces portal blood flow with a transitory increase in liver enzymes, reduces diuresis, diminishes pulmonary compliance, increases pressure in the airways, and obstructs cardiac function, reducing output due to an increase in systemic vascular resistance.

The patient therefore needs more intraoperative intervention to optimise mechanical ventilation. Devices for intermittent pneumatic compression of the lower limbs can be used to reduced venous stasis, the reverse Trendelenburg position plays a part in reducing operation time, and, finally, stabilising intravascular volume is beneficial.

In patients with previous cardiopulmonary diseases, invasive haemodynamic monitoring is needed using at least a radial arterial catheter to continually measure blood gas and arterial pressure [40].

It has been demonstrated that an alveolar recruitment manoeuvre carried out every 10 min with PEEP maintained at 10 cm/H_2O is able to improve oxygenation and levels of $PaCO_2$ in obese patients undergoing laparoscopic surgery for gastric bands [41].

However, no standardised and validated procedure for carrying out the recruitment manoeuvre has been demonstrated. Various random trials have been conducted using different values of controlled pressure, PEEP, and different dynamics of administration [42]. Even the most recent results appear diverse and, as a consequence, the meta-analysis has different results.

One possible technique is to use pressure-controlled ventilation (PCV) for periods of 2–3 min with PCV of 15 cm H_2O and incremental increases of PEEP up to 25–30 cm H_2O [42].

Ventilation strategies for lung protection in elective surgery in obese patients undergoing laparoscopic procedures can result in a comparable respiratory outcome to that seen in non-obese patients and can prevent VILI, even if there are greater complications and morbility.

14.3.6 Very Elderly Patients and 'Frailty'

Old age and correlated comorbidities in patients are the main prognostic factors related to surgical results, but not to complications [43].

A recent Italian study [44] on a group of elderly patients who had undergone a cholecystectomy (some as emergency surgery and others with various levels of urgency) confirmed the safety and effectiveness of the laparoscopic procedure and underlined the absence of statistically significant differences between the laparotomic group in terms of operation time, conversion rate, and the incidence of complications.

Frailty is an emerging concept that indicates a reduction in psychological and physical performance, resistance to stress, and in functional physiological reserves. A definition according to physiopathological parameters takes into account unintentional weight loss, tiredness, reduction in physical activity, a reduction in grip strength, and in walking speed [45].

This increases with age and is inversely proportional to the result of the surgical procedure and to morbility and postoperative mortality [46]. 'High risk' and 'frailty' are therefore two closely linked but not corresponding terms. All 'frail' patients should be considered 'high risk', but not all 'high-risk' patients are frail.

There is insufficient evidence in the literature to indicate or contraindicate one surgical technique over another.

14.4 Intraoperative Complications of Laparoscopy

The incidence of intraoperative complications depends on many factors: the most important ones are the patient's ASA score, the eventual urgency of the operation, intraoperative problems (blood loss and duration), and the experience of the professionals (surgeons and anaesthetists) [47].

There is currently little data in the literature on morbility and mortality and what exists is contradictory. In emergency surgery there is 10 % mortality, while in elective surgery there is 2.6 % mortality [47].

Below is a description of the typical intraoperative complications of laparoscopic procedures that often require a decision on the part of the surgeon–anaesthetist team.

14.4.1 Subcutaneous Emphysema

This is due to the insufflation of CO_2 in subcutaneous tissue, both due to accidental causes and as a collateral effect following laparoscopic procedures that involve it.

It can be identified by a crackling in the area involved, increased pressure in the airways, and/or an increase in $ETCO_2$ and $PaCO_2$ values. It is associated with hypercapnia and respiratory acidosis.

In the case of accidental insufflation [48], for example difficult insertion of the Veress needle, a passage can be created between the peritoneal cavity and subcutaneous tissues, producing a low-pressure channel that allows CO_2 to accumulate and then absorbed.

In other cases, during operations to repair inguinal hernias through laparoscopy, the diffusion of CO_2 from the peritoneal cavity may reach the mediastinum, due to the passage of gas through congenital lesions of the diaphragm, with the formation of pneumomediastinum and then subcutaneous emphysema in the cervical region.

Another cause of subcutaneous emphysema in the cervical region may be the opening of the peritoneum above the diaphragmatic hiatus during laparoscopic fundoplication to repair a hiatus hernia with the passage of high-pressure CO_2 in the mediastinum and then the cervical region.

In many cases, no action is involved during anaesthesiology management, as the emphysema spontaneously disappears as soon as the abdomen is deflated.

It should always be suspected during the procedure if there is an increase in $EtCO_2$.

Recommendations [48] for managing complications include:

- Repeated tests on the abdominal wall to check for the accumulation of gas.
- Ceasing the administration of nitrous oxide (N_2O) if in use, as it could favour the subcutaneous movement of gas.
- Using a CO_2 absorber.
- Increasing ventilation to contrast hypercapnia.
- Rapidly ending pneumoperitoneum and stopping CO_2 insufflation if the patient is unstable.
- Considering other causes of hypercapnia (bronchial intubation, pulmonary embolism of CO_2, malignant hyperthermia, or pneumothorax)

When the increase in the total volume of CO_2 expired (VCO_2) becomes such that hypercapnia can no longer be corrected by modifying ventilation, the laparoscopy should be interrupted to allow CO_2 to be eliminated and hypercapnia to be resolved. The procedure can begin again later using a reduced IAP. The patient should be mechanically ventilated until the hypercapnia is resolved [7].

If signs of cardiopulmonary instability persist, however, it is sometimes necessary to revert to an open procedure [49].

Subcutaneous emphysema, even in the cervical region, is not a contraindication for tracheal extubation at the end of the laparoscopy [50], but should be carried out after laryngoscopy or using protective techniques (positioning of tube exchangers) or should be deferred if the emphysema is massive, by placing the patient in intensive care.

14.4.2 Gas Embolism

This is the most dangerous complication that can occur during a laparoscopy. It can be caused by direct insufflation of CO_2 into a vein due to accidental insertion of the Veress needle or trocar, or may be due to the insufflation of gas in an abdominal organ [51].

It usually occurs when pneumoperitoneum is induced and the risk is greater in patients who have previously undergone abdominal surgery.

Intravascular insufflation of high-pressure carbon dioxide can cause an embolism in the vena cava and the right atrium of such a size that it obstructs venous return, immediately causing cardiac output to diminish and possible circulatory collapse [52].

Literature also contains cases of paradoxical embolism following the reopening of a foramen ovale, caused by increased pressure of the right ventricle [53].

In the case of small embolisms (with the insufflation of CO_2 up to 0.5 ml/kg), the use of a precordial Doppler probe or transesophageal echocardiography can confirm an early diagnosis.

In the case of larger embolisms (with insufflation of 2 ml/kg), intense hypotension may occur, together with an increase in central venous pressure, cyanosis, alterations in heart sounds, ECG changes in right leads, and arrhythmia leading to asystole in the most serious cases. It causes a V/Q mismatch, an increase in dead space, and hypoxemia [7].

Initially, there is a sudden increase of $ETCO_2$ that then diminishes with the reduction in cardiac output and pulmonary blood flow.

When gas embolism occurs, CO_2 insufflation should be stopped and the abdomen should be distended. If nitrous oxide is being administered this should be stopped. The patient should be placed in the Trendelenburg position lying on the left side, to allow gas to reach the apex of the right ventricle and thus avoid the entrance of the pulmonary artery. The patient should be hyperventilated with 100 % FiO_2 to correct the hypoxemia and promote the excretion of CO_2.

If these measures are not enough, it may necessary to position a central venous catheter or a catheter in the pulmonary artery to aspirate the gas. External cardiac massage may help break up the embolism into a bubble of a smaller diameter.

In the case of a massive embolism a cardiopulmonary bypass may be performed [54].

If a cerebral embolism of CO_2 is suspected, consider hyperbaric therapy [53].

Once the patient has been stabilised, pneumoperitoneum can carefully be created once more [54].

If the signs of cardiopulmonary imbalance remain, it may be necessary to revert to an open procedure [53].

14.4.3 Capnothorax

Embryonic residues between the serous membranes are potential pathways for communication between the peritoneal cavity, pleural cavity, and pericardium. These may open due to the increase in IAP as a result of pneumoperitoneum. Furthermore, defects or week spots in the diaphragm in the oesophageal hiatus or aortic hiatus may allow the passage of gas into the thorax. Pleural lesions around the gastroesophageal junction can also be possible complications of laparoscopic procedures. The spontaneous rupture of an existing emphysematic bubble is also a possibility. The same subcutaneous emphysema in the cervical region, which has previously been treated, can develop to generate a pneumothorax, as can all of the conditions listed above, with possible serious respiratory and haemodynamic alternations: a reduction in toracopulmonary compliance, an increase in pressure in the airways, an increase in $ETCO_2$ and $PaCO_2$, diminished SpO_2, hypotension, and—in the most serious cases—cardiac arrest [55].

As this is caused by CO_2, which is highly diffusible, if there is no associated thoracic trauma it will resolve itself spontaneously within 30–60 min [7].

If pneumothorax occurs due to the rupture of a pre-existing bubble, avoid PEEP and insert a chest tube.

14.5 Intraoperative Monitoring

Patients must be monitored according to SIAARTI [56] guidelines for any type of laparoscopic surgery carried out under general or loco-regional anaesthetic. Furthermore, special attention must be paid to certain aspects of monitoring during laparoscopic surgery:

- Capnometry. During general anaesthetic and deep sedation, patient ventilation must be continually monitored through capnometry. Clinical signs such as respiratory range, respiratory frequency, and auscultation of the chest can be combined with instrumental monitoring. Therefore, as well as $ETCO_2$, other fundamental parameters are those provided by the ventilator, such as maximum pressure of the airways and plateau pressure.

For example, in patients with altered cardiorespiratory functions, it may be necessary to monitor arterial blood pressure through an arterial cannula, also in order to frequently check arterial blood gas data, as the $PaCO_2/EtCO_2$ ratio may change. An arterial cannula is therefore recommended for ASA III, IV, and obese patients [56].

14.6 Postoperative Complications

The main postoperative complications, according to Bottger [47], seen in 12 % of patients treated, are heart failure, cerebrovascular complications, prolonged mechanical ventilation, the need for intensive care, bronchopneumonic and urinary infections. Cardiac complications and the need for prolonged mechanical ventilation are significantly linked to the patient's ASA, the length of the operation, and the need for transfusions.

On the basis of shorter postoperative recovery, reduced occurrence of complications and lower structural costs, Luz Moreira suggests a laparoscopic rather than a laparotomic approach to colectomies in ASA III–IV patients [57].

14.6.1 Postoperative Pulmonary Complications

In the immediate postoperative period, respiratory frequency and $ETCO_2$ in spontaneous respiration in a patient who has undergone laparoscopy are greater than in an open procedure. Exogenous CO_2 absorbed during pneumoperitoneum can create a greater risk of hypercapnia, including in the postoperative phase. The clinical picture is aggravated by the residual effects of anaesthetics and diaphragmatic dysfunction [58], which prevent the necessary ventilatory requirements of the patients, with the risk of not only hypercapnia but also respiratory insufficiency.

High-risk patients (the obese [59], elderly [60], smokers, and COPD [61]) suffer a greater reduction in expiratory volumes after a laparoscopy and are slower to recover pulmonary function than healthy subjects.

However, there is a great deal of literature to demonstrate that a laparoscopic procedure is associated with less alteration of pulmonary function in the postoperative period than a laparotomy [62, 63].

14.6.2 Deep Vein Thrombosis

Practice guidelines on pneumoperitoneum by the European Association for Endoscopic Surgery (EAES) in 2002 [26] state that during a laparoscopic procedure the reverse Trendelenburg position and increased IAP created during pneumoperitoneum cause a reduction in venous return in the lower extremities of over 40 %, with an increase in pressure in the femoral vein. This is why during long operations intraoperative devices are recommended for sequential pneumatic compression of the lower limbs, in order to reduce venous stasis.

14.7 Conclusions

It is now recognised that laparoscopic surgery is able to produce less postoperative immune response than open surgery, increasing the beneficial response of the body to surgical stress.

Anaesthetists and surgeons are destined to be faced with increasingly elderly and more fragile patients, with complex surgical histories, comorbidities, undergoing combination therapy, who would benefit from a less invasive technique.

Emergency laparoscopic surgery carried out on patients with a greater operatory risk is a challenge that should be faced appropriately and requires a process of learning and adaptation of specific surgical techniques (surgical instruments and mechanical respiration, etc.) in order to achieve a high level of competence on the part of the whole surgical team. Only this awareness, coupled with an awareness of absolute contraindications, can offer higher risk patients the advantages of laparoscopic procedures in emergency surgery.

References

1. Arati S, Ashutosh N (2010) Secrets of safe laparoscopic surgery: anaesthetic and surgical considerations. J Minimal Access Surg 6(4):91–94
2. Frederic JG et al (2006) Anesthesia for laparoscopy: a review. J Clin Anesth 18:67–78
3. Min S et al (2010) Carbon dioxide pneumoperitoneum, physiologic changes and anesthetic concerns. Ambulatory Surg 16(2):41–46
4. Rasmussen JP et al (1978) Cardiac function and hypercarbia. Arch Surg 113:1196–1200
5. Mäkinen MT, Yli-Hankala A (1996) The effect of laparoscopic cholecystectomy on respiratory compliance as determined by continuous spirometry. J Clin Anesth 8(2):119–122
6. Mullet CE et al (1993) Pulmonary CO_2 elimination during surgical procedures using intra or extraperitoneal CO_2 insufflation. Anesth Analg 76:622–626
7. Miller RD et al (2010) Anesthesia for laparoscopic surgery. In: Miller's Anesthesia, 7th edn. Elsevier, Philadelphia, PA, pp 4678–4718
8. Torri G, Calderini E (2013) Ventilazione artificiale meccanica, invasiva e non invasiva. Antonio Delfino Editore, pp 130–131
9. Maracaja-Neto LF et al (2009) Beneficial effects of high positive end-expiratory pressure in lung respiratory mechanics during laparoscopic surgery. Acta Anaesthesiol Scand 53:210–217
10. Bloomfield GL et al (1996) Effects of increased intra-abdominal pressure upon intracranial and cerebral perfusion pressure before and after volume expansion. J Trauma 40:936–941
11. Salihoglu Z et al (2002) Influence of the patient positioning on respiratory mechanics during pneumoperitoneum. MiddleEast J Anesthesiol 16:521–528
12. Burton A (1993) Precipitous decrease in oxygen saturation during laparoscopic surgery. Anesth Analg 1976:1177
13. Gutt CN et al (2004) Circulatory and respiratory complications of carbon dioxide insufflation. Dig Surg 21(2):95–105
14. Odeberg S et al (1994) Haemodynamic effects of pneumoperitoneum and the influence of posture during anaesthesia for laparoscopic surgery. Acta Anaesthesiol Scand 38(3):276–283
15. Hirvonen EA et al (2000) The adverse hemodynamic effects of anesthesia, head up tilt, and carbon dioxide pneumoperitoneum during laparoscopic cholecystectomy. Surg Endosc 14(3):272–277
16. Agresta F et al (2012) Laparoscopic approach to acute abdomen from the Consensus Development Conference of the Società Italiana di Chirurgia Endoscopica e nuove tecnologie

(SICE), Associazione Chirurghi Ospedalieri Italiani (ACOI), Società Italiana di Chirurgia (SIC), Società Italiana di Chirurgia d'Urgenza e del Trauma (SICUT), Società Italiana di Chirurgia nell'Ospedalità Privata (SICOP), and the European Association for Endoscopic Surgery (EAES). Surg Endosc 26:2134–2164
17. Gaieski DF (2015) Definition, classification, etiology, and pathophysiology of shock in adults. Wolters Kluwer. UpToDate review: http://www.uptodate.com/contents/definition-classification-etiology-and-pathophysiology-of-shock-in-adults
18. Vincent JL, De Backer D (2013) Circulatory shock. N Engl J Med 369:1726–1734
19. Goettler CE et al (2004) Laparoscopy in trauma. Curr Rev Gastrointest Minimally Invasive Endocrine Surg 61(6):554–559
20. SAGES Guidelines Committee, Board of Governors of the Society of American Gastrointestinal and Endoscopic Surgeons (SAGES) (2008) Diagnostic laparoscopy guidelines. Surg Endosc 22:1353–1383
21. Mobbs RJ, Yang MO (2002) The dangers of diagnostic laparoscopy in the head injured patient. J Clin Neurosci 9:592–593
22. Josephs LG et al (1994) Diagnostic laparoscopy increases intracranial pressure. J Trauma 36(6):815–818, discussion 818–819
23. Neudecker J et al (2002) The European Association for Endoscopic Surgery clinical practice guideline on the pneumoperitoneum for the laparoscopic surgery. Surg Endosc 16:1121–1143
24. Lentschener C et al (1996) Intra-ocular pressure changes during gynaecological laparoscopy. Anaesthesia 51:1106
25. Agrawal M et al (2013) A comparative study of four combinations of anesthetic drugs for assessing the intraocular pressure changes during gynaecological laparoscopic procedures. Anesth Essays Res 7(3):319–325
26. Lentschener C et al (2000) Effect of CO_2 pneumoperitoneum on early cellular markers of retinal ischemia in rabbits with alpha-chymotrypsin-induced glaucoma. Surg Endosc 14:1057
27. Bonatsos G et al (2001) Laparoscopic cholecystectomy in adults with sickle cell disease. Surg Endosc 15:816–819
28. Vichinsky EP et al (2000) Causes and outcomes of the acute chest syndrome in sickle cell disease. National Acute Chest Syndrome Study Group. N Engl J Med 342(25):1855–1865
29. Platt OS et al (1994) Mortality in sickle cell disease. Life expectancy and risk factors for early death. N Engl J Med 330:1639–1644
30. Portera CA et al (1995) Benefits of pulmonary artery catheter and transesophageal echocardiographic monitoring in laparoscopic cholecystectomy patients with cardiac disease. Am J Surg 169(2):202–206, discussion 206–207
31. Uranus S, Dorr K (2010) Laparoscopy in abdominal trauma. Eur J Trauma Emerg Surg 36:19–24
32. Choi YB et al (2003) Therapeutic laparoscopy for abdominal trauma. Surg Endosc 17:421–427
33. Mallat AF et al (2008) The role of laparoscopy in trauma: a ten-year review of diagnosis and therapeutics. Am Surg 74(12):1166–1170
34. http://epp.eurostat.ec.europa.eu/statistics_explained/index.php/Population_structure_and_ageing
35. Naitoh T et al (2013) Emergency laparoscopic cholecystectomy for a patient with an implantable left ventricular assist device: report of a case. Surg Today 43:313–316
36. Yacoub OF et al (1982) Carbon dioxide embolism during laparoscopy. Anesthesiology 57:533–535
37. Merkow RP et al (2009) Effect of body mass index on short-term outcomes after colectomy for cancer. J Am Coll Surg 208:53–61
38. Dumont L et al (1997) Changes in pulmonary mechanics during laparoscopic gastroplasty in morbidly obese patients. Acta Anaesthesiol Scand 41:408–413
39. Hedenstierna G et al (2005) The effects of anesthesia and muscle paralysis on the respiratory system. Intensive Care Med 31:1327–1335
40. Nguyen NT et al (2005) The physiologic effects of pneumoperitoneum in the morbidly obese-review. Ann Surg 241(2):219–226

41. De Baerdemaeker LE et al (2008) Comparison of volume-controlled and pressure-controlled ventilation during laparoscopy gastric banding in morbidly obese patients. Obesity Surg 18:680–685
42. Forgiarini Júnior LA et al (2013) Alveolar recruitment maneuver and perioperative ventilatory support in obese patients undergoing abdominal surgery. Rev Bras Ter Intensiva 25(4):312–318
43. Kim HO et al (2009) Outcome of laparoscopic cholecystectomy is not influenced by chronological age in the elderly. World J Gastroenterol 15:722–726
44. Ferrarese AG et al (2013) Elective and emergency laparoscopic cholecystectomy in the elderly: our experience. BMC Surg 13(Suppl 2):S21
45. Fried LP et al (2001) Frailty in older adults: evidence for a phenotype. J Gerontol A Biol Sci Med Sci 56(3):M146–M156
46. Rockwood K et al (1999) A brief clinical instrument to classify frailty in elderly people. Lancet 353:205–206
47. Böttger TC et al (2009) Modifiable surgical and anesthesiological risk factors for the development of cardiac and pulmonary complications after laparoscopic colorectal surgery. Surg Endosc 23:2016–2025
48. Pearce DJ (1994) Respiratory acidosis and subcutaneous emphysema during laparoscopic cholecystectomy. Can J Anaesth 41(4):314–316
49. Joshi GP (2001) Complications of laparoscopy. Anesthesiol Clin North America 19(1):89–105
50. Chien GL et al (1995) Pharyngeal emphysema with airway obstruction as a consequence of laparoscopic inguinal herniorrhaphy. Anesth Analg 80:201
51. De Plater RM, Jones IS (1989) Non-fatal carbon dioxide embolism during laparoscopy. Anaesth Intensive Care 17:359
52. Ostman PL et al (1990) Circulatory collapse during laparoscopy. J Clin Anesth 2:129
53. McGrath BJ (1989) Carbon dioxide embolism treated with hyperbaric oxygen. Can J Anaesth 36(5):586–589
54. Diakun TA (1991) Carbon dioxide embolism: successful resuscitation with cardiopulmonary bypass. Anesthesiology 74:1151
55. Jolis JL et al (1995) Pneumothorax during laparoscopic fundoplication: diagnosis and treatment with positive end-expiratory pressure. Anesth Analg 81:993
56. Bettelli G, Della Rocca G et al Gruppo di studio SIAARTI per la Sicurezza in Anestesia. Standard per il monitoraggio in anestesia (edizione 2012). http://www.siaarti.it/SiteAssets/Ricerca/Standard-per-il-monitoraggio-in-Anestesia/linee_guida_file_43.pdf
57. Da Luz Moreira A (2010) Laparoscopic versus open colectomy for patients with American Society of Anesthesiology (ASA) classification 3 and 4: the minimally invasive approach is associated with significantly quicker recovery and reduced costs. Surg Endosc 24:1280–1286
58. Sharma RR et al (1993) Diaphragmatic function before and after laparoscopic cholecystectomy. Anesthesiology 79:966
59. Joris JL et al (1998) Pulmonary function and pain after gastroplasty performed via laparotomy or laparoscopy in morbidly obese patients. Br J Anaesth 80:283
60. Tousignant G et al (1992) The effect of age on recovery of pulmonary function after laparoscopic cholecystectomy. Anesth Analg 74(2S):S321
61. Johnson D et al (1992) Postoperative respiratory function after laparoscopic cholecystectomy. Surg Laparosc Endosc 2(3):221–226
62. Bablekos GD et al (2014) Effects of laparoscopic cholecystectomy on lung function: a systematic review. World J Gastroenterol 20(46):17603–17617
63. Nguyen NT et al (2001) Comparison of pulmonary function and postoperative pain after laparoscopic versus open gastric bypass: a randomized trial. J Am Coll Surg 192:469

Imaging in Emergency Surgery 15

Claudia Rossi, Mariateresa Martino, Roberto Ronza, Roberto Rizzati, and Mariano Scaglione

15.1 Acute Cholecystitis

15.1.1 Rationale

- Helpful to diagnosis
- Assessment severity of disease
- To detect the cause: obstructive or non-obstructive
- Identify complications
- Differential diagnosis
- Follow-up: monitor treatment response

15.1.2 US

- First imaging examination in suspected biliary disease
- Useful to early diagnosis of acute uncomplicated cholecystistis
- Helpful to recognize the cause of disease [1, 2]

C. Rossi • M. Martino • R. Ronza
Dipartimento di Internistica, Clinica e Sperimentale "Magrassi-Lanzara" Seconda Università degli Studi di Napoli, Napoli, Italy
e-mail: cla-rossi@hotmail.it

R. Rizzati
Dipartimento di Radiologia, Ospedale Sant'Anna, Azienda Universitaria – Ospedaliera di Ferrara, Ferrara, Italy

M. Scaglione (✉)
Dipartimento di Radiologia, PO Pineta Grande, Castel Volturno, Italy
e-mail: mscaglione@tiscali.it

F. Agresta et al. (eds.), *Emergency Laparoscopy*,
DOI 10.1007/978-3-319-29620-3_15

- First signs of complications: gangrenous cholecystitis, emphysematous cholecystitis, perforation of the gallbladder, Mirizzi's syndome
- Follow-up

15.1.2.1 US Findings
- Distension of the gallbladder lumen [2]
- Gallbladder wall thickening with a" binary" shape
- Obstructing stone in the gallbladder neck or cystic duct
- US Murphy sign
- Hyperemic wall at color—Doppler
- Pericholecystic fluid
- Gaseous parietal, intraluminal, or extraparietal collection
- Aerobilia: hyperchoic images
- Intraluminal hemorrhage: hyperchoic areas
- Poor definition of the gallbladder

15.1.2.2 Advantages
- High accuracy
- Relative sensibility to study the main biliary duct

15.1.2.3 Disadvantages
- Less sensitivity in recognizing complications of acute cholecystitis
- Limitation to differentiate sludge and gallbladder wall thickening
- Less sensitivity to study the main pancreatic duct
- Frequent pitfalls: stones, duodenal artifacts, and other non-inflammatory conditions
- Obese patient
- Operator dependent

15.1.3 CT

- Second-line modality for acute cholecystitis
- Helpful to recognize early local and systemic complications
- Contrast-enhancement CT (CECT) is the "gold standard" in cases of acute abdomen [3]
- High sensitivity of CECT to detect peryglandular inflammatory changes [3, 4]

15.1.3.1 CT Findings
- Cholelithiasis: sensivity <70 %
- Gallbladder distension
- Gallbladder wall thickening
- Mural or mucosal hyperenhancement (halo sign)
- Pericholecystic fluid and inflammatory fat stranding
- Enhancement of the adjacent liver parenchyma due to reactive hyperaemia [3, 4]

- Complications [5]:
  - Gangrenous cholecystitis: sensitivity <30 %, specificity >95 %, intraluminal gas, irregularity of the gallbladder wall, abscess.
  - Emphysematous cholecystitis: site (intraparietal, intra-extraluminal) and large quantities of gas.
  - Gallbladder perforation: wall defect, pericholecystic fluid, and extraluminal stones.
  - Cholecysto-enteric fistula: most common with duodenum and colon. The passage of a stone is possible, through the fistula, in the intestinal lumen with secondary intestinal obstruction (Gallstone ileus).

15.1.3.2 Advantages

- Overview to evaluate local or systemic complications
- High specificity to evaluate acute inflammation with hyperenhancement of the wall, after contrast agent injection

15.1.3.3 Disadvantages

- Less sensitivity to show gallstones into gallbladder or bilary ducts
- Less sensitivity and low resolution to study gallbladder and biliary tree

15.1.4 MRI

- Magnetic Resonance (MR) and especially MRCP are the gold standard in cases of suspected acute biliary tract disease [6, 7]
- To confirm diagnosis of acute cholecystitis
- MRCP is useful to study the gallbladder and biliary ducts, particularly neck of gallbladder, and cystic duct
- To rule out coexisting bile duct stones in patients with known or suspected acute cholecysititis
- Provide same morphologic alterations as CT (i.e., inflammatory changes in the gallbladder wall and pericholecystic fat)
- More accurate than CT to evaluate other complications such as cholangitis, obstructive jaundice, and hemobilia [6]

15.1.4.1 MR Findings

- Gallbladder wall thickening: hyperintense signal (seq T2W FS)—very specific sign for the diagnosis of acute cholecystitis
- Pericholecystic and perihepatic fluid (C sign)
- Gallbladder distension
- Hyperenhancement of the wall: hyperintense signal (seq T1WFS post-contrast)
- Inflammatory fat stranding
- Complications:
  - Empyema: distended gallbladder by pus (hypointense signal in T2W)

  - Hemorrhagic cholecystitis: intraluminal and intramural hemorrhage (hypointense signal in T1W)
  - Emphysematous cholecystitis: parietal necrosis and endoluminal gas
  - Gallbladder perforation: wall discontinuity (seq T1W-T2W FS), greater sensitivity than TC [6, 7]

15.1.4.2 Advantages

- Accurate study of the biliary tree and main pancreatic duct
- Search for gallstone in the gallbladder neck or into cystic duct
- Differential diagnosis between acute and chronic cholecystitis
- Preferable in young adults and females
- No use of ionizing radiation
- High spatial resolution
- Multiplanar and multiparametric

15.1.4.3 Disadvantages

- To rule out systemic complications
- Motion and breathing artifacts
- Unavailability and expensive
- Long scanning time

15.1.5 Differential Diagnosis

- Choledocholithiasis
- Pancreatitis
- Peptic ulcer disease
- Acute hepatitis
- Liver abscess

15.2 Acute Pancreatitis

15.2.1 Rationale

- To rule out pancreatitis
- Early diagnosis and proper management: conservative treatment or surgery
- Assessment of severity of disease and complications
- To detect the cause
- Differential diagnosis
- Follow-up: monitor treatment response

15.2.2 CT

- CECT is the " gold standard" for the diagnosis of acute pancreatitis or to exclude other causes of abdominal pain (i.e., cholecystitis, bowel infarction, perforated ulcer, and other abdominal emergency) [8]
- Helpful to confirm the clinical hypothesis of acute pancreatitis [8, 9]
- Evaluate complications: peripancreatic collections and extrapancreatic necrosis.

15.2.2.1 CT Findings

Interstitial edematous pancreatitis-mild: no organ failure and no local or systemic complications

- Focal or diffuse parenchymal enlargement with normal enhancement of the entire pancreatic gland
- Changes of the pancreatic density because of edema
- Indistinct pancreatic margins owing to inflammation
- Surrounding retroperitoneal fat stranding
- No fluid collections; no necrosis of the pancreatic parenchyma [8]

Necrotizing pancreatitis: protracted clinical course, local complications, and high mortality

- Indistinct organ contour
- Alteration changes of the internal structure of the pancreatic parenchyma
- Pancreatic gland appears inhomogeneous and enlarged
- Focal areas of pancreatic necrosis
- Diffuse necrosis of the pancreatic gland
- Focal areas of hemorrhage
- Surrounding retroperitoneal fat stranding: larger than in interstitial oedematous pancreatitis
- Necrosis of peripancreatic tissue and pancreatic parenchyma (most common)
- Necrosis of only extrapancreatic tissue (less common)
- Necrosis of pancreatic parenchyma without peripancreatic collection [8]

15.2.2.2 Complications

- Early: acute fluid collection, hemorrhage, vascular complications, infected necrosis
- Late: pseudocysts, pancreatic/peripancreatic abscess [9]
  - Peripancreatic collections

    (A) Acute peripancreatic fluid collection (APFC)

      Early collection; can remain sterile or develop infection
      Purely liquid, homogeneous: low density at CT

Localization within the retroperitoneum and adjacent to the pancreas (anterior and posterior pararenal space, transverse mesocolon, small–bowel mesentery)
No wall

(B) Pseudocyst

Late collection
Purely liquid collection of pancreatic juice or fluid
Spherical-shaped semi-liquid fluid collections: low density on CT (0–25 HU)
Capsule of fibrous tissue: hyperdense and enhancement of capsule on CECT
Possible communication with pancreatic ductal system
Spontaneously resorb

(C) Acute necrotic collection (ANC)

Late collection, in the first 4 weeks of necrotizing pancreatitis
Contains both fluid and nonliquified necrotic material
No wall or capsule
Can be multifocal
Non-liquid densities on CT

(D) Walled-off Necrosis (WON)

Late collection
Development of ANC
Non-epithelialized wall

– Abscess

Pseudocyst with pus is defined as a pancreatic abscess, which has a (semi-)
Liquid center and a contrast-enhanced wall
Secondary infection: Intracystic air

– Infected Necrosis

Non-enhanced area on CECT

Vascular Complications

- Pancreaticoduodenal pseudoaneurysms
- Splenic or gastroduodenal artery thrombosis
- Mesenteric or portal venous thrombosis
- Hemorrhage

15.2.2.3 Advantages

- High sensivity and sensibility for diagnosis
- Differential diagnosis
- Evaluate complications: grading, quality, and quantity of pancreatic collections
- Careful study of the pancreas and adjacent organs
- Follow-up
- Availability
- Non-invasiveness and speed

15.2.2.4 Disadvantages

- Relative role to ascertain the acute pancreatitis (cholelithiasis, pancreas divisum)
- Low sensitivity in the study of the biliary tree and pancreatic ducts
- Low accuracy for differential diagnosis between necrosis and infected necrosis
- May be normal in mild cases
- Use of ionizing radiations

15.2.3 US

- High sensivity to recognize the cause of acute pancreatitis: obstructive or non-obstructive
- May reveal a normal-appearing gland in milder cases
- Follow-up

15.2.3.1 US Findings

- Focal or diffuse enlargement of the gland, with heterogeneous or low echogenicity
- Cause of the acute pancreatitis: cholelitiasis and gallstones into biliary ducts [10]
- Pancreatic and peripancreatic collection: anechoic or complex fluid mixed with solid components
- Used to monitor the patient with acute pancreatitis
- Guide percutaneous or endoscopic drainage for the collections
- Vascular complications (portal venous thrombosis)
- Hemorrhage

15.2.3.2 Advantages

- Cause of pancreatitis: gallstones and cholelitiasis
- Follow-up
- Availability
- Non-invasiveness
- Fast and cheap
- No use of ionizing radiations

15.2.3.3 Disadvantages

- Limited field of view of pancreas
- Obese patients
- Investigator's experience

15.2.4 MRI

- Superior than CT for characterization of fluid and/or solid necrotic areas into pancreatic parenchyma and peripancreatic tissue [10]
- Evaluate the integrity of the biliary system and pancreatic duct [10]
- To detect the cause of the acute pancreatitis
- Evaluate local complications [11]

15.2.4.1 MRI Findings

Interstizial Edematous Pancreatitis

- Enlarged pancreas or part of it: hypontense signal on T1W; hyperintense signal on T2W—T1 fat suppression post-contrast
- Peripancreatic inflammation: hyperintense signal on T2W-FS
- Cause of acute pancreatitis: gallstones and cholelitiasis on MRCP [10, 11]

Necrotizing Pancreatitis

- Necrotic areas: nonenhancing areas on T1W-FS post-contrast (particularly important is arterial phase) [11]
- Pancreatic and peripancreatic fluid collections
- Differential diagnosis between necrosis and infected necrosis
- Hemorrhage: areas hyperintense on T1W (subacute phase)

15.2.4.2 Advantages

- Accurate study of the biliary tree, pancreatic ducts, and pancreatic morphology [10]
- High spatial resolution
- Multiplanar and multiparametric study
- No use of ionizing radiation

15.2.4.3 Disadvantages

- Motion and breathing artifacts
- Relative unavailability in most hospitals and expensive
- Long scanning time

15.2.5 Differential Diagnosis

- Pancreatic ductal adenocarcinoma
- Autoimmune pancreatitis

- Peptic ulcer disease with posterior perforation
- Pancreatic lymphoma (diffuse pattern)

15.3 Acute Appendicitis

15.3.1 Rationale

- To rule out appendicitis
- Early diagnosis and proper management: conservative treatment or surgery
- Assessment severity of disease and complications
- To detect the cause: obstructive or non-obstructive [12]
- Differential diagnosis
- Follow-up

15.3.2 CT

- CECT is the "Gold standard", with high sensivity (98 %) and specificity (97 %) for the diagnosis of acute appendicitis [13, 14]
- Exclude alternative causes of abdominal pain, especially on right lower quadrant [12]
- Identify complicated appendicitis

15.3.2.1 CECT Findings

- Dilated appendix with distended lumen [13, 14]
- Increased intraluminal fluid
- Appendiceal wall thickening
- Hyperenhancement of the appendiceal wall
- Appendicolith
- Thickening of the caecal wall: caecal bar sign or arrowhead sign
- Enlarged mesenteric lymphonodes
- Periappendiceal inflammation: stranding of the adjacent fat and thickening of the lateroconal fascia or mesoappendix
- Extraluminal fluid [13, 14]
- Complications: inflammatory phlegmon, abscess, perforation, and generalized peritonitis

15.3.2.2 Advantages

- Differential diagnosis
- Image reconstruction and post-processing to maximize diagnostic efficiency and accuracy
- Identify complications
- Follow-up

15.3.2.3 Disadvantages

- Use of ionizing radiations

15.3.3 US

- First imaging examination in suspected acute appendicitis, particularly in young adults and females
- High safety and accuracy (lower than CT) [15]
- Graded-compression US allows successful examination of a patient who may have peritoneal irritation [15]
- Follow-up, in cases of nonsurgical right low pain [16]

15.3.3.1 US Findings

- Aperistaltic, noncompressible, dilated appendix
- US-McBurney's sign
- Appendicolith
- Distinct appendiceal wall layers
- Hyperechogenic pericaecal fat [16]
- Periappendiceal fluid
- Target appearance (axial section)
- Appendiceal abscess [16]

15.3.3.2 Advantages

- Differential diagnosis with gynecologic disorders
- Initial imaging approach especially in children, young people and women of childbearing age [15]
- Available
- Repeatable
- Non-invasiveness
- Fast and cheap
- Follow-up

15.3.3.3 Disadvantages

- Operator dependent
- Obese patients
- Difficult detection of the appendix in atypical sites

15.3.4 Differential Diagnosis

- Gynecologic conditions

15.4 Gynecologic Disorders

15.4.1 Rationale

- Identify causes of gynecological emergencies [17, 18]
- Differentiate surgical from non surgical gynecological emergencies
- Differential diagnosis with alternative causes of pelvic pain

15.4.2 US

First technique used for acute gynecologic emergencies

15.4.2.1 US Findings
- Free intrapelvic fluid
- Uterine echogenicity and enlargement
- Ovaries enlargement and echogenicity with multiple peripheric follicles
- Liquid or solid masses
- Ovaries displaced from its location with torsion of ovarian vessels [19]
- Hemorrhagic ovarian cyst or hemorrhagic corpus luteum

15.4.2.2 Advantages
- Provides an overview of uterus and ovaries
- Ability to evaluate the relationship of uterus and ovaries with the adjacent organs
- Possibility to use PD analysis to evaluate vascularization

15.4.2.3 Disadvantages
- Low spatial resolution because of deep position of genital organs
- Limited in women with abundant subcutaneous fat

15.4.3 Endovaginal US

It requires dedicated intracavitary transducers; technique of choice for acute gynecologic emergencies [20].

15.4.3.1 EVUS Findings
- Optimal visualization of endometrium and myometrium
- Size and location of ectopic pregnancy [21]
- Hemorrhagic ovarian cyst or hemorrhagic corpus luteum
- Presence of complications of PID such as tubo-ovaric abscess

15.4.3.2 Advantages

- Ability to perform a survey in obese women or with abdominal scars
- High spatial resolution
- High sensitivity for visualization of internal cavity

15.4.3.3 Disadvantages

- Changes of endometrium with ormonal phases
- May be difficult to differentiate benignant from malignant pathologies

15.4.4 MRI

MRI is a second technique used:

- To confirm or exclude US diagnosis
- To evaluate complications

15.4.4.1 MRI Findings

- Enlargement of uterus with alterations of signal
- Identification of endometrioma and its rupture [22]
- Hemorrhagic cyst associated with hemoperitoneum such as breaking of hemorrhagic corpus luteum, or ovarian cyst
- Characterization of masses such as liquid, solid, or mixed
- Differential diagnosis between acute from chronic bleeding
- Characterization of masses of pelvic inflammatory disease and its complications, such as tubo-ovaric abscess

15.4.4.2 Advantages

- High specificity for characterization and differential diagnosis of adnexial masses
- Allows a detailed anatomy
- High panoramicity with possibility to individuate extra-pelvic pathologies causing acute pelvic pain

15.4.4.3 Disadvantages

- Long scanning time
- Lower sensitivity than EVUS for visualization of internal cavity

15.5 Nonspecific Abdominal Pain

15.5.1 Rationale

- To rule out the cause of nonspecific pain
- To differentiate medical from surgical diseases
- To avoid unnecessary laparotomies

15.5.2 X-Ray Abdomen

X-ray abdomen is the first imaging technique [23];

15.5.2.1 X-Ray Findings

- Signs of pneumoperitoneum;
- Air-fluid levels, intestinal morphological changes, and behaviors;
- Signs of small- and large-bowel obstruction (LBO) or Ogilvie's syndrome
- Fecal stasis.

15.5.2.2 Advantages

- Provides an overview of abdominal cavity

15.5.2.3 Disadvantages

- Serial plain films help understand interstinal behaviours
- Low sensitivity to identify cause

15.5.3 CECT

CECT may provide additional information compared to plain film [24, 25]

15.5.3.1 CECT Findings

- May identify medical and surgical causes of abdominal pain
- To evaluate the enhancement of solid organ and hollow viscera
- To assess abdominal vessels
- To assess presence and characterization of masses

15.5.3.2 Advantages

- May identify both medical and surgical causes of abdominal pain [26]
- High prognostic negative value [27]

15.5.3.3 Disadvantages

- Use of ionizing radiations

15.6 Perforated Gastro-duodenal Ulcer

15.6.1 Rationale

- Evidence of free intraperitoneal air
- Definition of location of perforation

15.6.2 X-Ray Abdomen

First imaging exam. For positivity of exam, 1–2 ml of free gas are sufficient. At least 3 projections are needed:

- Postero-anterior and latero-lateral in orthostatism
- Postero-anterior in left lateral decubitus
- Anterior-posterior in supine decubitus

15.6.2.1 X-Ray Findings

- Free gas
- Presence of free air in perihepatic, perisplenic, along the course of falciform ligament or round ligament, or in Morrison space is indicative of perforation of gastroduodenal ulcera [28]

15.6.2.2 Advantages

- Fast and cheap
- Repeatable
- Performed also in supine patients

15.6.2.3 Disadvantages

- Use of ionizing radiations

15.6.3 CT

Most sensitivity method to research free gas [29, 30].

15.6.3.1 CT Findings

- Free air intraperitoneal
- Associated signs of paralitic ileus (horizontal loops, air-fluid levels)
- Spreading extraluminal contrast medium (rare, need oral contrast administration)
- Discontinuity and thickening intestinal wall (rare)
- Free intraperitoneal fluid

15.6.3.2 Advantages

- Sensitivity of 99 % in identify pneumoperitoneum
- It is able to recognize also small gas bubbles not visible to X-Ray abdomen
- Can recognize the site of perforation [31, 32]

15.6.3.3 Disadvantages

- Initial CT study may be negative for free air (covered perforation).

15.7 Large-Bowel Obstruction

15.7.1 Rationale

- To rule out LBO
- Identification of the cause
- Severity of LBO and possible complications
- Differential diagnosis

15.7.2 X-Ray Abdomen

- It is the first imaging study in patient suspected of having LBO
- two views at least in critical patient (supine position Antero-Posterior and Lateral views)
- When possible in both dependent (supine and prone) and nondependent (upright decubitus)
- The sensitivity of abdominal radiography for the detection of LBO is 84 %, and the specificity is only 72 % as a result of difficult to distinguish between obstruction and colonic pseudo-obstruction [33, 34]

15.7.2.1 X-Ray Findings

- Colon may be glossily dilated proximal to the site of obstruction "transition zone" with paucity or absence of gas distal to the obstruction site [35]
- Air-fluid levels
- Pneumatosis (unusual and difficult to detect)
- Portal venous gas (unusual and difficult to detect)
- Pneumoperitoneum
- Abnormal location of colonic segments (volvulus)

15.7.3 CT

- CECT is the gold standard for the evaluation of LBO
- Well-tolerated, rapid imaging study
- High sensitivity (96 %) and a specificity (93 %) [36, 37]

15.7.3.1 CT Findings

- Dilated large bowel proximal to the transition point and collapsed bowel distal to the site of obstruction [38]

  Colon Carcinoma LBO

  - Asymmetric and short-segment wall thickening

– Enhancing soft tissue narrowing the colonic lumen
– "Shoulder sign," central necrosis in a large obstructive mass
– Pericolonic fat infiltration (differential diagnosis with diverticulitis)
– Lymph nodes larger than 1 cm

Sigmoid Volvulus

– "Coffee bean" sign, apposition of the medial walls of the dilated loops forms the cleft of the bean
– "Bird beak" sign, tapering transition point
– The "inverted U" sign, dilated sigmoid extends into the upper quadrant
– "Northern exposure" sign, repositioning of the sigmoid colon out of the pelvis
– Absence of rectal gas;
– The point of twisting and the vessels (Whirl sign) [39, 40].

Cecal Volvulus

– Radiological findings

Marked distension of cecum
Bird beak sign, bowel tapers and meets at the site of twist
The whirl sign
Small-bowel dilatation, in incompetent valve
Signs of ischemia: wall thickening, mural hypoenhancement, pneumatosis

Diverticulitis

– Segmental, symmetric bowel wall thickening with hyperemia in a longer portion than colonic cancer
Pericolonic inflammation and fat stranding
Extramural abscesses or perforation as complications
Fluid in peritoneal spaces
Vascular engorgement [41]

Intussusception

– CT can identify the cause in more than 80 %. Colonic carcinoma is the most frequent cause in adults

Intraluminal Contents

– In old or weak patients, fecal impaction is frequent.
Very rare are hernias, inflammatory bowel disease, adhesions, or external compression.

Acute colonic pseudo obstruction (ACPO) or Ogilvie syndrome is a pseudo-obstruction without an exact pathophysiology. Distinguishing between LBO and pseudo-obstruction is challenging. On abdominal radiographs, colonic distension, involving the cecum, ascending colon, and transverse colon, is the hallmark of ACPO, but not pathognomonic. Repositioning the patient in right lateral decubitus results in air filling the distal colon.

Contrast enema may be made to evaluate a transition point. If diagnosis is unclear a CT may allow characterization of the entire large bowel with or without a transition point [42].

15.8 Small-Bowel Obstruction

15.8.1 Rationale

- To rule out small-bowel obstruction (SBO);
- To identify the severity of SBO and possible complications
- Determination of the transition point
- Identification of the cause of SBO
- Differential diagnosis

A diagnostic algorithm for evaluation of patients with suspected SBO is shown in Fig. 15.1 [43, 44].

15.8.2 X-Ray

- First imaging examination
- Its accuracy varies from 50 % to 70 % [33]
- At least three projections (supine, prone, and lateral decubitus)

15.8.2.1 Findings

- Dilated small bowel
- Dilated stomach
- Absence of rectal gas
- Multiple air-fluid levels (upright or left lateral decubitus radiography)

15.8.2.2 Advantages

- Availability
- Rapidity
- Non-invasiveness
- Follow-up

15.8.2.3 Disadvantages

- Rare identification of the cause [45]

15.8.3 US

- Not used in the United states, but it is frequently used in many other countries where the availability of CT is limited and expertise in sonography is high. Useful adjunct with plain film

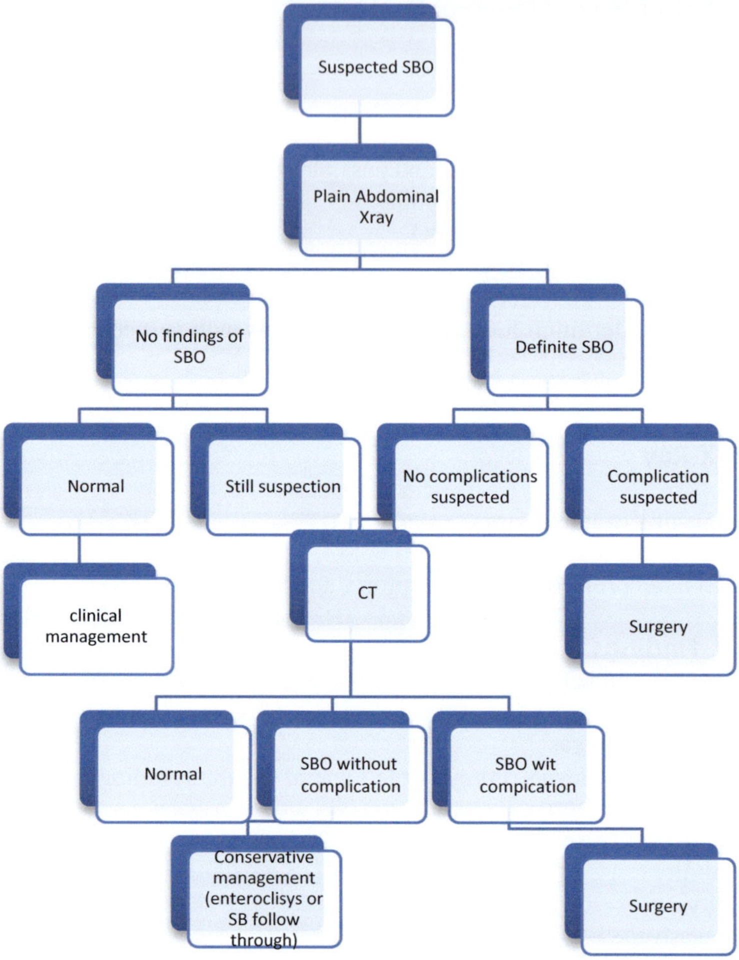

Fig. 15.1 This flow chart shows the imaging approach in patients with suspected small bowel obstruction

15.8.3.1 US Findings

- Dilated small-bowel loops
- Increased peristalsis of the dilated segments
- Bowel wall thickness
- Presence of extraluminal fluid

15.8.3.2 Advantages

- Availability
- Rapidity
- Non-invasiveness

- Presence or absence of peristalsis
- Presence of extraluminal fluid

15.8.3.3 Disadvantages

- Operator dependent
- Limitation in gas-containing structures
- Obese habit

15.8.4 CT

- CECT is the gold standard
- Confirm or exclude diagnosis of SBO
- Evaluation of severity and complications
- Identifies the cause [46]

15.8.4.1 Findings

- Small-bowel dilatation and colon not dilated
- Transition point from dilated to non-dilated small bowel
- Air-fluid levels
- Colon decompressed

  CT Findings of Ischemia
  - Bowel wall thickening
  - Fluid in mesentery or peritoneal cavity
  - Mesenteric edema
  - Abnormal bowel wall enhancement (increased or decreased)
  - Occlusion of mesenteric vessels
  - Engorged mesenteric veins
  - Whirl sign
  - Pneumatosis [47, 48]

15.8.4.2 Advantages

- Availability
- Non-invasiveness
- Fast exam
- Excellent evaluation of bowel wall, its vessels, and adjacent mesentery

15.8.4.3 Disadvantages

- No other disadvantage out of the use of ionizing radiation

15.9 Hernias

15.9.1 Rationale

- To evaluate the presence and the type of hernia
- To rule out the complications
- To guide the management
- Follow-up

15.9.2 US

- First-line imaging study for evaluation of non-acute adult groin hernia
- Frequently used in many European centers where the expertise in sonography is high

15.9.2.1 US Findings

- They differentiate between the multiple types of hernia and their contents
- Dilated small-bowel loops proximal to the hernia or in the sac
- Increased peristalsis of the dilated segments
- Bowel wall thickness
- Presence of extraluminal fluid in the sac or in peritoneal space
- Decreased vascularization.

15.9.2.2 Advantages

- Dynamic investigation assessment with and without Valsalva maneuver
- No ionizing radiation
- Evaluation of vessels flow

15.9.2.3 Disadvantages

- Operator dependent
- Limitation in gas-containing structures
- Obese habit
- Evaluation of internal hernias [49].

15.9.3 CT

- First-line imaging study in evaluation of hernia complications
- Fast and panoramic compared with other modalities

Imaging findings differ among the multiple types of hernia, but some signs are common to the same complication [50, 51]. The most common complications:

CT Findings of Bowel Obstruction
- Dilated bowel proximal to the hernia;
- Normal caliber or reduced caliber distal to the hernia
- Tapering of the afferent end efferent loop, at the hernia neck
- Dilation of herniated bowel loops
- Air-fluid levels in bowel proximal to the hernia
- Fecalization of small bowel proximal to obstruction [52, 53]

CT Findings of Incarceration
- Imaging can only suggest the diagnosis, when a small abdominal defect and a narrow neck are visualized.
- Incarceration predisposes to obstruction, ischemia, inflammation, or other complications

CT Findings of Strangulation
- Dilated fluid filled loops;
- U- or C-shaped loops of bowel entrapped within hernia sac
- Afferent and efferent have a "beak bird" signs in the transition point
- Wall thickening
- Abnormal mural hypo- or hyperattenuation and enhancement
- Mesenteric vessel engorgement
- Fat obliteration
- Mesenteric haziness
- Ascites and fluid within the sac [54]

CT Findings of Surgically Repaired Hernias Complications
- Hernia recurrence
- Fluid collections: contain serous fluid (seroma) or blood products (hematoma) are frequently in immediate postoperative period
- Infection: imaging confirms the presence and define the location of volume of collection and to guide drainage
- Mesh-related complications: inflammatory reactions and fibrosis;
- Testicular complications: testicular vessel ligation and testicular ischemia are the most feared complication and of inguinal hernia repair; ultrasound is the modality of choice for the study of vessel flow [55].

15.9.3.1 Advantages
- Availability
- Non-invasiveness
- The short duration of the examination
- Provide anatomic detail of abdominal wall and hernia sac and neck
- Accurate identification of hernia contents

- Differential diagnosis with other abdominal masses
- Evaluation of acute phase and complications
- Useful to evaluate surgically repaired abdominal wall hernias and their complications

15.9.3.2 Disadvantages

- Limited role in dynamic evaluation (Valsalva maneuver).
- Limited role in vessel flow study.

15.9.4 MRI

- MRI should be considered as possible alternative in young patients with symptoms, but only few studies support its use in wall hernia complications.
- Accurate view of musculoskeletal structures
- Very rare clinical use
- One indication is for pregnancy [56].

15.10 Abdominal Trauma

15.10.1 Rationale

- Early assessment and organ injury grading
- To guide patient toward appropriate management: NOM, intervention radiology, or surgery
- Follow-up

15.10.2 CT

- CECT is the "Gold standard" for early diagnosis, proper management, and outcome [57]
- Indication for hemodynamically stable or semi-stable patients [57, 58]
- Tailored protocols according to the mechanism: Abdominal CT survey to be incorporated into "Whole body CT protocols" for high-energy trauma (i.e., motor vehicle accidents)—two phases
- Conversely in direct or compressive trauma only one contrast-enhancement phase for abdominal evaluation can be performed—one phase
- Fast overview of the entire abdomen, skeleton, and vessels in a single scan acquisition
- "Whole body CT" is the fastest radiological investigation, for "complete" body coverage in multitrauma patient [59]
- Evaluation degree and extent of solid organ injuries [60, 61]
- Follow-up

15.10.2.1 CT Findings

- Hemoperitoneum or retroperitoneum
- Peritoneal or retroperitonel free fluid: mild (one peritoneal space), moderate (<3 peritoneal spaces), or massive (all peritoneal spaces) [57, 60]
- Pneumoperitoneum or retroperitoneum
- Sentinel clot sign (45–70 HU): blood located to the source of the hemorrhage [61]
- Nonclotted blood (30–40 HU): flow freely between peritoneal spaces
- Differentiate recent bleeding and chronic bleeding
- High sensivity for detecting small amounts of free peritoneal fluid
- Assessment degree of severity solid organ injuries
- Extent of injuries: diameter, length, depth [62]
- Capsular and parenchymal hematoma: hyperdense on acute/subacute phase (40–60 HU)
- Parenchymal lacerations: hypodense linear or starry area [60, 61]
- Differentiation between contained vascular injury (pseudoaneurysm, arterio-venous fistula) and arterial or venous active bleeding
- Posttraumatic hypoperfusion: hypovolemic shock complex, parenchymal infarct, shock bowel [7]

15.10.2.2 Advantages

- Proper management after abdominal trauma: treatment conservative or surgery
- Diagnosis of life-threatening injuries
- Image reconstruction and post-processing to maximize diagnostic efficiency and accuracy
- Follow-up
- Availability and speed
- Non-invasiveness

15.10.2.3 Disadvantages

- Questionable specificity for diaphragmatic, mesenteric, and hollow organ injuries
- Overestimation of solid organ injury

15.10.3 US-FAST

- Diagnostic modality of choice for evaluation of hemodynamically unstable patients
- Presence or absence of free peritoneal fluid in five spaces: pericardium, hepatorenal fossa, left subphrenic space, right and left paracolic gutters, and pouch of Douglas [63]
- Different role compared to CT in the clinical algorithm

15.10.3.1 Advantages

- Presence or absence of free peritoneal fluid
- Quantity and quality of peritoneal fluid
- Follow-up
- Available
- Non-invasiveness
- Fast and cheap

15.10.3.2 Disadvantages

- Is not predictor for a tailored surgery
- Does not indicate the need for intervention
- Rarely useful in bowel, pancreatic, and renal injuries
- No evaluation of retroperitoneal spaces
- Obese patient
- Investigator's experience

15.11 Mesenteric Ischemia

15.11.1 Rationale

- To rule out mesenteric ischemia;
- To identify the type of ischemia [64]:
  - *Arterial ischemia:* occlusion of AMS from embolic or thrombotic origin
  - *Vein ischemia:* occlusion of VMS
  - *Hypoperfusion* non-occlusive ischemia (NOMI)
- Differential diagnosis

15.11.2 CECT

CECT is the technique of reference with a sensitivity of 90 % [65].

15.11.2.1 CECT Findings

To evaluate [66]

- Mesentery
- Mesenteric vessels
- Thickness and enhancement of bowel loops
- Peritoneal cavity

15.11.2.2 CECT: Mesenteric Findings

- In arterial occlusion: bloodless for intense vasoconstriction
- In NOMI: bloodless for the reduced blood flow
- In vein occlusion: edematous for failure outflow

15.11.2.3 CECT: Mesenteric Vessel Findings

- In arterial occlusion: reduction of diameter or endoluminal defects [67];
- In vein occlusion: increase of diameter for venous engorgement
- In NOMI: reduction of diameter without endoluminal defect

15.11.2.4 CECT: Bowel loop Findings

- In arterial occlusion: thin loop; contrast-enhancement reduced or absent, or target sign in case of reperfusion
- In vein occlusion: thickened loop; contrast-enhancement increased, or target sign
- In NOMI: thin loop; contrast-enhancement reduced or absent, or target sign in case of riperfusion

15.11.2.5 Advantages [68, 69]

- Evaluate thrombotic or embolic origin of ischemia
- Identify type of acute ischemia;
- Evaluate late signs, such as intestinal, portal, and mesenteric pneumatosis or pneumoretroperitoneum.
- Necessary for early detection of NOMI with signs of organ hypoperfusion
- Assess signs of spastic, hypotonic, and paralytic ileus

15.11.2.6 Disadvantages

- Use of ionizing radiation

References

1. Smith EA, Dillman JR, Elsayes KM et al (2009) Cross-sectional imaging of acute and chronic gallbladder inflammatory disease. AJR Am J Roentgenol 192(1):188–196
2. Mirvis SE, Whitley NO, Miller JW (1986) The diagnosis of acute acalculous cholecystitis: a comparison of sonography, scintigraphy and CT. AJR Am J Roentgenol 147:1171–1175
3. Mirvis SE, Whitley NO, Miller JW (1987) CT diagnosis of acalculous cholecystitis. J Comput Assist Tomogr 11(1):83–87
4. Bennett GL, Rusinek H, Lisi V et al (2002) CT findings in acute gangrenous cholecystitis. AJR Am J Roentgenol 178(2):275–281
5. Shakespear JS, Shaaban AM, Rezvani M (2010) CT findings of acute cholecystitis and its complications. AJR Am J Roentgenol 194:6
6. Park MS, Yu JS, Kim YH et al (1998) Acute cholecystitis: comparison of MR cholangiography and US. Radiology 209:781–785
7. Altun E, Semelka RC, Elias J Jr et al (2007) Acute cholecystitis: MR findings and differentiation from chronic cholecystitis. Radiology 244:174–183
8. Balthazar EJ (2002) Acute pancreatitis: assessment of severity with clinical and CT evaluation. Radiology 223:603–613
9. O'Connor OJ, McWilliams S, Maher MM (2011) Imaging of acute pancreatitis. AJR Am J Roentgenol 197:2
10. Scaglione M, Casciani E, Pinto A et al (2008) Imaging assessment of acute pancreatitis: a review. Semin Ultrasound CT MR 29:322–340
11. Miller FH, Keppke AL, Dalal K (2004) MRI of pancreatitis and its complications: Part 1, Acute pancreatitis. AJR Am J Roentgenol 183:1637–1644

12. Birnbaum BA, Brooke Jeffrey R (1998) CT and sonography evaluation of acute right lower quadrant abdominal pain. AJR Am J Roentgenol 170:361–371
13. Choi D, Park H, Lee YR, Kook SH, Kim SK, Kwag HJ, Chung EC (2003) The most useful findings for diagnosing acute appendicitis on contrast-enhanced helical CT. Acta Radiol 44(6):574–582
14. Moteki T, Horikoshi H (2007) New CT criterion for acute appendicitis: maximum depth of intraluminal appendiceal fluid. AJR Am J Roentgenol 188(5):1313–1319
15. Lane MJ, Katz DS, Ross BA et al (1997) Unenhanced helical CT for suspected acute appendicitis. AJR Am J Roentgenol 168(2):405–409
16. Smith MP, Katz DS, Lalani T, Carucci LR, Cash BD, Kim DH et al (2015) ACR appropriateness criteria® right lower quadrant pain–suspected appendicitis. Ultrasound Q 31(2):85–91
17. Kamaya A, Shin L, Chen B, Desser TS (2008) Emergency gynecologic imaging. Semin Ultrasound CT MR 29(5):353–368
18. Vandermeer FQ, Wong-You-Cheong JJ (2009) Imaging of acute pelvic pain. Clin Obstet Gynecol 52(1):2–20
19. Varras M, Tsikini A, Polyzos D, Samara C, Hadjopoulos G, Akrivis C (2004) Uterine adnexal torsion: pathologic and gray-scale ultrasonographic findings. Clin Exp Obstet Gynecol 31(1):34–38
20. Qureshi IA, Ullah H, Akram MH, Ashfaq S, Nayyar S (2004) Transvaginal versus transabdominal sonography in the evaluation of pelvic pathology. J Coll Physicians Surg Pak 14(7):390–393
21. Hann LE, Bachman DM, McArdle CR (1984) Coexistent intrauterine and ectopic pregnancy: a reevaluation. Radiology 152(1):151–154
22. Brosens I, Puttemans P, Campo R, Gordts S, Kinkel K (2004) Diagnosis of endometriosis: pelvic endoscopy and imaging techniques. Best Pract Res Clin Obstet Gynaecol 18(2):285–303
23. Ahn SH et al (2002) Acute nontraumatic abdominal pain in adult patients: abdominal radiography compared with CT evaluation 1. Radiology 225(1):159–164
24. Rosen MP et al (2000) Impact of abdominal CT on the management of patients presenting to the emergency department with acute abdominal pain. Am J Roentgenol 174(5):1391–1396
25. Sala E et al (2007) A randomized, controlled trial of routine early abdominal computed tomography in patients presenting with non-specific acute abdominal pain. Clin Radiol 62(10):961–969
26. Taourel P et al (1992) Acute abdomen of unknown origin: impact of CT on diagnosis and management. Gastrointest Radiol 17(1):287–291
27. Siewert B et al (1997) Impact of CT on diagnosis and management of acute abdomen in patients initially treated without surgery. AJR Am J Roentgenol 168(1):173–178
28. Imuta M et al (2007) Multidetector CT findings suggesting a perforation site in the gastrointestinal tract: analysis in surgically confirmed 155 patients. Radiat Med 25(3):113–118
29. Furukawa A et al (2005) Gastrointestinal tract perforation: CT diagnosis of presence, site, and cause. Abdom Imaging 30(5):524–534
30. Yeung K-W et al (2004) CT evaluation of gastrointestinal tract perforation. Clin Imaging 28(5):329–333
31. Hainaux B et al (2006) Accuracy of MDCT in predicting site of gastrointestinal tract perforation. Am J Roentgenol 187(5):1179–1183
32. Kim SH et al (2009) Gastrointestinal tract perforation: MDCT findings according to the perforation sites. Korean J Radiol 10(1):63–70
33. Thompson WM, Kilani RK, Smith BB et al (2007) Accuracy of abdominal radiography in acute small-bowel obstruction: does reviewer experience matter? AJR Am J Roentgenol 188(3):W233–W238
34. Cappell MS, Batke M (2008) Mechanical obstruction of the small bowel and colon. Med Clin North Am 92(3):575–597, viii
35. Wittenberg J (1993) The diagnosis of colonic obstruction on plain abdominal radiographs: start with the cecum, leave the rectum to last. AJR Am J Roentgenol 161(2):443–444

36. Frager D, Rovno HD, Baer JW, Bashist B, Friedman M (1998) Prospective evaluation of colonic obstruction with computed tomography. Abdom Imaging 23(2):141–146
37. Godfrey EM, Addley HC, Shaw AS (2009) The use of computed tomography in the detection and characterization of large bowel obstruction. N Z Med J 122(1305):57–73
38. Horton KM, Abrams RA, Fishman EK (2000) Spiral CT of colon cancer: imaging features and role in management. RadioGraphics 20(2):419–430
39. Levsky JM, Den EI, DuBrow RA, Wolf EL, Rozenblit AM (2010) CT findings of sigmoid volvulus. AJR Am J Roentgenol 194(1):136–143
40. Hirao K, Kikawada M, Hanyu H, Iwamoto T (2006) Sigmoid volvulus showing "a whirl sign" on CT. InternMed 45(5):331–332
41. Horton KM, Corl FM, Fishman EK (2000) CT evaluation of the colon: inflammatory disease. RadioGraphics 20(2):399–418
42. Choi JS, Lim JS, Kim H et al (2008) Colonic pseudo obstruction: CT findings. AJR Am J Roentgenol 190(6):1521–1526
43. Nicolaou S, Kai B, Ho S, Su J, Ahamed K (2005) Imaging of acute small-bowel obstruction. AJR Am J Roentgenol 185(4):1036–1044
44. Rubesin SE, Gore RM (2008) Small bowel obstruction. In: Gore RM, Levine MS (eds) Textbook of gastrointestinal radiology, vol 1, 3rd edn. Saunders Elsevier, Philadelphia, PA, pp 871–899
45. Maglinte DD, Reyes BL, Harmon BH et al (1996) Reliability and role of film radiography and CT in the diagnosis of small bowel obstruction. AJR Am J Roentgenol 167(6):1451–1455
46. Furukawa A, Yamasaki M, Furuichi K et al (2001) Helical CT in the diagnosis of small bowel obstruction. RadioGraphics 21(2):341–355
47. Hayakawa K, Tanikake M, Yoshida S, Yamamoto A, Yamamoto E, Morimoto T (2013) CT findings of small bowel strangulation: the importance of contrast enhancement. Emerg Radiol 20(1):3–9
48. Barnett RE, Younga J, Harris B et al (2013) Accuracy of computed tomography in small bowel obstruction. Am Surg 79(6):641–643
49. Korenkov M, Paul A, Troidl H (1999) Color duplex sonography: diagnostic tool in the differentiation of inguinal hernias. J Ultrasound Med 18(8):565–568
50. Shadbolt CL, Heinze SB, Dietrich RB (2001) Imaging of groin masses: inguinal anatomy and pathologic conditions revisited. RadioGraphics 21:S261–S271
51. Aguirre DA, Santosa AC, Casola G, Sirlin CB (2005) Abdominal wall hernias: imaging features, complications, and diagnostic pitfalls at multi-detector row CT. RadioGraphics 25:1501–1520
52. Caoili EM, Paulson EK (2000) CT of small-bowel obstruction: another perspective using multiplanar reformations. AJR Am J Roentgenol 174:993–998
53. Boudiaf M, Soyer P, Terem C, Pelage JP, Maissiat E, Rymer R (2001) CT evaluation of small bowel obstruction. RadioGraphics 21:613–624
54. Yu CY, Lin CC, Yu JC, Liu CH, Shyu RY, Chen CY (2004) Strangulated transmesosigmoid hernia: CT diagnosis. Abdom Imaging 29:158–160
55. Crespi G, Giannetta E, Mariani F, Floris F, Pretolesi F, Marino P (2004) Imaging of early postoperative complications after polypropylene mesh repair of inguinal hernia. Radiol Med (Torino) 108:107–115
56. van den Berg JC, de Valois JC, Go PM, Rosenbusch G (1998) Groin hernia: can dynamic magnetic resonance imaging be of help? Eur Radiol 8:270–273
57. Becker CD, Mentha G, Terrier F (1998) Blunt abdominal trauma in adults: role of CT in the diagnosis and management of visceral injuries. Eur Radiol 8:553562
58. Soto JA, Anderson SW (2012) Multidetector CT of blunt abdominal trauma. Radiology 265(3)
59. Poletti PA, Wintermark M, Schnyer P, Becker CD (2002) Traumatic injuries: role of imaging in the management of the polytrauma victim. Eur Radiol 12:969–978
60. Shanmuganathan K, Mirvis SE (1998) CT scan evaluation of blunt hepatic trauma. Radiol Clin North Am 36:399–411

61. Moore EE, Cogbill TH, Jurkovich GJ, Shackford SR, Malangoni MA, Champion HR (1995) Organ injury scaling: spleen and liver (1994 revision). J Trauma 38(3):323–324
62. Mirvis SE, Shanmuganathan K, Erb R (1994) Diffuse small-bowel ischemia in hypotensive adults after blunt trauma (shock bowel): CT findings and clinical significance. AJR Am J Roentgenol 163(6):1375–1379
63. American Institute of Ultrasound in Medicine (2014) AIUM practice guideline for the performance of the focused assessment with sonography for trauma (FAST) examination. J Ultrasound Med 33(11):2047–2056
64. Furukawa A, Kanasaki S et al (2009) CT diagnosis of acute mesenteric ischemia from various ischemia. AJR Am J Roentgenol 192:408–416
65. Menke J (2010) Diagnostic accuracy of multidetector CT in acute mesenteric ischemia: systematic review and metanalysis. Radiology 256(1):93–101
66. Taourel P, Aufort S, Merigeaud S, Curros Doyon F, Devaux Hoquet M, Delabrousse E (2008) Imaging of ischemic colitis. Radiol Clin N Am 46:909–924
67. Wadman M, Block T, Ekberg O, Sky I, Elmstahl S, Acosta S (2010) Impact of MDCT with intravenous contrast on the survival in patients with acute superior mesenteric artery occlusion. Emerg Radiol 17(3):171–178
68. Yashura H (2005) Acute mesenteric ischemia: the challenge of gastroenterology. Surg Today 35:185–195
69. Kirkpatrick ID, Kroeker MA et al (2003) Biphasic CT with mesenteric CT angiography in the evaluation of acute mesenteric ischemia: initial experience. Radiology 229:91–98

Emergency Laparoscopy: The Nurse's Point of View 16

Monica Rolfo, Serena Langella, Valeria Esposito, Antonio Valenti, Angela Di Marco, and Alessandro Ferrero

16.1 Introduction

Laparoscopic surgery (LS) is increasingly used in the emergency setting [1]. It is of particular interest and efficacy for the diagnosis and treatment of acute conditions. In fact, emergency laparoscopy can be safely undertaken if there is an appropriate patient selection, the surgical team is adequately experienced, and there are sufficient resources to allow potentially more complex operations.

The advantages of LS are well established: better postoperative outcomes and pain management and significant reduction in the duration of hospital stay because of earlier recovery with decreasing of health and social costs [1].

The application of laparoscopy in emergency surgery involves several organization problems.

Firstly, surgeons should have large experience in laparoscopic techniques. Secondly, nurses should be trained in the management of surgical patients with acute diseases and all operators in the operating room (OR) must be confident with every technology and device required in LS.

Finally, the perioperative environment is multidimensional, dynamic, and composed of multidisciplinary teams. Moreover, providers of all specialties are facing with caring of patients with multiple risk factors in a complex condition. Even with a comprehensive knowledge of the most current strategies, the application of good communication skills within the surgical team remains a fundamental tool to achieve best practices. In this light, nurses contribute to the overall success

M. Rolfo, RN (✉)
Division of General and Oncology Surgery, Mauriziano "Umberto I" Hospital, Turin, Italy

Italian College of Nurses (IPASVI), Turin, Italy
e-mail: mrolfo@mauriziano.it

S. Langella, MD •V. Esposito, RN • A. Valenti, RN • A. Di Marco, RN • A. Ferrero, MD
Division of General and Oncology Surgery, Mauriziano "Umberto I" Hospital, Turin, Italy

F. Agresta et al. (eds.), *Emergency Laparoscopy*,
DOI 10.1007/978-3-319-29620-3_16

of the multidisciplinary management assuring a "communication bridge" among providers, patients, and caregivers.

It is well known that nurses play an important role in providing preoperative education, perioperative care, and postoperative evaluation [2]. Moreover, postoperative course is not only influenced by physiologic outcomes of disease but also addresses to the biopsychosocial responses on the health-illness continuum that are necessary to improve the quality of life even in emergent surgery.

In recent years, nursing responsibilities for decision-making in patients care have been expanded [3, 4]. The evolution of nursing is related to certain levels of education and practice to fill the important roles within the multi-professional team in the surgical area. In this light, the nurse leader should create learning opportunities and promote educational programs in order to improve the nurse practice in specialized surgical teams.

16.2 Preoperative Phase

16.2.1 Physical Preparation: Technical Skills

Before surgical interventions there are different preoperative procedures and activities in order to prepare the patient and his family for surgery. In case of emergent surgery this act must be done quickly because of acute condition.

Patient assessment and the definition of a care plan are designed to meet the physical, psychological, educational, social, and cultural needs. These aspects are the cornerstone of nursing activity. Another key point is the collaboration with the members of the surgical team in order to identify the best treatment for each case, according to clinical evidences and guidelines [5], and to define the future allocation of the patient in areas with different levels of intensity in the postoperative care (Fig. 16.1).

In the emergency setting, nurse should give importance to the areas of risk with major clinical implications [6]. Different scales of risk assessment have been reported [7]. These scales allow the use of rapid response to perform appropriate postoperative cares with a multidisciplinary approach.

Preoperative nurse management is targeted mainly to prevent infections and reduce the risk of perioperative complications. Based on the results obtained in reducing catheter correlate infections and pneumonia in patients artificially ventilated, the "care bundles" have been introduced. The concept of a care bundle was developed from evidence documenting that a structured approach performing 3–5 evidence-based collective interventions could improve patients' outcomes [8].

The care bundle approach is common to many guidelines for the prevention of surgical site infection (SSI). SSI is a well-known complication of general surgery occurring in about 3 % of all surgical procedures and in up to 20 % of patients undergoing emergency intra-abdominal procedures [9]. SSI adversely affects patient outcomes and healthcare costs. In a recent study, overall SSI rate was 4.09 % and colorectal surgery was associated with the highest SSI rate (9.43 %), in this setting was identified as an independent predictor [10]. Concerning the emergency LS, a mini-invasive approach resulted in a protective factor for SSI [11].

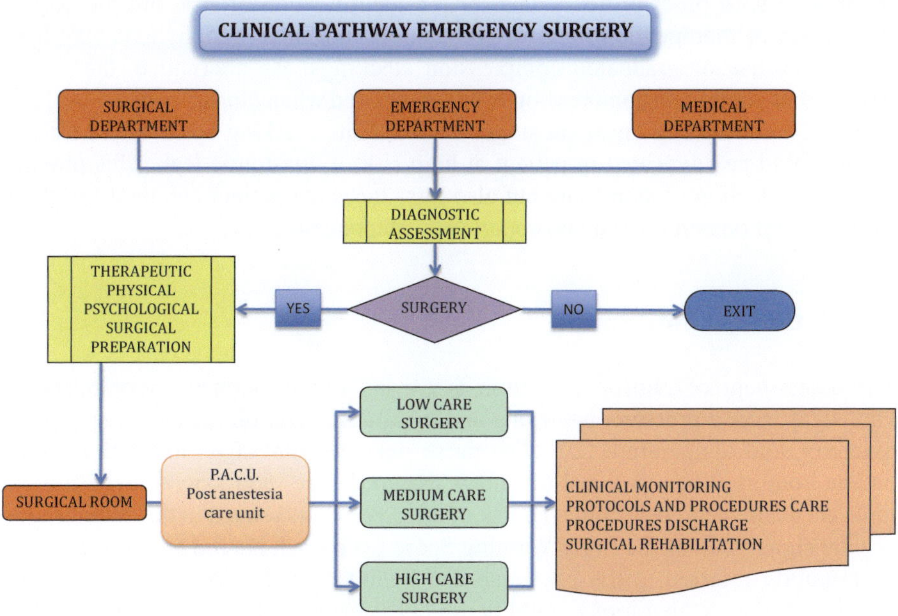

Fig. 16.1 Graphic representation of the clinical pathway in emergency surgery

A care bundle approach to SSI includes methods for preoperative removal of hair (when appropriate), rational antibiotic prophylaxis, avoidance of perioperative hypothermia, management of perioperative blood glucose, and effective skin preparation [12].

The skin of the surgical site must appear clean [13] and there is the possibility that the patient should be helped to meet the need for hygiene and showering without antiseptic. In particular, attention should be given to the cleanness of umbilical area. In fact, after LS it is described the infection of the umbilical site access with different rates depending on the type of intervention [15].

Regarding hair removal, the current evidences are in favor of trichotomy only in cases where the hairs in the area of incision could affect the operation [16]. Hairs should be removed with an electric shaver suitable for the purpose or with depilatory creams while the use of hand razor remains strongly discouraged. There is no specific report on the impact of trichotomy in emergency LS, but we could speculate that a possible conversion to laparotomy may justify the hair removal of the entire abdominal area. Removing jewelry, prosthesis for dentures, hearing and eye, and nail polish is always recommended.

At admission, patients should be evaluated for the risk of thromboembolism through appropriate flow chart. Operative time, prolonged pneumoperitoneum, and complexity of the surgical procedure and the surgical site are some of the risk factors to be considered in addition to the individual patient risks [17]. The nurse must collaborate with other professionals for the identification of risk and the correct application of therapeutic program. The embolic thrombus prophylaxis may have to pair the use of graduated compression stockings. As alternative, the use of intermittent pneumatic compression is recommended when clinically indicated [18].

Finally, concerning intestinal surgery, stomal site marking by a wound ostomy nurse should be advocated in patient at high risk of anastomic leak. This practice improves selection of stoma site but also introduces the patient and their family to stoma education empowering postoperative independence [19].

16.2.2 Clinical Monitoring

The assessment of clinical condition is carried out through the monitoring of vital signs: blood pressure, heart rate and breathing, pain, blood sugar level, pulse oximetry, and temperature [20]. The nurse puts the vital signs in relation to the patient comorbidities, surgical diagnosis assumed, age, and symptoms. Different tools are available to determine the risk of adverse events related to the deterioration of vital signs, such as the Early Warning Score [21]. Each altered parameter should be promptly referred to the physician and included in the documentation of the patient. This way, alterations could be quickly corrected improving postoperative outcomes. In particular, it is strongly recommended to obtain an optimal glycemic control since preoperative period [22] and a rapid correction of dehydration, especially in the elderly [23]. The evaluation of vital signs must be repeated at regular intervals until the transfer to the operating room.

Depending on the clinical condition, it could be necessary to place a nasogastric tube, urinary catheter, and to find one or more venous access (peripheral or central) before surgery.

The condition of fasting does not ever preclude the intake of preoperative oral therapy. This aspect is crucial to prevent possible postoperative consequences in particular in case of cardiac medications [24].

Patients under age or mental deficiency should always be accompanied by a caregiver. Before the transfer to the operating room (OR), nurse should verify that all these elements of the path are correct using a checklist [25]. When required by critical clinical conditions, patient is accompanied to the OR by nurse and/or doctor. Finally, dignity, comfort, and privacy of the patient should always be respected at all times and in every transfer of operational setting.

16.3 Operative Phase

The OR staff members participate in the intraoperative and postoperative stages of the multimodal approach to emergency LS. The OR is a complex reality that includes many operators with different roles and specialties often involved in critical situation. Furthermore, all providers must be confident with the highly available technologies. In fact, the team experience is proven to have a beneficial impact on overall surgery time [25]. In particular, the nursing team plays a highly important role in the success and speed of emergency LS.

The main objective of the nurse who accepts the patient in the OR is to understand the psychological state [26]. This way, an appropriate counseling offers the possibility to humanize the environment. During the conversation, nurses provide to minimize every source of stress, worry, and anxiety. This approach could be restricted in case of emergent surgery because of critical acute conditions compromising the conscious state.

Upon arrival to the OR, the circulating nurse will interview and identify the patient. At least two patient identifiers are used, and they should check medical record number, name, and date of birth. When appropriate, it is imperative for the patient to confirm the correct laterality (right or left side) of the injured organ. As suggested by others, the operative site could be marked while the patient is awake and alert and before sedative medication is administered.

After the patient is secured to the OR table with a safety belt, antithrombotic stockings and knee- or thigh-high sequential compression devices are placed on the lower extremities, to prevent venous stasis and reduce the risk of deep vein thrombosis and pulmonary embolism.

An indwelling urinary drainage catheter is inserted by either the circulating nurse or surgeon to decompress the bladder. When required, prophylactic intravenous antibiotics should be administered within 60 min from the initial skin incision. After the induction of general anesthesia, the patient is endotracheally intubated and an orogastric tube is placed to decompress the stomach. An arterial pressure line may be established for hemodynamic monitoring.

It has been demonstrated that a surgical safety checklist may reduce morbidity and mortality [27]. Haynes BN and colleagues collected data from a large prospective database on clinical processes and outcomes after noncardiac surgery. The rate of death was 1.5 % before the checklist was introduced and decreased to 0.8 % afterward ($P = 0.003$). Similarly, inpatient complications occurred in 11.0 % of patients at baseline and in 7.0 % after introduction of the checklist ($P < 0.001$) [28].

The main steps of surgical check list are conducted by nurse, anesthetist, and surgeon through three phases: Sign IN (before induction of anesthesia), Time OUT (before skin incision), and Sign OUT (before patient leave OR) according to WHO recommendations [29].

OR usually used for LS are often not designed for this purpose. Hence, all instrumental devices (screen, light, sources, electrocoagulators, insufflator) are located on dedicated trays. Because all these instruments take space, it is necessary to have room appositely prepared for this type of surgery, especially in emergency. Moreover, it is necessary to know highly technical details of sterilization methodology for all devices, which require more attention than conventional surgical instruments.

In this context, it appears to be fundamental a strict cooperation among all providers of surgical team. In order to facilitate the correct development of surgical procedures it is mandatory to adopt standardized protocols and checklists concerning preparation of OR, anesthetic machine, surgical bed, and laparoscopic column [30].

For the OR nurses, proper positioning is one of the key responsibilities to protect the safety and skin integrity of the patient under anesthesia. As reported [31], positioning of the patient was found to be particularly difficult for the prone (43.8 %), lithotomy (53.4 %), and lateral (65.5 %) positions. Moreover, lack of positioning competences and equipment for arm support, standardized equipment for leg support, and standard sizes of OR beds seemed to complicate positioning.

During LS, nurse must give attention to the control of pneumoperitoneum. It is well known that CO_2 insufflation could cause complications related to increased abdominal pressure and CO_2 retention. In order to avoid such complications, pressure limit of insufflator is 12 cm H_2O. Moreover, flow rate of CO_2 insufflation must be modulated during procedure starting slow at the beginning of operation and than progressively augmented [32].

An experienced OR nurse knows that any laparoscopic emergent procedure has the potential open conversion due to bleeding, unanticipated organ injury, or failure to progress as in the case of excessive intra-abdominal adhesions. Appropriate instrumentations and supplies necessary for laparotomy should be readily available in the room, but may be kept unopened and uncounted unless their use is required. During the procedure, the OR nurse must be vigilant to potential intraoperative complications. Laparoscopic instruments are placed on a mayo stand with the handles facing the surgeon to expedite transfer to the surgeon hands. A variety of laparoscopic thermal energy devices are also available. These devices have been shown to significantly decrease blood loss and operative time. Furthermore, hemostatic agents must be readily available to the surgical team should bleeding occur. Experienced circulating nurses can often anticipate the surgeon needs as they closely follow the steps of the procedure. During the procedure, the circulating nurse also monitors the level of the CO_2 tank and has reserve tanks available.

At the end of operation, the nurse assesses the patient's skin and temperature. The patient is then transported to the postanesthesia care unit (PACU). In the PACU, nurses play a key role in patient pain management and satisfaction. In fact, even at the early postoperative stage, nurses can directly affect the reduction of postoperative infections and ileus and facilitate the patient's safe and timely hospital stay. Interestingly, it has been reported [33] that the length of stay in the PACU correlates with pain intensity, nausea, and vomiting on arrival.

16.4 Postoperative Phase: From Hospitality to Discharge

16.4.1 Acceptance from Operating Room: Clinical Monitoring

Patients who have undergone emergency surgery are at risk for poor outcomes comparing to elective surgery [34]. The principal objectives of the immediate postoperative care are prevention of number and severity of complications [35] and restoring the physiological balance. Early detection and timely management of complications may reduce morbidity and mortality. After surgery, nurse first detects and evaluates signs and symptoms of the three major vital systems (nervous, respiratory, and cardiovascular). Afterward, the accommodation and the comfort of the patient are ensured. At this point, nurse starts recognition, measurement, and recording of clinical parameters: blood pressure, heart and respiratory rate, oximetry, glycemic index, pain, diuresis, characteristics and quantity of surgical drains (if placed), level of consciousness, body temperature, surgical wound, the presence of medical devices, and any symptoms reported by the patient. After LS particular importance covers the control of the presence of subcutaneous emphysema [36]. It is recommended to empty the urinary catheter and drains for precise postoperative monitoring. The nurse must verify the clinical documentation to check the surgical procedure and the type of anesthesia performed, any intraoperative problems, medications used, medical history and preoperative interventions performed, and not least the therapeutic prescriptions to be administered. All elements collected must lead the nurse to plan the subsequent appropriate care. Vital signs and clinical parameters of interest should be monitored every 1–2 h for at least the first 8 h. Moreover, nurse must continually check that the connections of the drainage pipes are correct and securely connected and the drains are working properly identifying significant bleeding or any appearance suggestive of complications (presence of bile, intestinal fluid, pus, urine air).

Fundamental to the success of any model of team-based care is the skill, reliability, and expertise of the individual members that comprise the team, including nurses. Additionally, the definition of a standard of care and the adoption of shared protocols and therapeutic procedures (defined by surgical team) may allow rapid intervention for the management of major alterations and most common postoperative symptoms (hypertensive crisis, hyperthermia, nausea or vomiting, pain, hyperglycemia). The postoperative delirium is one of the most common adverse events after emergency surgery especially in the elderly [37].The surgical approach (laparoscopic versus open) does not seem to influence this condition. Nevertheless, in the emergency setting nurses are frequently facing with patients affected by cognitive dysfunction. In this regard, the use of screening tools, such as The Nursing Delirium Screening Scale [38], lead to early recognition. This way, the interventions required are readily performed reducing the risk of injury and accelerating the return to normality.

16.4.2 Surgical Rehabilitation

After the initial 24 h, vital signs can be monitored every 4–8 h if the patient is stable. The incision and dressing should be monitored for the amount of drainage and signs of infection. The surgeon may order a dressing change during the first postoperative day; this should be done using sterile technique.

The patient should be monitored for any evidence of potential complications, such as leg edema, redness and pain (deep vein thrombosis), shortness of breath (bronchopneumonia and pulmonary embolism), dehiscence and infection of the incision, or ileus (intestinal obstruction), heart problems. The surgeon should be notified immediately if any of these occurs.

Particularly, in patients at higher risk of complication, rehabilitation exercises to prevent respiratory and thromboembolic complications should start early. When appropriate, preoperative education and maintaining previous levels of self-sufficiency increase the effectiveness of rehabilitative interventions [39]. The main objective of prevention is early mobilization from the bed [40]. If the patient is conscious, cooperative, and clinically stable mobilization can occur after only few hours after surgery, even after complex procedures [41]. Patients with limited mobility must be mobilized passively alternating on both sides several times a day, even for the prevention of pressure lesions, which is one of the main areas for action for nurses in this phase [42]. LS, even if performed in emergency, allows a rapid return to the levels of self-sufficiency when postoperative rehabilitation is rapid and constant [43]. Historically, the assumption of liquids and foods happens to the restarting of the intestinal functionality; nevertheless, this attitude was questioned by early rehabilitation programs in surgery having highlighted the absence of the benefit of fasting in various postoperative surgical procedures [41]. Few data are available about this aspect in emergency surgery, but a similar strategy should probably be chosen especially for minor procedures [44].

16.4.3 Therapeutic Education: The Role of the Nurse

The preoperative education is an important aspect of preparation for many surgical procedures. In particular, it has positive effects on fear [45] and anxiety [46] even prior to emergency surgery [47]. The contents of preoperative education may vary in different contexts, but generally include a presentation on the procedures and perioperative care, with respect to potential complications, management of the pain and other symptoms, device management, the mobilization, and respiration [48]. In the emergency setting, clinical conditions and degree of urgency may not enable a structured educational intervention. As previously reported [49], giving information just before surgery in urgency increases stress in anxious patients. In fact, education is best given at hospital admission. Nevertheless, therapeutic education on postoperative process is a high priority for patients and family members anticipating temporary changing needs as a result of the surgery. This stage of education usually happens preoperatively, preparing timely the patients at discharge. This way, the discharge is not an isolated event, but it becomes part of a process which begins at admission and actively involves patients and family during hospitalization [50].

However, for patients who underwent emergency surgery all the steps of this intervention are accomplished during the postoperative course.

A well-structured educational plan is based on the quality of given information, to reassure patients that initial fears and anxieties are a normal part of the healing process. It has been demonstrated that this approach could positively affect experience of postoperative pain, decrease preoperative state of anxiety, and promote exercise to prevent postoperative complications [51].

After surgery, nurse starts giving practical daily information as to the care of the surgical wound, both after laparoscopic and open surgery, diet, return to work, limits on activities, bowel movements, management of an eventual therapeutic regimen, and pain control. Before the discharge, other useful information should be given concerning the follow-up, such as the date, time, and location of their visits [52]. The best results are obtained associating oral information with other aids such as booklets or other information instrument. The delivery of written material has the advantage of ensuring a standardization of the educational process reducing the risk of the variability information based on different communication skills, knowledge, and resources of nurses.

The multidisciplinary team (surgeons, anesthetists, nurses, nutritionists, dietitians, and respiratory therapists) collaborates in the educational process. In this scenario, the role of nurse is essential giving proper planning instructions and educating patient and family.

16.4.4 Pain Management

The laparoscopic approach often results in lesser postoperative pain, shorter analgesia requirement, and earlier recovery. Nevertheless, in some cases early pain after laparoscopy can be comparable or even more severe than after open surgery. Pain intensity is maximal during the first postoperative hours and some patients need opioid analgesics to control it. Laparoscopy implicates insufflation of the abdominal cavity with carbon dioxide, and the remaining gas after pneumoperitoneum is one of the basics for postoperative pain, often described in the shoulder area and that it may persist for up to 72 h. However, pain after laparoscopic surgery is derived from multiple origins: nociceptive, incisional, and visceral pain; inflammatory pain in response to tissue trauma; and neuropathic pain in association with distension-induced neuropraxia. For this reason, a multimodal pain management protocol should be preferred. Moreover, persistent pain after laparoscopic surgery has also been reported. This condition could be partially explained by the influence of sociocultural and individual factors. Thus, these aspects should also be considered. Patient counseling on pain and pain management is important because it may increase the compliance and adherence to the selected analgesic treatments. Moreover, reaching patients early, even before surgery, leads to influence psychological variables such as presurgical anxiety. In fact, the impact of psychological intervention on the prevention of persistent pain is yet to be demonstrated, but this approach seems to be promising in terms of outcomes in the acute postsurgical time period in combination with multimodal preventive analgesia [53]. As previously reported by Fernandez et al., an acceptance-based psychological intervention along with the usual presurgical protocol for a laparoscopic cholecystectomy will produce healthier reactions to postsurgical pain and will reduce anxiety, duration of postsurgical hospitalization, and demand of analgesics. Unfortunately, data on the management of pain after laparoscopic emergency surgery are lacking. In this subset of patients, nurse can provide counseling mainly in the postoperative period [54]. There are multiple measures available to assess pain in adults. Each measure has its own strengths and weaknesses. Both the Visual Analog Scale (VAS) for Pain and the Numeric Rating Scale (NRS) for Pain are unidimensional single-item scales that provide an estimate of patients' pain intensity [55]. They are easy to administer, complete, and score. In particular, the pain NRS may be preferred for the patient care because of simpler scoring and its ability to be administered both verbally and in writing. Furthermore, by using specific pain assessment methods adapted for sensory and cognitive impairment, and language difficulties, pain can be managed effectively for most patients. During the postoperative course, nurses could apply strategies to involve patients in pain decision-making, which include educating patients to inform nurses when analgesia is required, offering patients' choices between analgesia, and evaluating the effectiveness of the treatments. Moreover, a collaborative relationship between nurses and clinicians improves communication to address complex pain management decisions. Finally, postoperative management requires substantial communication and collaboration between all members of the healthcare team to be successful.

In conclusion, the laparoscopic approach to emergency surgery is gaining widespread agreement. Nowadays, a multidisciplinary approach is mandatory for the successful management of patients who underwent emergency LS. The perioperative nursing in this setting is constantly changing and it requires knowledge, technical skills, leadership, and excellent communication abilities. In order to respond to the changing needs of the surgical patient, the nurse must constantly add knowledge and skills. These objectives could be accomplished through self-education practices and participating in educational opportunities.

References

1. Harji DP, Griffiths B, Burke D et al (2014) Systematic review of emergency laparoscopic colorectal resection. Br J Surg 101(1):e126–e133
2. Stobinski JX (2008) Perioperative nursing competency. AORN J 88(3):417–418, 421–436
3. Decreto Ministeriale 14 settembre 1994, n°739, GU 9 gennaio 1995 n°6: "Regolamento concernente l'individuazione della figura e del relativo profilo professionale dell'infermiere"
4. Legge 10 agosto 2000, n°251 GU 6 settembre 2000 n° 208: "Disciplina delle professioni infermieristiche, tecniche, della riabilitazione, della prevenzione nonché della professione ostetrica"
5. Møller TP, Münter KH, Østergaard D et al (2015) Exploring challenges and solutions in the preparation of surgical patients. Dan Med J 62:A5141
6. Visser A, Geboers B, Gouma DJ et al (2015) Predictors of surgical complications: a systematic review. Surgery 158(1):58–65
7. Carpenter CR, Shelton E, Fowler S et al (2015) Risk factors and screening instruments to predict adverse outcomes for undifferentiated older emergency department patients: a systematic review and meta-analysis. Acad Emerg Med 22(1):1–21
8. Tanner J, Padley W, Assadian O et al (2015) Do surgical care bundles reduce the risk of surgical site infection in patients undergoing colorectal surgery? A systematic review and cohort meta-analysis of 8,515 patients. Surgery 158(1):66–77

9. Barie PS (2002) Surgical site infections: epidemiology and prevention. Surg Infect (Larchmt) 3(Suppl 1):S9–S21
10. Isik O, Kaya E, Dundar HZ, Sarkut P (2015) Surgical site infection: re-assessment of the risk factors. Chirurgia (Bucur) 110(5):457–461
11. Hennessey DB, Burke JP, Ni-Dhonochu T et al (2016) Risk factors for surgical site infection following colorectal resection: a multi-institutional study. Int J Colorectal Dis 31(2):267–271
12. Leaper DJ, Tanner J, Kiernan M et al (2015) Surgical site infection: poor compliance with guidelines and care bundles. Int Wound J 12(3):357–362
13. Tanner J, Norrie P, Melen K (2011) Preoperative hair removal to reduce surgical site infection. Cochrane Database Syst Rev (11):CD004122
14. Webster J, Osborne S. (2015) Preoperative bathing or showering with skin antiseptics to prevent surgical site infection. Cochrane Database Syst Rev (1):CD004985
15. Sasmal PK et al (2015) Port site infection in laparoscopic surgery: a review of its management. World J Clin Cases 3(10):864–871
16. Lefebvre A, Saliou P, Lucet JC et al (2015) French study group for the preoperative prevention of surgical site infections. Preoperative hair removal and surgical site infections: network meta-analysis of randomized controlled trials. J Hosp Infect 91(2):100–108
17. Linee guida per la profilassi del tromboembolismo venoso nei pazienti ospedalizzati. SNLG. Aggiornamento anno 2015
18. Pavon JM, Adam SS, Razouki ZA et al (2016) Effectiveness of intermittent pneumatic compression devices for venous thromboembolism prophylaxis in high-risk surgical patients: a systematic review. J Arthroplasty 31(2):524–532
19. Baykara ZG et al (2014) A multicenter, retrospective study to evaluate the effect of preoperative stoma site marking on stomal and peristomal complications. Ostomy Wound Manag 60(5):16–26
20. Liddle C (2012) Preparing patients to undergo surgery. Nurs Times 108(48):12–13
21. Kyriacos U, Jelsma J, Jordan S (2011) Monitoring vital signs using early warning scoring systems: a review of the literature. J Nurs Manag 19(3):311–330
22. Schricker T, Lattermann R (2015) Perioperative catabolism. Can J Anaesth 62(2):182–193
23. Hooper L et al (2015) Clinical symptoms, signs and tests for identification of impending and current water-loss dehydration in older people. Cochrane Database Syst Rev 4, CD009647
24. Kluger MT, Gale S, Plummer JL et al (1991) Peri-operative drug prescribing pattern and manufacturers' guidelines. An audit. Anaesthesia 46(6):456–459
25. WHO (2009) WHO Guidelines for Safe Surgery 2009: Safe surgery saves lives. World Health Organization, Geneva
26. Malley A, Kenner C, Kim T et al (2015) The role of the nurse and the preoperative assessment in patient transitions. AORN J 102(2):181.e1–181.e9
27. Lingard L, Regehr G, Orser B et al (2008) Evaluation of a preoperative checklist and team briefing among surgeons, nurse, and anesthesiologists to reduce failures in communication. Arch Surg 143:12–18
28. Haynes AB, Weiser TG, Berry WR et al (2009) A surgical safety checklist to reduce morbidity and mortality in a global population. N Engl J Med 360(5):491–499
29. World Health Organization Surgical Safety Checklist, 1st edn. http://www.who.int/patientsafety/safesurgery/tools_resources/SSSL_Checklist_finalJun08.pdf ?ua=1. Accessed 30 Oct 2015
30. Lane-Fall MB et al (2015) The challenge of studying and improving perioperative teamwork, and yes, another checklist. Anesth Analg 121(4):852–853
31. Agostini J, Goasguen N, Mosnier H (2010) Patient positioning in laparoscopic surgery: tricks and tips. J Visc Surg 147(4):e227–e232
32. Kyle EB, Maheux-Lacroix S, Boutin A et al (2015) Complications of low compared to standard pneumoperitoneum pressures in laparoscopic surgery for benign gynecologic pathology: a systematic review protocol. Syst Rev 4:96
33. Ganter M, Blumenthal S, Dubendorfer S et al (2014) The length of stay in the post-anaesthesia care unit correlates whith pain intensity, nausea and vomiting on arrival. Perioper Med (Lond) 3(1):10

34. Ingraham AM, Cohen ME, Bilimoria KY et al (2010) Comparison of 30-day outcomes after emergency general surgery procedures: potential for targeted improvement. Surgery 148(2):217–238
35. Akinbami F, Askari R, Steinberg J et al (2011) Factors affecting morbidity in emergency general surgery. Am J Surg 201(4):456–462
36. Ott DE (2014) Subcutaneous emphysema–beyond the pneumoperitoneum. JSLS 18(1):1–7
37. De Castro SM, Ünlü Ç, Tuynman JB et al (2014) Incidence and risk factors of delirium in the elderly general surgical patient. Am J Surg 208(1):26–32
38. Gaudreau JD, Gagnon P, Harel F et al (2005) Fast, systematic, and continuous delirium assessment in hospitalized patients: the nursing delirium screening scale. J Pain Symptom Manage 29(4):368–375
39. Katsura M, Kuriyama A, Takeshima T et al (2015) Preoperative inspiratory muscle training for postoperative pulmonary complications in adults undergoing cardiac and major abdominal surgery. Cochrane Database Syst Rev 10, CD010356
40. Scottish Intercollegiate Guidelines Network (SIGN) (2010) Prevention and management of venous thromboembolism. Edinburgh: SIGN. (SIGN publication no. 122). Available from http://www.sign.ac.uk. Accessed 10 Dec 2010
41. Gustafsson UO et al (2012) Enhanced Recovery After Surgery Society. Guidelines for perioperative care in elective colonic surgery: Enhanced Recovery After Surgery (ERAS®) Society recommendations. Clin Nutr 31(6):783–800
42. Lupear SK, Overstreet M, Krau SD (2015) Perioperative nurses' knowledge of indicators for pressure ulcer development in the surgical patient population. Nurs Clin North Am 50(2):411–435
43. Rockall TA, Demartines N (2014) Laparoscopy in the era of enhanced recovery. Best Pract Res Clin Gastroenterol 28(1):133–142
44. Cestonaro T, Madalozzo Schieferdecker ME, Thieme RD et al (2014) The reality of the surgical fasting time in the era of the ERAS protocol. Nutr Hosp 29(2):437–443
45. Hathaway D (1986) Effect of preoperative instruction on postoperative outcomes: a meta-analysis. Nurs Res 35:269–275
46. Manataki A, Arnaoutoglou E, Papadopoulos G (2013) Patient's anxiety and fear of anesthesia: effect of education, and previous experience of anesthesia. A survey of 400 patients. J Anesth 27(1):104–108
47. Karanci AN, Dirik G (2003) Predictors of pre- and postoperative anxiety in emergency surgery patients. J Psychosom Res 55(4):363–369
48. Louw A, Diener I, Butler DS et al (2013) Preoperative education addressing postoperative pain in total joint arthroplasty: review of content and educational delivery methods. Physiother Theory Pract 29(3):175–194
49. Grieve RJ (2002) Day surgery preoperative anxiety reduction and coping strategies. Br J Nurs 11(10):647–678
50. White J, Dixon S (2015) Nurse led Patient Education Programme for patients undergoing a lung resection for primary lung cancer. J Thorac Dis 7(Suppl):2
51. Stern C, Lockwood C (2005) Knowledge retention from preoperative patient information. Int J Evid Based Healthc 3(3):45–63
52. Lithner M, Zilling T (1999) Pre- and postoperative information needs. Department of Surgery, Lund University Hospital, Lund, Sweden
53. Sjovall S, Kokki M, Kokki H (2015) Laparoscopic surgery: a narrative review of pharmacotherapy in pain management. Drugs 75:1867–1889
54. Fernandez MD, Luciano C, Valdivia-Solas S (2012) Impact of acceptance based nursing intervention on postsurgical recovery: preliminary findings. Span J Psychol 15(3):1361–1370
55. Hawker GA, Mian S, Kendzerska T et al (2011) Measures of adult pain. Arthritis Care Res 63(S11):S240–S252

Emergency Laparoscopy in the Elderly

17

From the Evidence to the Philosophy

Gian Luca Baiocchi, Luca Arru, Federico Gheza, Carlo Bergamini, Gabriele Anania, Fabio Cesare Campanile, Mauro Zago, Nazario Portolani, and Ferdinando Agresta

17.1 Introduction

The increasing age of the population is an ineluctable phenomenon, observed both in rich and emerging countries [1]. It is believed that the number of people older than 65 will be higher than those of children under 5 within a few years [2]. The number of octogenarians has risen by more than 50 % over the last 15 years [3]. People aged 85 and older will increase from 2.8 % in 2011 to 7.8 % in 2050, with an average life expectancy of 85.3 years for males and 90.5 years for females [1], with obvious implications, both for the health policies and from a clinical standpoint.

G.L. Baiocchi (✉) • F. Gheza • N. Portolani
Surgical Clinic, Department of Clinical and Experimental Sciences, University of Brescia, Via Cicognini, 6, 25127 Brescia, Italy
e-mail: gianluca.baiocchi@unibs.it

L. Arru
Service de Chirurgie Générale et Mini-Invasive, Centre Hospitalier de Luxembourg, Luxembourg City, Luxembourg, UK

C. Bergamini
SOD Chirurgia Generale 1, d'Urgenza e Mini-invasiva – AOU Careggi, Firenze, Italy

G. Anania
Department of Morfology, Surgery and Experimental Medicine, School of Medicine, University of Ferrara, Ferrara, Italy

F.C. Campanile
General Surgery Department, Ospedale Andosilla, Civita Castellana, VT, Italy

M. Zago
General Surgery Department, Minimally Invasive Surgery Unit, Policlinico San Pietro, Ponte San, Pietro, BG, Italy

F. Agresta
Department of General Surgery, Azienda ULSS19 del Veneto, Adria (RO), Italy

F. Agresta et al. (eds.), *Emergency Laparoscopy*,
DOI 10.1007/978-3-319-29620-3_17

Healthcare needs increase with age both in the elective and emergency setting [4]. However, while in the former the decision-making process can result from a comprehensive assessment, shared with the patients and their family, the urgency-emergency setting does not allow such a peaceful, quiet, and "settled" evaluation [5, 6]. The surgeon who deals with emergency surgery needs proper tools to quickly take the right decisions, based on solid data about the chances of success, and about the expectations of life after a successful procedure [7].

The elderly patient specificities heavily influence the diagnostic and therapeutic pathway. The diagnostic process is often more difficult and sometimes totally inconclusive, because of communication difficulties and peculiar biochemical and radiographic changes [8]. A retrospective Mayo Clinic analysis on 231 elderly patients with abdominal pain shows that temperature, physical examination, and basic blood tests have limited sensitivity in discriminating the surgical cases [9]. Another recent article reports that 75 % of elderly patients evaluated in the emergency room for abdominal pain were discharged with a final diagnosis of NSAP (nonspecific abdominal pain) [10]. In addition, the mortality is high, up to 44 % (for the most part due to abdominal and pulmonary septic complications) in a study that included only patients more than 80 years old [11]. In the series published by Arenal et al., mortality was 7 %, 8 %, and 9 % for appendectomy, cholecystectomy, and parietal surgery [3].

In this context, the use of minimally invasive surgical techniques is characterized by extreme uncertainty. While on one side a pragmatic approach considers as a good surgical practice a laparotomy for quick and essential damage control, leaving aside any aesthetic consideration; on the other side, it is likely that the principles of minimally invasive procedures would find especially in frail patients a very good indication. The emergency surgeon must quickly decide if and how to operate an elderly patient, and needs to know the clinical data about benefits and limitations of a minimally invasive approach.

This chapter aims to provide the emergency surgeon with the bibliographic elements on which to base its decisions [12], with specific reference to the use of the laparoscopic approach in urgent abdominal diseases in the elderly and frail patients (anyway, the simple chronological age is a parameter by itself inadequate to define a patient at increased risk; thus, in this chapter the term "old/frail" will be used).

The following questions are answered:

- *Who's the old/frail patient?*
- *What are the clinical pictures of potential emergency abdominal surgery in old patients? When is it right not to operate an old/frail patient despite life-threatening condition?*
- *Should a minimally invasive approach be a priori ruled out in old/frail patients?*
- *May a minimally invasive approach be beneficial in old/frail patients?*
- *What are the essential conditions to approach acute abdomen in old/frail patients by minimally invasive surgery?*
- *Should the indication for laparotomy conversion be different in old/frail patients?*

- *What are the acute abdominal diseases potentially treatable by laparoscopy in old/frail patients?*
- *Outcomes analysis*

17.2 Who Is the Old Patient?

Though it is now accepted that the chronological age determines the clinical choices less than the so-called biological age, it is possible to identify some demographic cutoff and group patients into homogeneous risk classes. In particular, it is defined "old-young" a patient aged 70–80, "old" a patient aged 80–90, and "old-old" a patient over the age of 90 years. From a medical perspective, however, the most relevant definition for clinical choices is that of "frail" patients. It is defined by this way: a clinical situation that predisposes to increased morbidity and mortality, assessed over some parameters that can be easily determined such as the speed of walking, the level of physical activity, and cognitive capacity [13, 14]. There are no clinical scores validated for frail patients with acute abdominal disease to be treated surgically. However, it may be useful to take into account some other scores, initially designed for different clinical settings [15, 16]. This score takes into account the following parameters: anorexia, weight loss, BMI, motility, neuropsychological problems (dementia, depression), number of daily medications, chronological age, and comparison with peers.

17.3 What Are the Clinical Pictures of Potential Emergency Abdominal Surgery in Frail Patients?

At least one-fourth of the patients with acute abdomen are more than 50 years [17]. In this group of patients, the diagnostic path is often aggressive and is often completed with a CT scan [18]. CT scan is generally characterized by a good ability to identify the source of the problem. Several retrospective papers have investigated the incidence of abdominal diseases requiring urgent surgical treatment in elderly patients. In principle, 40–50 % of cases are obstructive syndromes, 30–40 % peritonitis, 5 % visceral ischemia, and 10 % hemorrhagic issues. In particular, inguinal hernia and colorectal cancer are the most frequent causes of obstruction; perforated acute diverticulitis and acute cholecystitis are the most frequent causes of peritonitis, while acute appendicitis is less frequent. It must also be taken into account that in the abovementioned retrospective Spanish series, 53 % of cholecystitis and 44 % of appendicitis were gangrenous [3]. Acute appendicitis is characterized by delay in treatment, high perforation rate, and unfavorable outcome [19]. Colorectal obstructions represent a significant cause of morbidity and mortality: a retrospective study in a tertiary referral university center included 292 patients operated on in the period 2000–2006. The overall mortality was 15 % and morbidity was 35 % [20]. Conversely, the incidence of small bowel obstruction does not seem to be age dependent. Finally, trauma requiring surgery is generally related to a low-speed impact (fall in the bathroom or in the garden), while traffic accidents are rare [3]. Two studies, retrospectively targeting patients >80 and >90 years old, confirm that incarcerated hernias, colorectal cancer, and peritonitis from perforated diverticulitis or gangrenous cholecystitis are the leading causes of surgery in elderly patients [11, 21]. In another recent retrospective study including 456 patients older than 65 years who underwent emergency surgery between 2006 and 2009 in Finland, 32 %, 13 %, 11 %, and 11 %, respectively, had acute cholecystitis, incarcerated hernia, colorectal cancer, and acute appendicitis [22].

17.4 When Is It Right Not to Operate a Frail Patient Despite Life-Threatening Condition?

Answering to this question is extremely complex, and there are few scientific studies that have attempted to justify the answer on strong clinical data [2]. In the decision, clinical issues (chance of recovery, procedure-related risks, available therapeutic alternatives), ethical aspects (who decides that a patient should die?), philosophical observations (which life is worth living?), and health policy considerations (what resources is it right to employ against a limited life expectancy?) need to be considered. Therefore, in this area it is really difficult to give appropriate instruments for clinical choices. We should evaluate, in order: (1) the degree of patient consciousness (if dignity of life equals to a clear conscience, and the propriety of informed consent requires formally a conscious signature, it is rather hard to justify invasive procedures in a frail unconscious patient); (2) the "*quod vitam*" prognosis, besides the acute disease for which the patient is actually observed (with particular reference to oncologic, cardiac, and pulmonary terminal diseases: it is hard to justify a life-saving intervention in a patient with a few months prognosis); (3) the success rate of the procedure (with particular reference to abdominal sepsis and severe ischemia); and (4) the wish of the patients and families. There have been some attempts to identify preoperative data helpful to determine the real impact associated with urgent intervention [23]; globally, it is known that, in the last period of life, intensive treatments often prolong the suffering of the patient [24], and the hospitalization, even more in the ICU, worsens his quality of life and restricts the psychosocial well-being of the patient and his family [5].

17.5 Should a Minimally Invasive Approach Be a Priori Ruled Out in Frail Patients?

The answer to this question is very easy: no. No anesthetic or surgical elements, based on frailty only, formally contraindicate a laparoscopic procedure. It is, however, true that in everyday practice this indication is often disregarded: in the series published by Ukkonen of 460 patients aged over 65, 80.7 % had a straight laparotomy [22]. This is in apparent conflict with an already broad literature, testifying that even complex surgical procedures can be performed, in the elective setting, with equal safety in elderly patients [25–27].

17.6 May a Minimally Invasive Approach Be Beneficial in Frail Patients?

Also the answer to this question is very easy: yes. While considerations related to cosmetics clearly lose their value in frail patients, the benefits of a minimally invasive approach in terms of postoperative pain, wound infections, mobilization, transit, and nutrition resumption could be of even greater relevance in these patients. In a retrospective Korean study, 30 patients over 65 who underwent laparoscopic appendectomy were compared to 47 patients undergoing an open procedure for acute appendicitis: the incidence of complications was strongly in favor of the laparoscopic group (7 % vs. 32 %, $P<0.01$), while all the other parameters, including costs, were equal [28]. Another paper on the same subject considered a much larger population (65,464 elderly patients with acute appendicitis) and concluded that for both perforated and non-perforated appendicitis, the laparoscopic approach allowed a reduction of complications (15 % vs. 23 % and 36 % vs. 46 %, in laparoscopic vs. open appendectomy, in perforated and non-perforated appendicitis, respectively), mortality, costs, and length of stay (3.0 vs. 4.8 and 5.8 vs. 8.7 days, respectively) [29]. However, also negative trials were published. Shin and colleagues, for example, evaluated the incidence of postoperative delirium in 130 patients undergoing open and laparoscopic (elective) gastrectomy. The evaluation was conducted through perspective, dedicated questionnaires, administered in the third postoperative day. Though the incidence and severity of delirium (31 % vs. 41 %) and the cognitive impairment rate (38 % vs. 42 %) were all in favor of the laparoscopic approach, none of these differences was significant. This may obviously be due just to a limited sample size [30]. Indeed, other studies have suggested, but not proven, an advantage associated with the laparoscopic approach on postoperative cognitive function [31].

17.7 What Are the Essential Conditions to Approach Acute Abdomen in Frail Patients by Minimally Invasive Surgery?

Undoubtedly, among these cannot be missed: (a) the patient suitability to anesthesia:, laparoscopy involves well-known pathophysiological changes, due to both the pneumoperitoneum (decreased venous return and increased respiratory pressures) and the extreme positions required for the proper conduct of the operation (trendelenburg or lateral rotation). Such changes may be particularly significant in frail patients [32]. (b) The availability of proper materials (the logistics in emergency may be different from those in the elective setting, for the presence of an unaccustomed auxiliary team, unusual operating room, or instruments). (c) The presence of a surgical team with sufficient expertise in minimally invasive procedures. Indeed, in the frail patients it is of paramount importance not to accept technical compromises that could make surgery more difficult, slower, and less effective. In younger patients, the advantages of minimally invasive approach, also aesthetic, could make a greater fatigue and a prolongation of the surgical times justified. On the contrary, the antiplatelet therapy is not considered among the essential conditions: the hypothesis that it increases the bleeding risks just in laparoscopy and not in laparotomy has been largely disavowed [33].

17.8 Should the Indication for Laparotomy Conversion Be Different in Frail Patients?

Generally speaking, yes. Besides the obvious and universally accepted reasons for conversion in laparotomy (bleeding difficult to control, jatrogenic injury difficult to repair, judgment of substantial ineffectiveness of the procedure), in frail patients the element to which it must be paid greater attention is the duration of the intervention. The operation should be converted to laparotomy when the presumed operative time for laparoscopy is significantly longer than for laparotomy and this could have a negative adverse impact on the condition of the patient. Given a protracted operative time of 30–60 min more than that of a presumptive open surgery, we suggest to cautiously convert into laparotomy and proceed with an effective conclusion of the intervention. In the retrospective Finnish study, the conversion rate was of 25.9 %, thus considerably higher than that expected in the general population [22].

17.9 What Are the Acute Abdominal Diseases Potentially Treatable by Laparoscopy in Frail Patients?

Certainly, it is cholecystectomy for acute cholecystitis, which keeps the known benefits of minimally invasive surgery and does not differ in anything from the already accepted rules of laparoscopic surgery in young patients. It is likely appendectomy, especially in relation to a greater diagnostic accuracy, which takes into account the fact that acute appendicitis is relatively rare in the elderly, while numerous alternative diseases could be the cause of symptoms [34]. In the same way, it is the conservative therapy by washing-drainage of complicated Hinchey stage 3 acute diverticulitis. Considering that in elderly patients a terminal colostomy has lesser chance of being converted in the following months [35], the simple peritoneal washing and drainage may be an attractive option; instead, in Hinchey stage IV, laparoscopy is formally contraindicated in elderly patients, and laparotomic resection-anastomosis protected by lateral oostomy would be preferable to the Hartmann procedure (of course if the general conditions allow a longer lasting intervention). A prospective randomized study of 62 patients aged over 60 years has shown that the rate of recanalization is higher with primary anastomosis and diversion by loop ileostomy [36]. The perforation of peptic ulcer is a not as a great indication to laparoscopy: the concern for a malignant nature of the ulcer, at least in the stomach, and the reported limited effectiveness of laparoscopic repair compared to open repair, make this intervention to be proposed with less conviction [37]. The same applies to the small bowel occlusion: the difficult standardization of times and results of laparoscopic viscerolysis makes the price to pay to laparoscopy (potential less efficacy, increased surgical time, possible underestimation of suffering intestinal loop, and increased iatrogenic injury) not justifiable in frail patients. The indications for the laparoscopic approach to strangulated inguinal and ventral hernia do not change in the elderly. On the contrary, minimally invasive surgery in our opinion should not be considered in nonspecific abdominal pain (which must be ruled out with imaging techniques without the concerns on radiotoxicity rightfully arising for young patients) [38], in gynecological pathology (virtually absent in women after menopause), and in blunt abdominal trauma. In the same way, it appears to make no sense to treat obstructing colorectal cancer with a laparoscopic approach. Since the strategy of colonic stent as a bridge to elective surgery was recently questioned because of high morbidity and mortality associated with iatrogenic perforation [39], the best strategy for frail patients remains at the moment the Hartmann procedure, to be done quickly and effectively by laparotomy. The alternative of primary anastomosis with diversion may be considered, similarly to diverticular peritonitis. Rare anecdotal cases of laparoscopic management of postsurgical complications are, however, described also in elderly patients (Shadis, for example, report a case of laparoscopic treatment of anastomotic fistula in an 86-year-old patient [40]). A special discussion should be reserved to the case of mesenteric ischemia, because of the high incidence of this pathology in the elderly. Although the clinical scenario in which all the conditions making a laparoscopic exploration useful for settling the hypothesis of intestinal ischemia are very limited, this strategy, potentially feasible also in critically ill patients in the ICU, still looks more appealing in the frail patient, and it deserves to be taken into account.

17.10 Outcomes

The expected mortality after emergency abdominal surgery in elderly/frail patients is obviously high. In the series of Ukkonen mortality is reported as high as 14.2 % at 30 days, with 31.9 % morbidity [22]. Adverse prognostic factors were age, atrial fibrillation, low BMI, laparoscopic surgery, ASA 3 or 4, and a history of cancer. Similar data are reported by the National Surgical Quality Improvement Project (30-day mortality and morbidity 22.3 % and 42.1 %, respectively) [41] and by the Spanish series (all-cause mortality 22 %, 24 % for patients >80 years [3]). ASA score, the delay between the onset of symptoms and treatment, and the chance to make only a palliative treatment (e.g., defunctioning stoma) were negative prognostic factors in this paper. An Italian study still under peer review shows that only one out of four patients >90 years operated in urgency is alive 2 years later.

Thus, in the overall management of the frail patient undergoing emergency surgery, it takes maximum relevance a perioperative management paying specific attention to the need of these patients. In particular, the prevention of postoperative delirium (which affects 35–70 % of elderly patients after gastrointestinal surgery) [30], the adequate (opioid-sparing) pain therapy, and a proper communication strategy represent essential elements to restore the patient's living conditions antecedents to the acute event [42]. The problem is indeed not only to save the patient life but also to look at the following life conditions. As concerns rehabilitation, a number of papers reported as indicators for recovery of everyday autonomy a number of scores for daily activity. Lawrence and colleagues in a prospective cohort study of 372 consecutive patients >60 year old showed that, after major abdominal surgery, the return to previous autonomy takes up to 3 months for normal daily activities and up to 6 months for more complex intellectual task. Preoperative depression is another problem with very difficult treatment [43].

17.11 Conclusions

The more protective system for the emergency surgeon who should take the decision to approach an elderly patient by open or laparoscopic surgery in the emergency setting would provide a simple list of essential requirements, in the absence of even one of which the indication shall not to be considered correct. We propose the following flow chart, which lends itself to a practical use to guide a cumbersome and complex choice, often to be taken in a short time and without the decision support of other colleagues.

1. The patient is conscious?
2. The patient has a life perspective, regardless of the urgent disease, of at least 3 months?
3. The current disease could be treated surgically?
4. If not treated in emergency, it would have clinically meaningful consequences?
5. The patient and family require and accept the intervention?
6. If it was not a frail patient, the approach would be minimally invasive?
7. The suspected disease is appendicitis, cholecystitis, Hinchey 3 diverticulitis (accepted indication)? Is it peptic ulcer, incisional or other incarcerated hernia, suspected intestinal ischemia (doubtful indication)?
8. The anesthesiologist agrees to the use of laparoscopy?
9. Are there environmental conditions for safe operation?
10. Has the team experience of minimally invasive surgery?
11. The expected duration of the intervention is not greater than 60 min than the expected duration of the open intervention?

If the answer to all these items is YES, the operation can be performed by laparoscopy.

References

1. Ageing well: a global priority (2012) Lancet 379(9823):1274. http://dx.doi.org/10.1016/S0140-6736(12)60518-2
2. Søreide K, Desserud KF (2015) Emergency surgery in the elderly: the balance between function, frailty, fatality and futility. Scand J Trauma Resusc Emerg Med 23:10. doi:10.1186/s13049-015-0099-x
3. Arenal JJ, Bengoechea-Beeby M (2003) Mortality associated with emergency abdominal surgery in the elderly. Can J Surg 46:111–116
4. Laurell H, Hansson LE, Gunnarsson U (2006) Acute abdominal pain among elderly patients. Gerontology 52(6):339–344, Epub 2006 Aug 11
5. Cooper Z, Courtwright A, Karlage A, Gawande A, Block S (2014) Pitfalls in communication that lead to nonbeneficial emergency surgery in elderly patients with serious illness: description of the problem and elements of a solution. Ann Surg 260(6):949–957. doi:10.1097/SLA.0000000000000721
6. Pappas A, Toutouni H, Gourgiotis S, Seretis C, Koukoutsis I, Chrysikos I, Gemenetzis G, Matzoukas I, Karavitis G, Lagoudianakis E (2013) Comparative approach to non-traumatic acute abdominal pain between elderly and non-elderly in the emergency department: a study in rural Greece. J Clin Med Res 5(4):300–304. doi:10.4021/jocmr1424w, Epub 2013 Jun 21
7. National Confidential Enquiry into Patient Outcome and Death (NCEPOD). An age old problem: a review of the care received by elderly patients undergoing surgery. The National Confidential Enquiry into Patient Outcome and Death. 2010info@ncepod.org.uk, http://www.ncepod.org.uk/
8. Launay-Savary MV, Rainfray M, Dubuisson V (2015) Emergency gastrointestinal surgery in the elderly. J Visc Surg. pii: S1878-7886(15)00123-X. doi:10.1016/j.jviscsurg.2015.09.016 [Epub ahead of print]
9. Parker JS, Vukov LF, Wollan PC (1996) Abdominal pain in the elderly: use of temperature and laboratory testing to screen for surgical disease. Fam Med 28(3):193–197
10. Tran BK, Espolio Desbaillet Y, Groebli Y, Della SV (2012) Abdominal pain among elderly patients in the emergency department. RevMed Suisse 8:1548–1552
11. Green G, Shaikh I, Fernandes R, Wegstapel H (2013) Emergency laparotomy in octogenarians: a 5-year study of morbidity and mortality. World J Gastrointest Surg 5:216–221
12. OCEBM Levels of Evidence Working Group. *The Oxford 2011 levels of evidence*. Oxford Centre for Evidence-Based Medicine. http://www.cebm.net/index.aspx?o=5653
13. Fried LP, Tangen CM, Walston J et al (2001) Frailty in older adults: evidence for a phenotype. J Gerontol A Biol Sci 56:M146–M156
14. Sternberg SA, Wershof Schwartz A, Karunananthan S, Bergman H, Mark Clarfield A (2011) The identification of frailty: a systematic literature review. J Am Geriatr Soc 59:2129–2138
15. Soubeyran P, Bellera C, Goyard J et al (2011) Validation of the G-8 screening tool in geriatriconcology: the ONCODAGE project. J Clin Oncol 2001:29 (suppl; abstr 9001; 2011 ASCO Annual Meeting)
16. Bellera CA, Rainfray M, Mathoulin-Pélissier S et al (2012) Screening older cancer patients: first evaluation of the G-8 geriatric screening tool. Ann Oncol 23:2166–2172
17. Hastings RS, Powers RD (2011) Abdominal pain in the ED: a 35 year retrospective. Am J Emerg Med 29(7):711–716
18. Reginelli A, Russo A, Pinto A, Stanzione F, Martiniello C, Cappabianca S, Brunese L, Squillaci E (2014) The role of computed tomography in the preoperative assessment of gastrointestinal causes of acute abdomen in elderly patients. Int J Surg 12(Suppl 2):S181–S186. doi:10.1016/j.ijsu.2014.08.345, Epub 2014 Aug 23
19. Kraemer M, Franke C, Ohmann C, Yang Q, Acute Abdominal Pain Study Group (2000) Acute appendicitis in late adulthood: incidence, presentation, and outcome. Results of a prospective multicenter acute abdominal pain study and a review of the literature. Langenbecks Arch Surg 385(7):470–481

20. McGillicuddy EA, Schuster KM, Davis KA, Longo WE (2009) Factors predicting morbidity and mortality in emergency colorectal procedures in elderly patients. Arch Surg 144(12):1157–1162. doi:10.1001/archsurg.2009.203
21. Racz J, Dubois L, Katchky A, Wall W (2012) Elective and emergency abdominal surgery in patients 90 years of age or older. Can J Surg 55:322–328
22. Ukkonen M, Kivivuori A, Rantanen T, Paajanen H (2015) Emergency abdominal operations in the elderly: a multivariate regression analysis of 430 consecutive patients with acute abdomen. World J Surg 39(12):2854–2861
23. Amrock LG, Neuman MD, Lin HM, Deiner S (2014) Can routine preoperative data predict adverse outcomes in the elderly? Development and validation of a simple risk model incorporating a chart-derived frailty score. J Am Coll Surg 219(4):684–694. doi:10.1016/j.jamcollsurg.2014.04.018, Epub 2014 Jun 3
24. Wright AA, Zhang B, Ray A et al (2008) Associations between end-of-life discussions, patient mental health, medical care near death, and caregiver bereavement adjustment. JAMA 300:1665–1673
25. Koh FH, Wong J, Tan JK, Tan KK, Cheong WK, Lieske B (2015) Laparoscopic colorectal surgery is safe and benefits octogenarian patients with malignant disease: a matched case-control study comparing laparoscopic and open colorectal surgery. Int J Colorectal Dis 30(7):963–968. doi:10.1007/s00384-015-2252-4, Epub 2015 May 24
26. Grailey K, Markar SR, Karthikesalingam A, Aboud R, Ziprin P, Faiz O (2013) Laparoscopic versus open colorectal resection in the elderly population. Surg Endosc 27(1):19–30. doi:10.1007/s00464-012-2414-1, Epub 2012 Jun 30
27. Kurian AA, Suryadevara S, Vaughn D et al (2010) Laparoscopic colectomy in octogenarians and nonagenarians: a preferable option to open surgery? J Surg Educ 67(3):161–166 [PubMed]
28. Baek HN, Jung YH, Hwang YH (2011) Laparoscopic versus open appendectomy for appendicitis in elderly patients. J Korean Soc Coloproctol 27(5):241–245. doi:10.3393/jksc.2011.27.5.241, Epub 2011 Oct 31
29. Masoomi H, Mills S, Dolich MO, Ketana N, Carmichael JC, Nguyen NT, Stamos MJ (2012) Does laparoscopic appendectomy impart an advantage over open appendectomy in elderly patients? World J Surg 36(7):1534–1539. doi:10.1007/s00268-012-1545-9
30. Shin Y-H, Kim D-K, Jeong H-J (2015) Impact of surgical approach on postoperative delirium in elderly patients undergoing gastrectomy: laparoscopic versus open approaches. Korean J Anesthesiol 68(4):379–385. doi:10.4097/kjae.2015.68.4.379
31. Tan CB, Ng J, Jeganathan R, Kawai F, Pan CX, Pollock S, Turner J, Cohen S, Chorost M (2015) Cognitive changes after surgery in the elderly: does minimally invasive surgery influence the incidence of postoperative cognitive changes compared to open colon surgery? Dement Geriatr Cogn Disord 39(3–4):125–131. doi:10.1159/000357804, Epub 2014 Nov 27
32. Peden CJ (2011) Emergency surgery in the elderly patient: a quality improvement approach. Anaesthesia 66:440–445
33. Joseph B, Rawashdeh B, Aziz H, Kulvatunyou N, Pandit V, Jehangir Q, O'Keeffe T, Tang A, Green DJ, Friese RS, Rhee P (2015) An acute care surgery dilemma: emergent laparoscopic cholecystectomy in patients on aspirin therapy. Am J Surg 209(4):689–694. doi:10.1016/j.amjsurg.2014.04.014, Epub 2014 Jun 27
34. Omari AH, Khammash MR, Qasaiheh GR et al (2014) Acute appendicitis in the elderly: risk factors for perforation. World J Emerg Surg 9:1–6
35. Salem L, Flum DR (2004) Primary anastomosis or Hartmann's procedure for patients with diverticular peritonitis? A systematic review. Dis Colon Rectum 47:1953–1964
36. Oberkofler CE, Rickenbacher A, Raptis DA et al (2012) A multicenter randomized clinical trial of primary anastomosis or Hartmann's procedure for perforated left colonic diverticulitis with purulent or fecal peritonitis. Ann Surg 256:819–826, discussion 826–827
37. Mouly C, Chati R, Scotté M, Regimbeau JM (2013) Therapeutic management of perforated gastroduodenal ulcer: literature review. J Visc Surg 150:333–340

38. Esses D, Birnbaum A, Bijur P, Shah S, Gleyzer A, Gallagher EJ (2004) Ability of CT to alter decision making in elderly patients with acute abdominal pain. Am J Emerg Med 22(4):270–272
39. Cirocchi R, Farinella E, Trastulli S et al (2013) Safety and efficacy of endoscopic colonic stenting as a bridge to surgery in the management of intestinal obstruction due to left colon and rectal cancer: a systematic review and meta-analysis. Surg Oncol 22:14–21
40. Shadis R, Zebley DM, Kim SY, Hofmann MT, Fassler SA (2011) Laparoscopic repair of colonic anastomotic leak in an elderly patient. JSLS 15(4):555–557. doi:10.4293/108680811X13176785204553
41. Scarborough JE, Pappas TN et al (2012) Failure-to-pursue rescue: explaining excess mortality in elderly emergency general surgical patients with preexisting do not-resuscitate orders. Ann Surg 256:453–461
42. Griffiths R, Beech F, Brown A, Dhesi J, Foo I, Goodall J, Harrop-Griffiths W, Jameson J, Love N, Pappenheim K, White S, Association of Anesthetists of Great Britain and Ireland (2014) Peri-operative care of the elderly 2014: Association of Anaesthetists of Great Britain and Ireland. Anaesthesia 69(Suppl 1):81–98. doi:10.1111/anae.12524
43. Lawrence VA, Hazuda HP, Cornell JE et al (2004) Functional independence after major abdominal surgery in the elderly. J Am Coll Surg 199:762–772

MIX
Papier aus verantwortungsvollen Quellen
Paper from responsible sources
FSC® C105338

If you have any concerns about our products,
you can contact us on
ProductSafety@springernature.com

In case Publisher is established outside the EU,
the EU authorized representative is:
Springer Nature Customer Service Center GmbH
Europaplatz 3, 69115 Heidelberg, Germany

Printed by Libri Plureos GmbH
in Hamburg, Germany